SYNOPSIS OF

ORAL PATHOLOGY

SYNOPSIS OF
ORAL PATHOLOGY

S. N. BHASKAR, B.D.S., D.D.S., M.S., Ph.D.

Major General, U.S. Army (Ret.);
formerly Chief, U.S. Army Dental Corps;
Diplomate, American Board of Oral Pathology;
Diplomate, American Board of Oral Medicine;
Monterey, California

SIXTH EDITION

with 716 *illustrations*

The C. V. Mosby Company

ST. LOUIS • TORONTO • LONDON   1981

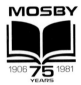

MOSBY

1906 **75** 1981
YEARS

A TRADITION OF PUBLISHING EXCELLENCE

SIXTH EDITION

The C. V. Mosby Company
11830 Westline Industrial Drive, St. Louis, Missouri 63141

Library of Congress Cataloging in Publication Data

Bhaskar, S   N
  Synopsis of oral pathology.

  Bibliography: p.
  Includes index.
  1. Teeth—Diseases.   2. Mouth—Diseases.
I. Title.   [DNLM: 1. Mouth diseases—Pathology.
2. Tooth diseases—Pathology.   WU 140 B575s]
[RK307.B48 1981]   617'.522'07   80-39514
ISBN 0-8016-0685-3

C/CB/B   9   8   7   6   5   4   03/D/305

To the memory of

my first and most devoted teachers,

Maya D. Bhaskar

and

Jagan N. Bhaskar

my mother and father

Preface

Oral pathology teaches the student about the cause, development, gross and microscopic alterations, natural history, and final outcome of disease. It forms the basis for correct diagnosis and therapy. No other subject in dental education imparts greater confidence to the student or assures better treatment for the patient.

The first edition of this book was written to provide the student and the practicing dentist with all necessary information about oral pathology without the burden of minutiae and superfluous detail. The response from dentists and dental students around the world would indicate that all five editions of the book have accomplished this goal.

In this sixth edition, the initial purpose of the book has not changed. The subject matter has been brought up to date, and new figures have been added.

As a dentist engaged in clinical practice, I deeply appreciate the needs and the concerns of the patients, as well as the challenges and the responsibilities that constantly face all clinicians. It is my fervent hope, therefore, that this subject and especially this book will make it easier for the clinician to diagnose oral diseases quickly and to treat them with confidence.

S. N. Bhaskar

Acknowledgment

Regardless of how old a man is and what his accomplishments are, he always owes a deep debt of gratitude to his parents and to some of his teachers. To his parents, he is indebted for their teaching of all the worthwhile values of human life; and to a select group of teachers, he is indebted for their encouragement and nurturing of these values. I am deeply grateful, therefore, to my mother and father, who taught me with affection; and I dedicate this book to them and to their memory. Of my many outstanding teachers, now a part of the legend of dentistry, I will always remember Drs. Isaac Schour, Balint Orban, Harry Sicher, and Joseph P. Weinmann. It is especially to Professor Weinmann, a teacher, a dear friend, and a scientist of outstanding talent and deep humility, who taught with patience and who was willing to share all his knowledge, that I am in deepest debt.

Innumerable dentists in the United States, teachers, practitioners and students alike, have told me, through letters and spoken words, about the assistance the past editions of this book have provided them in their professional lives. Without such encouragement and support, the very purpose of this book would be lost. I express, therefore, my deep gratitude to all my professional colleagues in the United States and abroad.

A number of my students, now prominent oral pathologists in their own right, offered criticism and advice for the last edition. I wish to express my thanks to all of them and especially to Drs. Peter Tsaknis, James C. Adrian, John Nelson, Duane Cutright, and Thomas Payne for helpful advice and assistance.

No man can accomplish much without the help, support, and understanding of his family. The patience and support of my wife, Norma, and sons, William, Philip, and Thomas, are therefore acknowledged with the deepest of affection.

Contents

PART I

ORAL DIAGNOSIS

One of the most important purposes of oral pathology is to give the student the ability to correctly diagnose oral lesions. There are more than 200 different types of diseases that afflict the oral cavity, and many of these can only be diagnosed through microscopic examination. The clinical appearance and history of oral lesions, however, can often give the clinician a reliable provisional diagnosis on which to plan further management of the patient. Oral diagnosis is based on a sound knowledge of oral pathology and is essential for good clinical practice.

The purpose of this part of the book, therefore, is to present oral pathology in a manner that is meaningful to the clinician. The lesions of the oral cavity are classified according to their clinical appearance, and such information that will aid the clinician in making a rational assessment of a given lesion is furnished. Details about microscopic features and theories about histogenesis of lesions have been omitted.

The pathology of the oral regions is presented in tabular form under the following headings:

Surface lesions of oral mucosa

1. White lesions
2. Vesicular lesions
3. Ulcerations
4. Pigmented lesions

Soft tissue growths of oral cavity

1. Firm, nonhemorrhagic growths
2. Hemorrhagic or easily bleeding growths
3. Compressible growths
4. Papillary or cauliflower-like growths

Lesions of jaws

1. Radiolucent lesions
2. Radiopaque lesions
3. Partly radiolucent and partly radiopaque lesions

Lesions of salivary glands

1. Swellings

WHITE LESIONS OF ORAL MUCOSA

The following conditions appear as white surface lesions of the oral mucosa (Table 1, pp. 8 to 13):

Desquamative gingivitis

Benign hyperkeratosis (pachyderma oris; pachyderma oralis; focal keratosis)

Leukoplakia with dyskeratosis (and verrucous leukoplakia)

Carcinoma in situ

Squamous cell carcinoma

White sponge nevus (naevus spongiosis albus mucosae; white folded gingivostomatitis; congenital leukokeratosis mucosae oris)

Hereditary benign intraepithelial dyskeratosis (red eye)

Lichen planus

Stomatitis nicotina

White hairy tongue (lingua villosa alba)

Candidiasis (moniliasis; thrush)

Fordyce's disease

Chemical burn

Geographic tongue

Epstein's pearl (Bohn's nodule)

Allergic reactions

VESICULAR LESIONS OF ORAL MUCOSA

Vesicular lesions of the oral mucosa are short-lived. They rupture soon after formation and leave superficial ulcers. The following lesions appear either as vesicles that soon form ulcers or as ulcers that may be erroneously thought to have had a vesicular beginning (Table 2, pp. 14 to 19):

Primary herpetic gingivostomatitis

Secondary herpetic lesion

Aphthous ulcer

Periadenitis mucosa necrotica recurrens (Sutton's disease; Mikulicz's ulcer)

Herpes zoster (shingles)

Erythema multiforme (Stevens-Johnson syndrome; ectodermosis erosiva pluriorificialis)

Behçet's syndrome

Reiter's syndrome

Pemphigus vulgaris

Benign mucous membrane pemphigus (pemphigoid)

Smallpox and chickenpox

Herpangina

Hand-foot-and-mouth disease

Epidermolysis bullosa

Allergic reactions (stomatitis medicamentosa; stomatitis venenata)

Mucocele

ULCERATIONS OF ORAL MUCOSA

In the presence of an ulcer, a number of possibilities should be considered. It will be noted that all vesicular lesions of the oral mucosa terminate in ulcers and are included among the following (Table 3, pp. 20 to 29):

Traumatic ulcer
Desquamative gingivitis
Vincent's stomatitis (necrotizing ulcerative gingivitis)
Eosinophilic granuloma
Erosive lichen planus
Candidiasis (moniliasis; thrush)
Primary herpetic gingivostomatitis
Secondary herpetic lesion
Aphthous ulcer
Periadenitis mucosa necrotica recurrens (Sutton's disease; Mikulicz's ulcer)
Herpes zoster (shingles)
Erythema multiforme (Stevens-Johnson syndrome; ectodermosis erosiva pluriorificialis)
Behçet's syndrome
Reiter's syndrome
Pemphigus vulgaris
Benign mucous membrane pemphigus (pemphigoid)
Smallpox and chickenpox
Herpangina
Hand-foot-and-mouth disease
Stomatitis venenata
Stomatitis medicamentosa
Squamous cell carcinoma and other malignant epithelial tumors
Lymphomas and leukemias
Chancre (syphilis)
Mucous patch (syphilis)
Tuberculosis
Histoplasmosis
Infectious mononucleosis
Riga-Fede disease
Pterygoid ulcer (Bednar's aphtha)

PIGMENTED LESIONS OF ORAL MUCOSA

Pigmentation of the oral mucosa is produced by any one of the following conditions (Table 4, pp. 30 to 33):

Black hairy tongue
Amalgam tattoo
Addison's disease
Normal pigmented patches
Jeghers' (Peutz-Jeghers) syndrome
Melanotic macule
Nevus
Melanoma
Heavy metal poisoning (bismuth, mercury, lead, silver)
Postmenopausal state
Drug ingestion (tranquilizers, oral contraceptives)
Varicosity
Malnutrition

FIRM, NONHEMORRHAGIC SOFT TISSUE GROWTHS OF ORAL CAVITY

A firm, nonbleeding growth of oral soft tissue usually indicates one of the following lesions (Table 5, pp. 34 to 37):

Fibromatosis
Torus (exostosis; peripheral osteoma) and related lesions
Irritation fibroma
Peripheral fibroma and peripheral fibroma with calcification
Myxoma (fibroma with myxomatous degeneration)

Neurofibroma and schwannoma (neurilemoma)
Lipoma
Granular cell myoblastoma
Sialadenitis
Tumor of salivary gland

HEMORRHAGIC OR EASILY BLEEDING SOFT TISSUE GROWTHS OF ORAL CAVITY

Soft tissue growth of the oral tissues that bleed easily could represent any one of the following lesions (Table 6, pp. 38 to 41):

Parulis (periodontal abscess; gumboil)
Eosinophilic granuloma
Epulis fissuratum
Peripheral giant cell granuloma
Pyogenic granuloma

Pregnancy tumor (granuloma gravidarum)
Squamous cell carcinoma and other malignant tumors
Lymphomas (lymphosarcoma; reticulum cell sarcoma) and leukemias

COMPRESSIBLE SOFT TISSUE GROWTHS OF ORAL CAVITY

The following lesions present as compressible growths of the oral soft tissues (Table 7, pp. 42 to 45):

Eruption cyst
Mucocele (mucous retention cyst; retention phenomenon)
Mucous cyst
Ranula
Gingival cyst
Nasoalveolar cyst

Epidermoid cyst (dermoid, epidermal, dermal)
Cavernous and capillary hemangioma
Lymphangioma
Cystic hygroma (cystic lymphangioma; hygroma cysticum colli)

PAPILLARY OR CAULIFLOWER-LIKE SOFT TISSUE GROWTHS OF ORAL CAVITY

The following papillary or cauliflower-like lesions occur in the oral cavity (Table 8, pp. 44 to 47):

Verrucous leukoplakia
Verruca vulgaris
Condyloma acuminatum
Papilloma

Pseudoepitheliomatous hyperplasia (keratoacanthoma)
Inflammatory papillary hyperplasia
Verrucous carcinoma

RADIOLUCENT LESIONS OF JAWS

The radiolucent lesions of the jaws can be subdivided into eight groups as follows (Table 9, pp. 48 to 61):

Lesions at apex of tooth

Dental granuloma
Radicular cyst
Residual cyst
Periapical (dentoalveolar) abscess
Apical scar
Cementoma (first stage)

Lesions in midline of maxilla

Median palatine cyst
Median alveolar cyst
Globulomaxillary cyst
Nasoalveolar cyst
Incisive canal cyst
Cyst of palatine papilla

Lesion in place of missing tooth

Primordial cyst

Lesions around crown of impacted tooth

Dentigerous cyst
Ameloblastoma
Odontogenic adenomatoid tumor (adenoameloblastoma)
Odontogenic fibroma and myxoma

Soap bubble–like radiolucencies

Multilocular cyst
Aneurysmal bone cyst
Ameloblastoma
Giant cell granuloma (central)
Cherubism (early stage) or familial intraosseous fibrous swelling of jaws
Myxoma (nonodontogenic)

Multiple but separate radiolucent lesions

Cherubism (early stage) or familial intraosseous fibrous swelling of jaws
Multiple myeloma
Eosinophilic granuloma
Hand-Schüller-Christian disease
Letterer-Siwe disease
Hyperparathyroidism (brown node, giant cell lesion)
Metastatic tumor

Lesions that destroy cortical plate

Metastatic tumor
Primary malignant tumor
Osteomyelitis

Lateral periodontal cyst
Traumatic cyst
Idiopathic bone cavity
Osteomyelitis

Hematopoietic marrow
Gingival cyst
Physiologic osteoporosis
Hemangioma (central)

RADIOPAQUE LESIONS OF JAWS

A radiopaque area of the jaw may represent any one of the following lesions (Table 10, pp. 62 to 67):

Cementoma (third stage)
Compound odontoma
Complex odontoma
Ossifying fibroma (fibrous dysplasia)
Osteoma and torus
Osteogenic sarcoma
Chondrosarcoma
Metastatic tumor
Paget's disease (osteitis deformans)

Osteopetrosis (Albers-Schönberg disease; marble bone disease)
Leontiasis ossea
Caffey's disease (infantile cortical hyperostosis)
Garré's osteomyelitis
Condensing osteitis
Root fragment or foreign body
Chronic sclerosing osteomyelitis

PARTLY RADIOPAQUE AND PARTLY RADIOLUCENT LESIONS OF JAWS

The following lesions usually present as partly radiopaque and partly radiolucent areas (Table 11, pp. 66 to 69):

Cementoma (second stage)
Ameloblastic fibro-odontoma
Cystic odontoma
Ossifying fibroma (fibrous dysplasia)
Osteogenic sarcoma
Chondrosarcoma

Metastasis from carcinoma of prostate or breast
Paget's disease (osteitis deformans)
Condensing osteitis
Chronic sclerosing osteomyelitis

SWELLINGS OF SALIVARY GLANDS

A swelling in the area of a major or minor salivary gland may represent any one of the following lesions (Table 12, pp. 70 to 73):

Mucocele (mucous retention cyst; retention phenomenon)
Ranula
Mumps (infectious parotitis)
Cat-scratch disease
Sarcoidosis (Besnier-Boeck-Schaumann disease)
Mikulicz's disease (benign lympho-epithelial lesion)

Sjögren's syndrome (sicca syndrome [*sicca*, dry])
Fatty infiltration
Hypertrophy
Sialadenitis
Benign tumor
Malignant tumor

• • •

The information included in Tables 1 to 12 is not precise. In a sense, it is crude—but only as crude as an eye is to a microscope. There are exceptions to many points given; but when intelligently applied to a given oral lesion, this information can aid the clinician in making a reasonably accurate diagnosis.

Table 1. White lesions of oral mucosa

Lesion	Usual location	Usual age and sex	Clinical features
Desquamative gingivitis	Free and attached gingiva	Over 40 yr; female	Multiple white areas that can be rubbed off by finger pressure; red, inflamed mucous membrane
Benign hyperkeratosis (pachyderma oris; etc.)	Anywhere on oral mucosa, especially lip and cheek	Adulthood; male	White lesion, flat or raised, may be rough; usually single; duration, weeks to months; cannot be wiped off
Leukoplakia with dyskeratosis (and verrucous leukoplakia)	Anywhere on oral mucosa, usually lip, tongue, cheek, and floor of mouth	Adulthood, usually fourth decade and later; male	White lesion, flat or elevated, may be fissured, rough, or smooth; any size; asymptomatic; may be increasing in size; may present as ulcer or as mottled or red area; duration varies; cannot be wiped off
Carcinoma in situ	Anywhere on oral mucosa	Adulthood; male	Same as in leukoplakia
Squamous cell carcinoma	Lip, tongue, floor of mouth, and cheek, in that order of frequency	Adulthood; male	About 4%-6% present as white plaques; may be flat, elevated, or fissured; may be associated with lymph node enlargement in neck
White sponge nevus (naevus spongiosis albus mucosae; etc.)	Large area of oral mucosa or entire mucosa	Present from childhood; either	Hereditary disease; present in number of members of same family; may appear in one area and then spread; asymptomatic; mucosa appears parboiled; cannot be wiped off

Microscopic features	Treatment	Prognosis	Page ref.
Separation of epithelium from connective tissue at basement membrane	Symptomatic; hormones; corticoids; vitamins	Fair	186
Epithelium covering mucosa shows thick layer of keratin; epithelial cells normal	If cause removed lesion should disappear in about 3 wk; may be excised	Excellent	374
Epithelial covering shows thick layer of keratin, as seen in benign hyperkeratosis; also, epithelial cells show abnormalities called dyskeratosis (p. 379); basement membrane intact	Total excision with wide margin	Untreated lesion becomes squamous cell carcinoma; if totally excised, prognosis good; better prognosis in lesions of lip and cheek than in those of floor of mouth or base of tongue	375
Only difference between this lesion and leukoplakia is presence of dyskeratotic cells in almost all layers; basement membrane intact; carcinoma in situ differs from leukoplakia only in degree	Total, wide excision	Same as in leukoplakia; prognosis only fair in lesions of floor of mouth and base of tongue	380
Epithelial covering shows keratinization; numerous dyskeratotic cells, many of which invade underlying tissues; basement membrane violated	Wide excision	Good for lip lesion; poor for lesions of floor of mouth and base of tongue	380 and 539
Thickening of epithelial covering; superficial layers of epithelial cells swollen and fail to stain	None; lesions harmless and should not be treated	Excellent	380

9

Continued.

Table 1. White lesions of oral mucosa—cont'd

Lesion	Usual location	Usual age and sex	Clinical features
Hereditary benign intra-epithelial dys-keratosis (red eye)	Generalized on oral mucosa	Present from child-hood; either	White spongy mucosa; corners of mouth may be involved; white plaques on cornea and conjunc-tivitis, giving red eye appear-ance
Lichen planus	Cheek; may be on tongue or lip or else-where on oral mucosa	Adulthood; either	White or gray-white lacy lesion or gray-white patch; cannot be wiped off; may be associated with scaly papules on skin; oral lesion may precede skin lesion; believed to be of psychosomatic origin
Stomatitis nic-otina	Palate	Adulthood; male	Reddening of palatal mucosa that later becomes white; sur-face studded with numerous nipplelike elevations, center of which shows pinpoint orifice of palatal gland duct; patients usu-ally pipe smokers; cannot be wiped off
White hairy tongue (lin-gua villosa alba)	Dorsum of tongue	Adulthood and later; male	Long, white, hairlike elongation of filiform papillae; asympto-matic or accompanied by pain and enlargement of tongue
Candidiasis (moniliasis; thrush)	Anywhere on oral mucosa	Two ex-tremes of life; also debilitated persons and those receiving antibiotics; either	Multiple white, curdlike patches on oral mucosa; can be scraped off but leave bleeding surfaces; lesions heal in one area to ap-pear elsewhere; may appear as red, raw oral mucosa
Fordyce's dis-ease	Cheek, level of occlusal plane of teeth	Adulthood; either	White or yellowish granules; may coalesce to appear as white or yellow plaque; asymp-tomatic; condition very common

Microscopic features	Treatment	Prognosis	Page ref.
Similar to those in white sponge nevus; also presence of benign dyskeratosis	None	Excellent	384
Epithelial ridges sawtooth shaped; epithelium may show keratinization; connective tissue under epithelium shows clearly demarcated lymphocytic infiltration; basement membrane edematous	None; spontaneous regression occurs in few months	Excellent	387
Epithelial covering has layer of keratin; mucous glands underlying epithelium show inflammation and obstruction of ducts by squamous metaplasia	Discontinuation of smoking	Excellent	390
Marked elongation of filiform papillae; some inflammatory infiltrate of subepithelial tissue	None; brushing of tongue as frequently as possible	Excellent	392
White patch consisting of necrotic epithelium in which numerous fungi *(Candida albicans)* can be seen	Administration of topical or systemic nystatin	Usually excellent; generalized infection extremely rare and usually secondary	396
Numerous or few sebaceous glands in subepithelial tissues; each gland appears clinically as granule	None	Excellent	397

11

Continued.

Table 1. White lesions of oral mucosa—cont'd

Lesion	Usual location	Usual age and sex	Clinical features
Chemical burn	Anywhere on oral mucosa, usually in retromolar area, where patient puts aspirin tablets to alleviate pain due to impacted third molars	Any age; either	White or grayish white necrotic lesion; very short duration; painful; caused by aspirin, camphor, phenol, etc.
Geographic tongue	Dorsum of tongue	Adulthood; female	Irregular red patches of desquamation that heal on one side but spread on other; however, surrounding area of tongue appears white—partly due to contrast and partly due to elongation of filiform papillae; allergic reactions on tongue may give rise to similar lesions
Epstein's pearl (Bohn's nodule)	Anywhere on oral mucosa, especially mandibular and maxillary alveolar mucosa	Newborn; either	Multiple white, ricelike lesions of mucous membrane; seen in almost 85% of newborn infants
Allergic reactions	Anywhere on oral mucosa, especially cheek	Any age	May be white patches that peel off on pressure; usually associated with toothpaste or mouthwash

Microscopic features	Treatment	Prognosis	Page ref.
Epithelium and part of underlying tissue necrotic; peripherally, edema and neutrophilic infiltration	None except symptomatic; healing occurs quickly, and necrotic tissue sloughs off	Excellent	398
Desquamated areas show loss of papillae and inflammatory cells in lamina propria; white areas appear as elongation of filiform papillae	None except good oral hygiene	Excellent	400 and 443
Each ricelike lesion has keratin-containing cyst that lies very near mucosal surface	None	Excellent; lesion disappears spontaneously in few weeks	400 and 639
Edema; desquamation of epithelium; lymphocytic infiltrate	Removal of cause	Excellent	None

Table 2. Vesicular lesions of oral mucosa

Lesion	Usual location	Usual age and sex	Clinical features
Primary herpetic gingivostomatitis	Entire oral mucosa	1-3 yr, but may be older; either	Headache, pain, sore mouth, irritability, drooling, enlargement of cervical nodes, fever; oral mucosa becomes red with numerous vesicles that rupture and form painful ulcers
Secondary herpetic lesion	Lips, hard palate, and attached gingiva	Adulthood; either	Localized single or groups of vesicles; associated with fever, stress, trauma, menstruation, etc.; vesicles soon rupture, leaving painful ulcers; vesicles on skin of lips do not ulcerate but form scabs
Aphthous ulcer	Anywhere on oral mucosa except anterior hard palate and gingiva	Adulthood or later; female	Single or group of vesicles that rupture, leaving ulcers; lesions recurrent; more common in winter and spring; physical and emotional stress contributory factors; probably caused by alpha hemolytic *Streptococcus*
Periadenitis mucosa necrotica recurrens (Sutton's disease; Mikulicz's ulcer)	Salivary gland–bearing areas of oral and laryngeal mucosa	Adulthood; either	Single or multiple nodules or vesicles that rupture, leaving deep ulcers; ulcers deeper than those of herpetic lesions; lesions heal with scar formation; while one lesion heals, another appears elsewhere; cause same as that for aphthous ulcers
Herpes zoster (shingles)	Lip, buccal mucosa, tongue, and soft palate; follows areas of sensory nerve distribution	Adulthood; male	Oral lesions extremely rare; resemble herpes simplex vesicles; vesicles rupture, leaving ulcers

Microscopic features	Treatment	Prognosis	Page ref.
Hyperemia and edema in subepithelial tissue accumulations of fluid in epithelial covering; formation of vesicles; later, vesicles rupture, leaving ulcers that show secondary inflammation of underlying connective tissue	Symptomatic	Excellent; ulcers heal spontaneously without scarring in 7-14 days	403
Same as in primary herpetic gingivostomatitis	Symptomatic	Excellent; lesions heal spontaneously in 7-14 days; recurrences to be expected	405
Same as in other vesicles	Symptomatic, or 250 mg tetracycline in 5 ml water as mouthwash later to be swallowed, 3 or 4 times daily; soothing mouthwash (p. 412)	Good	410
Ulceration and necrosis; infiltration of underlying mucous glands by neutrophils, plasma cells, and lymphocytes	Symptomatic; in severe cases 250 mg tetracycline in 5 ml water as mouthwash later to be swallowed, 3 or 4 times daily; soothing mouthwash (p. 412)	Spontaneous healing in 3-6 wk; scarring	412
Same as in herpes simplex and other vesicles	Symptomatic	Good	413

15

Continued.

Table 2. Vesicular lesions of oral mucosa—cont'd

Lesion	Usual location	Usual age and sex	Clinical features
Erythema multiforme (Stevens-Johnson syndrome; ectodermosis erosiva pluriorificialis)	Anywhere on skin and mucous membrane	Early adulthood; either	Oral lesions consist of multiple red macules, papules, and vesicles that rupture, leaving many painful ulcers; lesions appear in 1-2 days and heal spontaneously; skin lesions usually present, and therefore diagnosis not difficult; etiology of disease not definitely known but believed to be allergic; many variants (p. 417)
Behçet's syndrome	Mouth, genitals, eyes, and skin	10-30 yr; male	Multiple aphthalike ulcers; presence of oral, ocular, and genital lesions distinguishing feature
Reiter's syndrome	Skin and oral mucosa	20-30 yr; male	Vesicles and ulcers of oral and penile mucosa; urethritis, arthritis, and conjunctivitis
Pemphigus vulgaris	Anywhere on oral mucosa	40-70 yr; either	Oral lesions consist of multiple bullae that may precede, accompany, or follow skin lesions; bullae rupture rapidly, leaving painful ulcers; Nikolski's sign positive
Benign mucous membrane pemphigus (pemphigoid)	Oral mucosa and conjunctiva	Over 40 yr; either	Bullous lesions that become ulcers; patients in general good health; involvement of other mucous membranes
Smallpox and chickenpox	Anywhere on oral mucosa	Childhood; either	Oral lesions consist of single or clusters of small vesicles that rupture, leaving shallow ulcers; skin lesions always present, and diagnosis not difficult
Herpangina	Soft palate, tonsil, uvula, and pharynx	Childhood; either	Vesicles on oral mucosa that soon rupture, leaving ulcers; associated with fever and malaise

Microscopic features	Treatment	Prognosis	Page ref.
Depend on stage of disease; essentially consist of ulceration, edema, and infiltration of lamina propria by eosinophils, plasma cells, and lymphocytes	Symptomatic	Good; disease self-limiting; lesions heal spontaneously; may recur	415
Nonspecific ulcer	Symptomatic	Good	417
Not specific; ulceration and inflammatory cells	Symptomatic	Good	418
Intraepithelial accumulation of fluid; degeneration of epithelial cells; mild subvesicular edema and inflammation; Tzanck cells seen in bullae	Symptomatic only; cortisone of temporary value	Poor; disease fatal in more than 50% of patients	418
Intraepithelial and subepithelial accumulation of fluid	Symptomatic	Good, but eye lesions may produce blindness	421
Typical of vesicle and later of ulcer	Symptomatic	Excellent; disease self-limiting; lesions heal spontaneously	422
Typical of vesicle and later of ulcer	Symptomatic	Excellent; disease self-limiting; lesions heal spontaneously	424

Continued.

Table 2. Vesicular lesions of oral mucosa—cont'd

Lesion	Usual location	Usual age and sex	Clincal features
Hand-foot-and-mouth disease	Hard palate, tongue, buccal mucosa	Under 5 yr; either male or female	Multiple ulcers and vesicles of oral mucosa; skil lesions; fever, malaise, anorexia, and diarrhea; caused by coxsackievirus
Epidermolysis bullosa	Skin and oral mucosa	Infancy and early childhood; either	Bullae of skin and mucosa; some types fatal
Allergic reactions (stomatitis medicamentosa; stomatitis venenata)	Anywhere on oral mucosa	Any age; either	Stomatitis medicamentosa represents allergic reaction, whereas venenata represents contact allergy; lesions may consist of areas of erythema or vesicles and bullae; appear rapidly (hours to days); history of contact with allergen; in stomatitis medicamentosa, skin lesions may be present; vesicles rupture, leaving ulcers
Mucocele	Lip, cheek, and tongue	Any age; either	Small clear or bluish vesicle

Microscopic features	Treatment	Prognosis	Page ref.
Nonspecific ulcer and vesicle	Symptomatic	Excellent	424
Same as in other vesicles	Symptomatic	Fair to grave, depending on type	426
Same as in herpangina	Discontinuation of allergen (drugs, toothpastes, mouthwashes, lipsticks, etc.)	Excellent	426
Mucus-containing cyst lined by granulation tissue	Excision	Good	429

Table 3. Ulcerations of oral mucosa

Lesion	Usual location	Usual age and sex	Clinical features
Traumatic ulcer	Anywhere on oral mucosa; those related to dentures in vestibular mucosa, ridges, and palate	Any age; either	Solitary lesion; painful; short duration; cause usually apparent (e.g., ill-fitting denture)
Desquamative gingivitis	Gingiva	Postmenopause; female	Usually multiple areas of gray mucosa that are necrotic and peel off, leaving superficial ulcers; some cases have red, raw appearance
Vincent's stomatitis (necrotizing ulcerative gingivitis)	Gingiva	Early adulthood; either	Lesions start as reddening and ulceration of interdental papillae; ulcers produce cuplike destruction of papillae; necrosis, fetid breath, pain, fever, and malaise
Eosinophilic granuloma	Gingiva	Adulthood; male	Ulceration, necrosis, pain, loose teeth, and fetid breath
Erosive lichen planus	Cheek	Adulthood; either	Condition rare; solitary or multiple lesions; appears as superficial ulcer surrounded by white lines or plaque of usual type of lichen planus
Candidiasis (moniliasis; thrush)	Anywhere on oral mucosa	Two extremes of life; also in debilitated persons and in those receiving antibiotics; either	Multiple small white patches; white surface may be lifted or rubbed off, leaving superficial ulcerations of irregular size and shape

Microscopic features	Treatment	Prognosis	Page ref.
Loss of epithelial covering; infiltration of exposed connective tissue by neutrophils, plasma cells, and lymphocytes	Removal of cause; otherwise symptomatic	Excellent	None
Nonspecific superficial ulceration	Lesions refractory to treatment, but disease does not endanger life; cortisone, estrogens, vitamin B complex have been tried	Good	186
Ulceration of mucosa with necrosis of superficial layer; tissue under ulcer shows edema and infiltration by neutrophils and lymphocytes	Scaling and improvement of oral hygiene; debridement of area with hand or ultrasonic devices; soothing mouthwashes; rest; fluids	Good	189
Eosinophils and histiocytes	Surgical excision or low dosage of radiation	Varies; some lesions regress and others progress	356
Ulceration and dense lymphocytic infiltration of upper layers of mucosa; surrounding epithelium shows sawtooth ridges, etc.	None except symptomatic; healing spontaneous	Excellent	389
Ulceration of mucosa; presence of *Candida albicans* near surface; connective tissue under ulcer shows neutrophils, plasma cells, and lymphocytes	Topically or systemically administered nystatin	Good unless disease generalized	396

21

Continued.

Table 3. Ulcerations of oral mucosa—cont'd

Lesion	Usual location	Usual age and sex	Clinical features
Primary herpetic gingivostomatitis	Generalized over mucous membrane	Childhood, usually 1-3 yr; either	Multiple small ulcers of short duration that begin as vesicles but rupture rapidly; preceded by fever, lymphadenopathy, irritability, drooling, headache; present over many areas of mucosa; have yellow-gray membrane
Secondary herpetic lesion	Lips, hard palate, and attached gingiva	Adulthood; either	Lesion starts with itching, followed by reddening and formation of vesicle that ruptures, leaving ulcer; limited to one area; painful; associated with trauma, menstruation, or psychosomatic disturbances
Aphthous ulcer	Oral mucosa except gingiva and anterior hard palate	Adulthood or later; female	Single or multiple ulcers; recurrent; associated with stress; probably caused by alpha hemolytic *Streptococcus*
Periadenitis mucosa necrotica recurrens (Sutton's disease; Mikulicz's ulcer)	Salivary gland–bearing areas of oral and laryngeal mucosa	Adulthood; either	Lesion solitary; starts as painful nodule that soon ulcerates; ulcer craterlike, larger and deeper than herpetic lesion
Herpes zoster (shingles)	Cheek, tongue, and soft palate	Adulthood; male	Ulcers that follow sensory nerve distribution
Erythema multiforme (Stevens-Johnson syndrome; etc.)	Anywhere on oral mucosa	Early adulthood; either	Oral lesions multiple; may start as macules, then becomes vesicles, and finally ulcers; bleeding and crusting of blood on lips may be seen; skin lesions usually also present; believed to be of allergic origin

Microscopic features	Treatment	Prognosis	Page ref.
Essentially same as in traumatic ulcer	Symptomatic to alleviate pain; lesions heal in 7-14 days without scarring	Excellent	403
Same as in primary herpetic gingivostomatitis	Symptomatic; lesions heal in 7-14 days but may recur	Excellent	405
Typical of ulcer	Symptomatic; soothing mouthwashes; tetracyclines	Excellent	410
Ulcer seen lying over salivary gland–bearing portion of mucous membrane	Only symptomatic; ulcers heal spontaneously but slowly and leave scars	Excellent, but lesion annoying and painful; unlike herpetic lesions, heal with scarring	412
Vesicle and later ulcer	Symptomatic	Good	413
Essentially same as in nonspecific ulcer	Symptomatic to alleviate pain and seconday infection	Good; disease self-limiting but annoying	415

Continued.

Table 3. Ulcerations of oral mucosa—cont'd

Lesion	Usual location	Usual age and sex	Clinical features
Behçet's syndrome	Mouth, genitals, eyes, and skin	10-30 yr; male	Aphthalike lesions; presence of oral, ocular, and genital lesions distinguishing feature
Reiter's syndrome	Skin and oral mucosa	20-30 yr; male	Vesicles and ulcers of oral and penile mucosa; urethritis, arthritis, and conjunctivitis
Pemphigus vulgaris	Anywhere on oral mucosa and skin	Middle age or older; either	Oral lesions multiple bullae that soon rupture, leaving large, painful, superficial ulcers; skin lesions usually accompany oral ulcers
Benign mucous membrane pemphigus (pemphigoid)	Anywhere on oral mucosa and on conjunctiva	Over 60 yr; either	Bullous lesions that become ulcers; patient in good health
Smallpox and chickenpox	Anywhere on oral mucosa	Childhood; either	Single or multiple, small, superficial ulcers that start as vesicles; skin lesions always present
Herpangina	Soft palate, uvula, pharynx, and tonsil	Childhood; either	Disease may start with fever, vomiting, and aches; multiple vesicles appear that soon rupture, leaving ulcers; caused by coxsackievirus
Hand-foot-and-mouth disease	Hard palate, tongue, buccal mucosa	Under 5 yr; either	Multiple ulcers and vesicles of oral mucosa; skin lesions; fever, malaise, anorexia, and diarrhea; caused by coxsackievirus
Stomatitis venenata	Anywhere an oral mucosa, especially lip	Any age; either	Single or multiple ulcers of short duration that may start as vesicles; history of allergy and application or local use of substance to which patient is sensitive
Stomatitis medicamentosa	Anywhere on oral mucosa	Any age; either	Same as in stomatitis venenata except that allergen taken systemically

Microscopic features	Treatment	Prognosis	Page ref.
Nonspecific ulcer	Symptomatic	Good	417
Nonspecific ulcer	Symptomatic	Good	418
Essentially same as in ulcer	Symptomatic and palliative	Poor; disease fatal in 50% of patients	418
Intraepithelial and sub-epithelial vesicles and later ulcer	Symptomatic	Good but blindness possible	421
Same as in nonspecific ulcer	None	Good for smallpox; excellent for chicken-pox	422
Same as in primary herpetic gingivostomati-tis	Symptomatic; le-sions heal sponta-neously	Excellent	424
Nonspecific ulcer and vesicle	Symptomatic	Excellent	424
Ulceration and inflam-mation	Removal of aller-gen; symptomatic	Excellent	426
Same as in stomatitis venenata	Discontinuation of offending drug; symptomatic	Excellent	426

Continued.

Table 3. Ulcerations of oral mucosa—cont'd

Lesion	Usual location	Usual age and sex	Clinical features
Squamous cell carcinoma and other malignant epithelial tumors	Any part of oral cavity, usually on lower lip, tongue, and floor of mouth	Fourth decade or later; male	Solitary indurated ulcer of long duration; about 60% present as ulcers
Lymphomas and leukemias	Gingiva	Any age; either	Primary lymphoma may start in oral cavity; oral tissues invariably infiltrated in leukemias; generalized enlargement of gingiva with multiple ulcerations, bleeding, foul odor, and loosening of teeth; varied systemic symptoms
Chancre (syphilis)	Lip, usually upper; sometimes tongue	Adulthood; either	Solitary lesion; 1-4 wk in duration; ulcer with indurated border
Mucous patch (syphilis)	Anywhere on oral mucosa	Adulthood; either	Multiple small, shallow ulcers with gray surface; usually associated with skin eruption; onset with fever, malaise, and sore throat
Tuberculosis	Tonsillar area and soft palate	Any age; either	Rare; usually single chronic ulcer; often secondary to pulmonary tuberculosis

Microscopic features	Treatment	Prognosis	Page ref.
Ulceration; connective tissue shows infiltration by nests, islands, clusters, and sheets of pleomorphic dyskeratotic epithelium; one or more cervical nodes may be enlarged due to metastases	Wide excision; in cervical node metastasis, radical surgical procedure on cervical tissues; in inoperable cases, radiation	Depends on location, size, type of tumor, and age and health of patient	539
In addition to ulcerations, dense infiltration of subepithelial tissues by atypical cells of lymphoid or myeloid series	In lymphosarcoma, wide local excision, but recurrence and metastases common; in leukemias, only supportive and symptomatic oral treatment	Poor	558 and 561
Ulceration of mucous membrane with very dense infiltration by plasma cells and lymphocytes; edema of tissues underlying ulcer	Local only; symptomatic	Good	674
Ulceration; under darkfield illumination or with special stains, numerous spirochetes may be seen	Local only; symptomatic	Fair	675
Ulceration; connective tissue shows circumscribed areas that consist of epithelioid cells and giant cells; some granulomas show central areas of necrosis; lymphocytic infiltration surrounds granulomas	Surgical excision; in lesions secondary to pulmonary tuberculosis, chemotherapeutic and antibiotic agents	Fair	676

Continued.

Table 3. Ulcerations of oral mucosa—cont'd

Lesion	Usual location	Usual age and sex	Clinical features
Histoplamosis	Tongue and gingiva	Adulthood, usually in Mississippi valley; either	Multiple nodules that ulcerate usually associated with fever, malaise, and enlargement of lymph nodes, liver, and spleen
Infectious mononucleosis	Anywhere on oral mucosa	Second and third decades; either	Oral lesions multiple; consist of numerous small ulcers that appear before generalized manifestation of disease; 80% of patients show oral lesions before any other manifestation
Riga-Fede disease	Lingual frenum and tip of tongue	Infancy, either	Ulcer of lingual frenum and tip of tongue due to natal and neonatal teeth
Pterygoid ulcer (Bednar's aphtha)	Soft palate	Newborn, either	Ulcer on soft palate near greater palatine foramen

Microscopic features	Treatment	Prognosis	Page ref.
Underneath ulcer, dense collection of histiocytes with numerous intracytoplasmic, pinpoint-sized spores of *Histoplasma capsulatum*	None except symptomatic; amphotericin B of value	Poor	679
Same as in ulcer	Symptomatic; soon after oral lesions appear, lymph nodes enlarge and other aspects of disease become apparent	Good	696
Same as in nonspecific ulcer	Removal of tooth (if accessory tooth or if symptomatic)	Excellent	None
Same as in nonspecific ulcer	Disappears spontaneously	Excellent	None

Table 4. Pigmented lesions of oral mucosa

Lesion	Usual location	Usual age and sex	Clinical features
Black hairy tongue	Dorsum of tongue	Adulthood; either	Brown to black hairy appearance of dorsum of tongue
Amalgam tattoo	Anywhere on oral mucosa	Any age; either	Small black or bluish pigmentation; usually in vicinity of amalgam filling
Addison's disease	Cheek, lip and gingiva but may be elsewhere	Adulthood; either	Brown-gray or black pigmented patches associated with pigmentation of skin and other systemic manifestations of disease
Normal pigmented patches	Gingiva	Any age; either	Multiple areas of pigmentation on gingiva present from childhood in dark-complexioned individuals
Jeghers' (Peutz-Jeghers) syndrome	Anywhere, especially cheek, palate, and lip	Infancy and later; either	Numerous small brown patches on mucosa; asymptomatic; do not increase in size; associated with similar lesions around mouth, nose, and eyes; symptoms of intestinal polyposis
Melanotic macule	Anywhere, especially lip, gingiva, cheek, and palate	Adulthood; male	Solitary, discrete, gray, brown, blue, or black, nonelevated lesions 0.1-2 cm in size
Nevus	Palate	Any age; either	Usually raised, smooth-surfaced lesions

Microscopic features	Treatment	Prognosis	Page ref.
Hypertrophy of filiform papillae; inflammation of underlying mucosa	Brushing of tongue as frequently as possible	Excellent	441
Connective tissue under epithelium shows numerous black microscopic granules deposited on fibers and around blood vessels; in addition, pieces of amalgam may be present	Excision if necessary	Excellent	430
Melanin pigment in basal layer of epithelium	None for oral lesions	Poor	430 and 671
Melanin pigment in basal layer of epithelium	None	Excellent	433
Melanin pigment in basal layer of epithelium	None for oral lesions	Depends on outcome of intestinal lesions	433
Melanin pigment in basal layer of epithelium and/or upper layers of the lamina propria	None	Excellent	434
Depends on type: junctional, compound, intradermal, or blue	Excision	Good	436

Continued.

Table 4. Pigmented lesions of oral mucosa—cont'd

Lesion	Usual location	Usual age and sex	Clinical features
Melanoma	Maxillary mucosa, mandibular mucosa, cheek, tongue, and floor of mouth, in that order of frequency	30 yr or older; men about twice as frequently as women	Area of pigmentation that increases in size for weeks to years; may be elevated or nonelevated; usually painless; in late stages, ulcerative destruction of bone and loosening of teeth; evidence of metastases in nodes or bones usually present
Heavy metal poisoning (bismuth, mercury, lead, silver)	Free gingiva, but may be elsewhere, especially in silver poisoning (argyria)	Adulthood; either	Gray to black pigmentation of free gingiva, but pigmentation also may be present elsewhere on mucous membrane, particularly in argyria; history of exposure to heavy metals through use of drugs or some other means; systemic symptoms common; gray pigmentation of skin, as in argyria; excessive salivation may be seen
Postmenopausal state	Attached gingiva	Over 40 yr; female	Brown or black pigmentation of attached gingiva
Ingestion of tranquilizers	Attached gingiva	Adulthood; either	Brown or black pigmentation of attached gingiva caused by tranquilizers
Ingestion of oral contraceptives	Attached gingiva	Adulthood; female	Multiple light brown or gray areas of pigmentation
Varicosity	Ventral surface of tongue	Old age; either	Bluish area; can be blanched with pressure
Malnutrition	Anywhere on oral mucosa	Any age; either	Multiple black or brown patches; other evidences of malnutrition present

Microscopic features	Treatment	Prognosis	Page ref.
Usually large epithelial cells lying in clusters but noncohesive; melanin pigment in both intracellular and extracellular locations; however, microscopic picture varies widely	Wide excision, with radical neck procedure if indicated	Grave	441 and 550
Deposition of fine black or brown granules on collagen fibers, particularly around blood vessels	Prophylaxis; if possible, elimination of contact with offending metal	Good	441 and 663
Melanin pigment in basal layer of epithelium	None	Good	441
Melanin pigment in basal layer of epithelium	None	Good	441
Pigmentation in basal layer of epithelium	None	Excellent	441
Dilated veins	None unless large, in which case surgical excision or ligation	Excellent	441
Melanin pigment in basal layer of epithelium	Removal of cause	Good	441

Table 5. Firm, nonhemorrhagic soft tissue growths of oral

Lesion	Usual location	Usual age and sex	Clinical feature
Fibromatosis	Gingiva	Any age; either	Multiple generalized enlargements of gingiva; smooth-surfaced, firm lesions; cover part of teeth; may produce migration of teeth; long duration; may be hereditary or result from ingestion of phenytoin
Torus (exostosis; peripheral osteoma) and related lesions	Midline of palate and mandible	Adulthood; female	Hard, nodular enlargement in midline of palate (torus palatinus) or on lingual surface of mandible in area of premolars (torus mandibularis); long duration; slow growth
Irritation fibroma	Anywhere on oral mucosa, expecially cheek, tongue, and lip	Third decade and later; either	Solitary firm, smooth-surfaced, pedunculated or sessile, elevated growth of long duration; usually associated with some local mild, persistent trauma
Peripheral fibroma and peripheral fibroma with calcification	Gingiva	Any age; either	Solitary sessile, firm to hard lesion; may have smooth or cobblestone surface
Myxoma (fibroma with myxomatous degeneration)	Anywhere on oral mucosa	Any age; either	True myxoma in oral cavity extremely rare; so called "myxomas" are fibromas with myxomatous degeneration; pedunculated or sessile lesions of long duration
Neurofibroma and schwannoma (neurilemoma)	Tongue, lip, palate, and cheek	Any age; either	Sessile or deep-seated and freely movable lesion; solitary except in multiple neurofibromatosis, in which multiple lesions of skin and tongue common; long duration; smooth surface

cavity

Microscopic features	Treatment	Prognosis	Page ref.
Growth consists entirely of collagen; covered by stratified squamous epithelium that shows long, thin ridges	Gingivectomy and scaling; recurrences common	Good	182
Exophytic lesion with periphery of cortical bone and center of trabecular bone and fibrous marrow; entire lesion covered by normal mucosa	Excision	Excellent	311
Lesion covered by stratified squamous epithelium; consists of dense collagen	Local excision curative	Excellent	485
Tumor covered by stratified squamous epithelium; consists of connective tissue that sometimes shows foci of calcification	Local excision usually curative, but lesion may recur	Excellent	485
Lesions show dense connective tissue with areas of myxomatous degeneration	Excision	Excellent	485 and 489
Neurofibroma and schwannoma may be distingusihed microscopically, but essentially similar lesions; consist of fibroblastic and Schwann cell proliferation	Excision	Excellent	512

35

Continued.

Table 5. Firm, nonhemorrhagic soft tissue growths of oral

Lesion	Usual location	Usual age and sex	Clinical features
Lipoma	Cheek and floor of mouth	Any age; either	Rare growth; yellowish or normal color; pedunculated or deep seated; long duration
Granular cell myoblastoma	Tongue	Any age; either	Elevated sessile, or deep-seated lesion; long duration
Sialadenitis	Floor of mouth	Adulthood; male	History of pain and swelling in area of submaxillary gland associated with eating; evidence of salivary stone possible; firm enlargement in area of submaxillary and sublingual glands
Tumor of salivary gland	Palate, lip, cheek, and tongue, in that order of frequency	Any age; either	Various types of tumor; elevated or deep-seated lesion of long or short duration; in swelling of oral tissues, tumor of salivary gland must be considered

cavity—cont'd

Microscopic features	Treatment	Prognosis	Page ref.
Usually circumscribed growth consisting of normal fat cells	Excision	Excellent	519
Lesion composed of characteristic large granular cells; covering epithelium shows marked hyperplasia and mimics carcinoma	Excision	Excellent	520
Gland shows fibrosis, atrophy of acini, and in-filtration by plasma cells and lymphocytes	Excision	Excellent	588
Depends on type	Wide excision	Depends on type	597

Table 6. Hemorrhagic or easily bleeding soft tissue growths of

Lesion	Usual location	Usual age and sex	Clinical features
Parulis (periodontal abscess; gumboil)	Gingiva and alveolar mucosa	Any age; either	Solitary soft, red, circumscribed enlargement of gingiva or alveolar mucosa; incision reveals pus; associated with periodontal disease
Eosinophilic granuloma	Maxillary or mandibular gingiva	Adulthood; male about five times as frequently as female	Soft tissue lesion usually associated with underlying lesion in bone; consists of swelling, ulceration, necrosis, and pain in involved gingiva; loosening of teeth; fetid breath
Epulis fissuratum	Maxillary or mandibular fornix	Middle age or older; either	Red, exuberant tissue associated with ill-fitting denture flange in mucobuccal or mucolabial fold; may be ulcerated and often shows gutter where denture fits
Peripheral giant cell granuloma	Gingiva, especially interdental papilla	20-50 yr; male about twice as frequently as female	Pedunculated or broad-based, smooth or lobulated, hemorrhagic, easily bleeding lesion; duration, week to months; sometimes occurs after tooth extraction
Pyogenic granuloma	Gingiva and tongue, but may occur anywhere on oral mucosa	Any age; either	Hemorrhagic, pedunculated or sessile, smooth-surfaced or lobulated growth that bleeds easily and often shows bloody crust; may look like raspberry; duration, weeks to months

Microscopic features	Treatment	Prognosis	Page ref.
Swelling covered by stratified squamous epithelium; consists of circumscribed aggregate of pus	Drainage and correction of periodontal disturbance that is primary cause of lesion	Excellent	201
Characteristic infiltration of involved area by histiocytes and dense aggregates of eosinophilic leukocytes	Surgical removal or low doses of radiation	Varies; some regress or do not recur after excision, whereas others progress	356
Connective tissue with dense infiltration by plasma cells and lymphocytes; surface covered by stratified squamous epithelium but may be ulcerated in an area	Removal and correction of ill-fitting denture; surgical excision if mass large; small lesions may regress after removal of denture	Excellent	492
Tumor composed of many small blood vessels, abundant fibroblasts, and many giant cells; shows hemosiderin and bleeding	Excision	Excellent	497
Lesion usually pedunculated and only partly covered by stratified squamous epithelium; mainly composed of small blood vessels; connective tissue that separates blood vessels shows edema and infiltration by neutrophils, plasma cells, and lymphocytes	Excision; if incomplete, recurrence possible	Excellent	498

Continued.

Table 6. Hemorrhagic or easily bleeding soft tissue growths of

Lesion	Usual location	Usual age and sex	Clinical features
Pregnancy tumor (granuloma gravidarum)	Gingiva, especially interdental papilla	Adulthood; female	Same as in pyogenic granuloma; occurs only on gingiva; starts about third month of pregnancy and grows up to parturition
Squamous cell carcinoma and other malignant tumors	Anywhere in oral cavity	Any age; either	Rapidly growing, easily bleeding soft tissue growth
Lymphomas (lymphosarcoma; reticulum cell sarcoma) and leukemias	Gingiva	Any age; either	Lymphomas may be primary in oral cavity and appear as ulcers or hemorrhagic growths of short duration; leukemias invariably produce generalized enlargements of gingiva that may later ulcerate; bleeding frequent

Microscopic features	Treatment	Prognosis	Page ref.
Same as in pyogenic granuloma	After childbirth, lesion may regress spontaneously; recurrence in same location in subsequent pregnancy likely; excision after parturition recommended	Excellent	502
Depends on type; squamous cell carcinoma most common	Wide excision of primary lesion as well as metastatic growth; radiation in inoperable cases	Fair to grave, depending on location, size, grade, type of tumor, and age of patient	539
Dense infiltration of connective tissue by abnormal cells of lymphocytic and reticulum cell series	In lymphomas, surgical excision; recurrence and spread common; in leukemias, treatment only symptomatic	Grave	558

Table 7. Compressible soft tissue growths of oral cavity

Lesion	Usual location	Usual age and sex	Clinical features
Eruption cyst	Alveolar ridge	Childhood; either	Compressible, sometimes blue lesion overlying erupting tooth
Mucocele (mucous retention cyst; retention phenomenon)	Usually lip and tongue but may be anywhere on oral mucosa	Any age; either	Solitary vesicular, compressible, translucent, sometimes bluish lesion; history of week or more; ruptures, discharges mucoid secretion, and recurs
Mucous cyst	Floor of mouth; less often, cheek, lip, and tongue	Adulthood; either	Rare; resembles mucocele; no evidence of trauma to gland
Ranula	Floor of mouth	Adulthood; either	Compressible enlargement in floor of mouth; may elevate tongue and interfere with speech; associated with submaxillary or sublingual gland
Gingival cyst	Buccal gingiva in mandibular canine and premolar area	Adulthood; either	Rare, small, asymptomatic lesion; compressible when large; may appear as small radiolucency
Nasoalveolar cyst	Upper lip and base of nostril	Adulthood; either	Compressible soft tissue growth in upper lip; may produce periosteal bone resorption
Epidermoid cyst (dermoid, epidermal, dermal)	Floor of mouth but may be elsewhere	Early adulthood or later; either	Compressible enlargement in floor of mouth; elevates tongue and interferes with speech; slow growth; long duration

Microscopic features	Treatment	Prognosis	Page ref.
Cyst lined by squamous epithelium	None or incision	Excellent	226
Cyst containing mucus and lined by granulation tissue; associated gland may show interstitial inflammation; in early stages, mucus diffusely dispersed in connective tissue	Local excision	Excellent; if associated gland not removed, recurrence most likely	461
Cyst lined by epithelium	Excision	Excellent	463
Large mucus-containing cyst with lining of granulation tissue	Excision or removal of roof of cyst (marsupialization)	Excellent	463
Cyst lined by squamous epithelium	Excision	Excellent	464
Cyst lined by squamous or respiratory epithelium	Excision	Excellent	237
Keratin-containing cyst lined by keratinized stratified squamous epithelium; wall of cyst may contain sebaceous glands and, rarely, sweat glands and hair follicles	Excision	Excellent	466

Continued. 43

Table 7. Compressible soft tissue growths of oral cavity—cont'd

Lesion	Usual location	Usual age and sex	Clinical features
Cavernous and capillary hemangioma	Cheek, tongue, and lip	Childhood and adulthood; either	Bluish, red, or purple lesion diffuse and compressible; grows slowly or remains stationary in size; asymptomatic except when large; bleeds on trauma; may produce macroglossia and macrocheilia
Lymphangioma	Tongue and cheek	Childhood and adulthood; either	Multiple vesicular excrescences; compressible; translucent; long duration and asymptomatic except when large; lesions of tongue may produce macroglossia and interfere with speech and deglutition
Cystic hygroma (cystic lymphangioma; hygroma cysticum colli)	Floor of mouth	Infancy; either	Extensive compressible unilateral growth extending upward from neck; grows progressively; involved areas replaced by tumor; normal structures grossly displaced or destroyed

Table 8. Papillary or cauliflower-like soft tissue growths of oral

Lesion	Usual location	Usual age and sex	Clinical features
Verrucous leukoplakia	Anywhere on oral mucosa	Middle age or older; male	Rough, elevated, solitary white lesion
Verruca vulgaris	Lip, cheek, and tongue	Adulthood; either	Sessile, white, cauliflower-like lesion; solitary but sometimes multiple
Condyloma acuminatum	Anywhere on oral mucosa	Adulthood; either	Very rare; papillary growth with broad base; multiple lesions

Microscopic features	Treatment	Prognosis	Page ref.
Numerous large, thin-walled, blood-containing channels in connective tissue of mucosa	Escharotics, electrocautery, or surgical excision; some will regress spontaneously	Usually excellent	502
Numerous large, thin-walled spaces that contain clear homogeneous lymph; my occur in conjunction with hemangiomas	Excision only treatment	Good, depending on site and size of tumor	507
Numerous large lymph-containing cavernous spaces	Excision	Poor	510

cavity

Microscopic features	Treatment	Prognosis	Page ref.
Epithelium thrown in folds; shows hyperkeratosis and dyskeratosis but no invasion	Wide excision	Depends on location; good prognosis in lesions of lip	380
Epithelium thrown into numerous folds; shows keratinization and parakeratosis; epithelial cells normal	Excision	Excellent	475
Papillary lesion covered by parakeratotic thick layer of stratified squamous epithelium	Excision	Excellent	475

Continued.

Table 8. Papillary or cauliflower-like soft tissue growths of oral

Lesion	Usual location	Usual age and sex	Clinical features
Papilloma	Anywhere on oral mucosa	Adulthood; either	Pedunculated, white, cauliflower-like growth on long duration
Pseudoepitheliomatous hyperplasia (keratoacanthoma)	Lip	Middle age or older; male	Verrucous lesion; rough; grows rapidly to about 1 cm in size; duration, few weeks
Inflammatory papillary hyperplasia	Palate	Middle age or older; either	Lesion associated with ill-fitting dentures; usually seen on palate; presents as multiple papillae on mucosa; due to food impaction between papillae; inflammation common, and area appears red
Verrucous carcinoma	Alveolar ridge and palate	Old age; male	White, cauliflower-like, exophytic growth; patients usually tobacco chewers

Microscopic features	Treatment	Prognosis	Page ref.
Papillary lesion with covering of stratified squamous epithelium that may be keratinized; epithelial papillae carry thin connective tissue stalks	Excision at base	Excellent	477
Epithelium thrown in folds and keratinized; in center of lesion, curettage reveals mass of keratin; normal epithelium extends to and covers sides of lesion; must be distinguished from squamous cell carcinoma, which it closely mimics	Excision	Excellent; spontaneous regression may occur	481
Each papilla consists of connective tissue infiltrated by plasma cells and lymphocytes; covered by hyperplastic stratified squamous epithelium	Removal and correction of ill-fitting denture; early lesions may regress if denture temporarily removed; surgical excision in extensive involvement	Excellent	483
Papillary lesion consisting of folded epithelium; latter usually keratinized and shows dyskeratosis; underlying connective tissue invaded by tumor cells	Wide excision	Better than that of squamous cell carcinoma, nonverrucous type	545

Table 9. Radiolucent lesions of jaws

Lesion	Usual location	Usual age and sex	Clinical and radiographic features
Lesions at apex of tooth			
Dental granuloma	Either jaw	Any age; either	Asymptomatic, circumscribed radiolucency at apex of nonvital tooth
Radicular cyst	Either jaw	Any age; either	Same as in dental granuloma
Residual cyst	Edentulous space; apical area of extraction site	Any age; either	Usually solitary, asymptomatic, circumscribed radiolucency located in edentulous space; history of extraction in area
Periapical (dentoalveolar) abscess	Either jaw	Any age; either	Usually solitary, diffuse or fairly well-circumscribed area of radiolucency; swelling, redness, pain, and fever may be associated symptoms; one or more teeth in area nonvital; associated tooth very sensitive to percussion
Apical scar	Apical area	Adulthood; either	Tooth with root canal filling and apical surgery; asymptomatic; apical radiolucency
Cementoma (first stage)	Anterior mandibular teeth	Over 30 yr; female	Asymptomatic, usually multiple, small periapical areas of radiolucency in incisor region; teeth vital; must be distinguished from periapical cysts and granulomas
Lesions in midline of maxilla			
Median palatine cyst	Midline of palate only	Adulthood; either	Solitary area of radiolucency in midline of palate behind incisive papilla; asymptomatic or may produce swelling in palate

48

Microscopic features	Treatment	Prognosis	Page ref.
Connective tissue with neutrophils, plasma cells, and lymphocytes	Root canal treatment or extraction of involved tooth	Excellent	161
Cystic cavity lined by stratified squamous epithelium; connective tissue wall contains plasma cells, lymphocytes, and foam cells	Root canal treatment with or without apicoectomy	Excellent	165
Same as in radicular cyst; represents radicular cyst left in jaw after extraction of tooth	Enucleation	Excellent	169
Connective tissue with dense neutrophilic infiltration, edema, plasma cells, and lymphocytes; surrounding areas of bone marrow show similar changes and necrotic osteocytes	Drainage; extraction of offending tooth	Excellent	172
Dense scar tissue	None	Excellent	172
In early stage, lesion consists of young fibrous connective tissue; few foci of cementum may also be seen	None necessary	Excellent	266
Cyst lined by stratified squamous or respiratory epithelium	Enucleation	Excellent	233

Continued.

Table 9. Radiolucent lesions of jaws—cont'd

Lesion	Usual location	Usual age and sex	Clinical and radiographic features
Median alveolar cyst	Anterior to incisive papilla	Adulthood; either	Solitary circumscribed radiolucent area in anterior part of midline of palate; asymptomatic or may produce swelling; neighboring teeth vital
Globulomaxillary cyst	Between lateral incisor and canine	Adulthood; either	Solitary pear-shaped radiolucency between lateral incisor and canine; neck or "pear" toward crowns; cyst produces divergence of roots of canine and lateral incisor; may produce swelling on palatal or labial sides; teeth vital
Nasoalveolar cyst	Upper lip at base of nostril	Adulthood; either	Rare; usually causes no radiolucency; sometimes bone destruction from periosteal side produces radiolucency in lateral incisor area
Incisive canal cyst	Behind maxillary anterior teeth	Adulthood; either	Solitary circumscribed, often heart-shaped area of radiolucency behind maxillary incisors; asymptomatic or may produce swelling in palate; all teeth in area vital
Cyst of palatine papilla	Incisive papilla	Adulthood; either	Swelling in area of incisive papilla; sometimes produces radiolucency, as does incisive canal cyst

Lesion in place of missing tooth

Lesion	Usual location	Usual age and sex	Clinical and radiographic features
Primordial cyst	Mandible, especially third molar and premolar areas	Adulthood; either	Solitary well-circumscribed radiolucent area; asymptomatic or may produce enlargement; cyst arises in place of normal or supernumerary tooth

Lesion around crown of impacted tooth

Lesion	Usual location	Usual age and sex	Clinical and radiographic features
Dentigerous cyst	Most often mandibular third molar and maxillary canine areas	Adulthood; either	Solitary well-defined area of radiolucency associated with crown of impacted or unerupted normal or supernumerary tooth; enlargement of jaw and migra-

50

Microscopic features	Treatment	Prognosis	Page ref.
Cyst lined by stratified squamous or respiratory epithelium	Enucleation	Excellent	233
Cyst lined by stratified squamous or respiratory epithelium	Enucleation	Excellent	235
Cyst lined by ciliated or squamous epithelium	Enucleation	Excellent	237
Cyst lined by stratified squamous or respiratory epithelium; connective tissue wall contains nerves and mucous glands	Enucleation	Excellent	238
Same as in incisive canal cyst	Enucleation	Excellent	238
Cyst lined by stratified squamous epithelium	Enucleation and curettage	Excellent	218
Epithelium-lined cystic lesion around crown of impacted tooth; connective tissue wall of cyst may show foci of ame-	Enucleation and curettage; latter necessary because some ameloblastomas arise	Good	220

51

Continued.

Table 9. Radiolucent lesions of jaws—cont'd

Lesion	Usual location	Usual age and sex	Clinical and radiographic features
	but may be elsewhere		tion of teeth may be present; cortex intact
Ameloblastoma	Mandible, especially posterior part of body and ramus	Over 30 yr; male	Solitary or multicystic soap bubble–like area of radiolucency; long duration; slow growth; asymptomatic or may produce marked enlargement and deformity; migration of teeth; cortex of jaw seldom destroyed; teeth in area vital
Odontogenic adenomatoid tumor (adeno-ameloblastoma)	Maxillary canine area	10-20 yr; female	Solitary area of well-defined radiolucency usually associated with crowns of impacted teeth; growth slow; asymptomatic or may produce enlargement
Odontogenic fibroma and myxoma	Mandibular third molars and maxillary canines	Under 20 yr; either	Solitary area of radiolucency; well-defined borders; associated with crowns of impacted teeth; often small but may expand cortex; teeth vital

Soap bubble–like radiolucencies

Lesion	Usual location	Usual age and sex	Clinical and radiographic features
Multilocular cyst	Either jaw	Adulthood; either	Extremely rare; multicystic radiolucency; may have soap bubble–like appearance; enlargement of jaw; cortex intact
Aneurysmal bone cyst	Mandible more often than maxilla	Under 20 yr; either	Solitary or honeycombed well-demarcated cystic lesion; cortex often expanded but not destroyed; history of trauma; may be swelling, migration of teeth, and slight tenderness; associated teeth vital; exploration reveals defect filled with hemorrhagic spongy tissue

52

Microscopic features	Treatment	Prognosis	Page ref.
loblastic proliferation	in these cysts		
Islands and cords of epithelium with tall, columnar peripheral cells and central cells resembling stellate reticulum	Depends on individual patient and varies from local conservative excision to radical resection of jaw	Good to fair, depending on lesion; recurrence common; lesion may metastasize, but this is extremely rare	252
Tumor encapsulated or circumscribed; consists of ductlike structures lined by columnar cells; between ducts, abundant amount of epithelium; foci of calcification may also be associated with lesion	Enucleation	Excellent; lesion benign and, unlike ameloblastoma, does not recur	259
Fibroblastic proliferation with foci of odontogenic epithelium; in odontogenic myxoma, abundant myxomatous tissue	Curettage	Excellent; odontogenic myxoma must be distinguished from true myxoma	269
Multiple cysts lined by stratified, sometimes keratinized, epithelium; cysts may contain keratin	Curettage	Good, but lesion may recur	226
Lesion not true cyst; shows numerous blood-containing spaces; tissue between blood pools consists of giant cells, fibroblasts, and blood vessels and shows foci of hemosiderin	Curettage curative; recurrences rare	Excellent	242

53

Continued.

Table 9. Radiolucent lesions of jaws—cont'd

Lesion	Usual location	Usual age and sex	Clinical and radiographic features
Ameloblas-toma (p. 52)			
Giant cell granuloma (central)	Mandible more than maxilla	Under 20 yr; female more frequently than male	Solitary clear-cut or soap bubble–like lesion of jaw; expansive, with cortex destruction possible; history of trauma; regional teeth may show migration
Cherubism (early stage) or familial intraosseous fibrous swelling of jaws	Mandible, especially posterior region	Childhood; either	Hereditary disease that begins in early childhood and produces bilateral enlargement of posterior part of mandible; multicystic, slowly enlarging bilateral lesion; expands but does not destroy cortex; regional teeth and tooth germs migrate; lesion may involve anterior part of mandible or maxilla; teeth in region vital; lesion painless; disease present in number of members of same family
Myxoma (nonodonto-genic)	Either jaw	Second to fourth decade; either	Single or soap bubble–like radiolucency; slow growth, migration of teeth; teeth in area retain vitality

Multiple but separate radiolucent lesions

Lesion	Usual location	Usual age and sex	Clinical and radiographic features
Cherubism (p. 54)			
Multiple myeloma	Mandible more than maxilla; premolar and molar area, angle, and ramus	After middle age; male	In about one third of patients, jaws involved; jaw lesion may be earliest manifestation; clear-cut multiple areas of complete radiolucency; may be pain, pressure, numbness, swelling, and mobility of teeth; solitary lesions may occur in jaws

Microscopic features	Treatment	Prognosis	Page ref.
Giant cells, blood vessels, and fibroblastic proliferation; hemosiderin and foci of bone formation	Curettage	Excellent	295
Fibrous connective tissue with foci of bone formation and giant cells	None; lesion grows in size for 4-6 yr, then becomes static; gradually growth of mandible catches up with deformity	Excellent	306
Myxomatous tissue; no evidence of odontogenic epithelium	Wide excision	Good	298
Dense mass of plasma cells	Symptomatic; surgical; radiation	Grave	322

Continued.

Table 9. Radiolucent lesions of jaws—cont'd

Lesion	Usual location	Usual age and sex	Clinical and radiographic features
Eosinophilic granuloma	Either jaw	Second or third decade; either	Sharp, clear-cut areas of complete radiolucency; if around teeth, latter appear to be "hanging in air"; associated soft tissue or oral mucosa shows ulceration and necrosis; pain, malaise, and other systemic symptoms; teeth in area vital
Hand-Schüller-Christian disease	Either jaw	Childhood; male	Same as in eosinophilic granuloma; many other systemic manifestations
Letterer-Siwe disease	Mandible and maxilla	Under 3 yr; either	Multiple jaw radiolucencies; enlargement of spleen, liver, and lymph nodes; rapid deterioration of general health
Hyperparathyroidism (brown node, giant cell lesion)	Either jaw	Middle age or older; female more frequently than male	Rare, but oral lesions may be first manifestation of disease; consist of diffuse or clear-cut areas of radiolucency; teeth vital
Metastatic tumor	Either jaw	Middle age or older; either	Radiolucent area usually solitary but may be multiple; asymptomatic or associated with pain and numbness; history of tumor elsewhere, or jaw radiolucency may be primary symptom

Microscopic features	Treatment	Prognosis	Page ref.
Histiocytes and eosinophils; destruction of bone	Surgical excision or low dosage of radiation	Fair to good, depending on other sytemic and skeletal involvement	356
Histiocytes, some of which contain cholesterol and appear large and foamy	Symptomatic; radiation	Poor	360
Proliferation of histiocytes	Symptomatic; corticosteriods	Poor	361
Same as in giant cell granuloma, but these lesions recur after repeated removal	Removal of hyperplastic or neoplastic parathyroid gland	Fair to good	667
Depends on type of tumor; usually primary sites are breast, kidney, large bowel, and prostate; prostatic and breast tumors may produce radiopacity	Treatment of primary site and of jaw lesion depends on type of tumor, duration, age of patient, and numerous other factors	Poor to grave	330

Continued.

Table 9. Radiolucent lesions of jaws—cont'd

Lesion	Usual location	Usual age and sex	Clinical and radiographic features
Lesions that destroy cortical plate			
Metastatic-tumor (p. 56)			
Primary malignant tumor	Either jaw	Any age; either	Rare, rapidly growing radiolucency; may produce loosening of teeth and resorption of roots; single area of radiolucency; destruction of cortex
Osteomyelitis	Any area of jaws; however, more common in mandible	Any age; either	Diffuse radiolucency; may destroy the cortex; any or all of following symptoms present: pain, swelling, pus, draining sinuses, loose and painful devitalized teeth or tooth in area, history of trauma, sequestration of necrotic bone, leukocytosis, fever
Miscellaneous radiolucencies			
Lateral periodontal cyst	Periodontal ligament; buccal, lingual, mesial, or distal	Any age; either	Solitary small, circumscribed lesion in periodontal ligament; tooth may be vital or nonvital; lesion rare
Traumatic cyst	Mandible between canine and ramus	Early adulthood; either	Solitary well-circumscribed cystic lesion; upper border often appears scalloped; history of trauma; lesion asymptomatic or may produce enlargement of jaw; may be pain; teeth in area vital; cortex intact; exploration reveals cavity to be empty or to contain very little blood-stained fluid
Idiopathic bone cavity	Mandible	Adulthood; either	Asymptomatic radiolucency below inferior dental canal just anterior to mandibular angle

Microscopic features	Treatment	Prognosis	Page ref.
Depends on type	Radical local excision	Fair	316
Necrosis of bone; bone resorption; infiltration of marrow spaces by neutrophils, plasma cells, and lymphocytes	Drainage, antibiotics, removal of sequestra; in extensive cases, bone grafts	Good	362
Cystic lesion lined by stratified squamous epithelium	Enucleation; if associated with devitalized tooth, root canal treatment or extraction	Excellent	169
Cyst lined by extremely thin layer of connective tissue; absence of epithelial lining; usually difficult to obtain specimen for microscopic study	Curettage; lesion fills in with clot and heals	Excellent	239
Fibrous tissue or salivary gland or fat	None	Excellent	241

Continued.

Table 9. Radiolucent lesions of jaws—cont'd

Lesion	Usual location	Usual age and sex	Clinical and radiographic features
Osteomyelitis (p. 58)			
Hemato-poietic marrow	Premolar and molar areas of mandible	Middle age or older; either	Asymptomatic radiolucency
Gingival cyst	Premolar and canine areas of mandible	Adulthood; either	Rare, small, asymptomatic radiolucency in mandibular canine or premolar areas; gingiva enlarged; palpation usually reveals small cystic lesion
Physiologic osteoporosis	Premolar and molar areas of mandible	Old; either	Ill-defined areas of radiolucency; asymptomatic
Hemangioma (central)	Mandible more than maxilla	Young; either	Single or honeycomb-like radiolucency; loosening of teeth; area may be warmer than normal; expansion may be present

Microscopic features	Treatment	Prognosis	Page ref.
Usual features of red bone marrow	None	Excellent	364
Cyst lined by stratified squamous epithelium; cyst present in gingiva but produces bone resorption from gingival side	Enucleation	Excellent	464
Reduction in number of bone trabeculae	None	Excellent	367
Marrow with many blood vessels or spaces	Resection; small lesion may be sclerosed	Poor	313

Table 10. Radiopaque lesions of jaws

Lesion	Usual location	Usual age and sex	Clincal and radiographic features
Cementoma (third stage)	Mandible anterior teeth	Over 30 yr; female	Multiple small, asymptomatic periapical areas of radiopacity; teeth vital
Compound odontoma	Either jaw	Any age; either	Radiopacity that remains static for years and in which toothlike structures can be vaguely or distinctly seen
Complex odontoma	Either jaw	Any age; either	Irregular, asymptomatic radiopacity of limited growth; teeth vital
Ossifying fibroma (fibrous dysplasia)	Either jaw	Childhood and adulthood; either	Single radiopacity; long duration; painless; may be expansile
Osteoma and torus	Either jaw	Any age; either	Circumscribed radiopaque area of slow growth
Osteogenic sarcoma	Mandible	Under 30 yr; male	Radiopacity of rapid growth; usually extends beyond cortex; radiographs may show sunray effect, which consists of radiopaque streaks that extend away from cortex; loosening of teeth; pain; numbness; root resorption
Chondrosarcoma	Either jaw	Over 25 yr; either	Rare; radiopacity usually extends beyond confines of jaw; paresthesia; pain; loosening of teeth
Metastatic tumor	Either jaw	Old age; either	Extremely rare; irregular areas of radiopacity; solitary or multiple; usually from metastasis of prostatic carcinoma and, less often, breast cancer; loosening of teeth; paresthesia; pain

Microscopic features	Treatment	Prognosis	Page ref.
Dense mass of cementum	None	Excellent	266
Few or many toothlike structures composed of dentin, enamel, and cementum	Excision unless danger of fracture during removal	Excellent	279
Irregular, disorganized mass of hard dental tissue	Excision unless danger of fracture during removal	Excellent	279
Fibrous tissue with bone	Excision	Good	302
Normal mature lamellated bone	Excision	Excellent	310 and 311
Atypical trabeculae of bone; osteoid, atypical osteoblasts, and giant cells	Wide radical excision or radiation followed by excision	Poor	316
Cartilage and cartilage-like tissue; atypical chondrocytes	Wide, radical excision	Fair to poor	320
Depends on primary site	Treatment of primary lesions; excision of metastasis	Poor	330

Continued.

Table 10. Radiopaque lesions of jaws—cont'd

Lesion	Usual location	Usual age and sex	Clinical and radiographic features
Paget's disease (osteitis deformans)	Maxilla slightly more frequently than mandible	Over 45 yr; male	Single or multiple areas of irregular cotton wool appearance; in early stages, lesion may have ground-glass appearance; hypercementosis on regional teeth; teeth vital; spacing of teeth; systemic symptoms; lesions in other bones; enlarging skull
Osteopetrosis (Albers-Schönberg disease; marble bone disease)	Both jaws	Childhood; either	Rare; marked radiopacity of entire skeleton; blindness, deafness, anemia, fractures, and many other systemic manifestations; retarded eruption of teeth
Leontiasis ossea	Maxilla	Childhood; either	Very rare disease; diffuse radiopacity of maxilla and zygomatic and other bones of upper face; blindness, deafness, and other symptoms of pressure on cranial nerves
Caffey's disease (infantile cortical hyperostosis)	Mandible	Under 6 mo; either	Mandible commonly involved in this generalized disease; irritability, swelling, and cortical thickening over mandible; radiographs negative in early stages but later show faint radiopacity and thickening of cortex
Garré's osteomyelitis	Mandible	Childhood and adolescence; either	Radiopaque bulge at cortical surface of mandible; associated with carious tooth, often first molar
Condensing osteitis	Mandible	Any age; either	Usually solitary but may be multiple radiopacities; associated with periapical area of carious teeth, broken roots, or endentulous jaws; asymptomatic or with sporadic symptoms of pain and drainage

64

Microscopic features	Treatment	Prognosis	Page ref.
Dense trabecular bone with numerous areas of bone apposition and resorption; fibrous marrow	None	Poor	340
Numerous trabeculae of bone; fibrous marrow	None	Poor	344
Dense bone trabeculae	None	Grave	346
New, widely spaced trabeculae of immature bone separated by edematous connective tissue	Antibiotics; lesion regresses within year	Excellent	347
New bone formation; fibrous marrow with infiltration by plasma cells and lymphocytes	Extraction of offending tooth, after which deformity may disappear	Excellent	347
Dense bone; fibrous marrow with infiltration by plasma cells and lymphocytes	Removal of cause; some lesions may be left untreated, whereas others require excision	Excellent	350

Continued.

Table 10. Radiopaque lesions of jaws—cont'd

Lesion	Usual location	Usual age and sex	Clinical and radiographic features
Root fragment or foreign body	Either jaw	Any age; either	Asymptomatic; radiopacity resembling roots of teeth; foreign bodies such as amalgam appear as total radiopacites
Chronic sclerosing osteomyelitis	Mandible	Fourth decade or later; female	Multiple radiopaque areas in jaw; molar and premolar areas; few months to few years in duration; usually asymptomatic; alkaline phosphatase normal

Table 11. Partly radiopaque and partly radiolucent lesions of

Lesion	Usual location	Usual age and sex	Clinical and radiographic features
Cementoma (second stage)	Anterior teeth of mandible	Over 30 yr; female	Asymptomatic; usually multiple small periapical areas of radiolucency and radiopacity; teeth vital; must be distinguished from periapical cyst and granuloma
Ameloblastic fibro-odontoma	Maxilla	Under 20 yr; female	Irregular, slowly growing area of radiopacity associated with varying degree of radiolucency
Cystic odontoma	Either jaw	Any age; either	Complex or compound odontoma surrounded by or associated with radiolucency that appears to increase in size slowly

Microscopic features	Treatment	Prognosis	Page ref.
Consistent with root tip or appropriate foreign matter	None unless associated with inflammation and radiolucency	Excellent	None
Dense lamellated bone with many basophilic lines; may resemble Paget's disease; fibrous marrow	None; if secondarily infected, surgical excision	Good	350

jaws

Microscopic features	Treatment	Prognosis	Page ref.
Fibrous connective tissue with foci of cementum	Unless secondarily infected, none necessary	Excellent	266
Areas of dentin and enamel; abundant to little soft tissue that consists of ameloblastic epithelium and tissue resembling dental papilla	Local excision	Excellent	276
Complex or compound odontoma associated with epithelium-lined cyst	Local enucleation and curettage	Excellent	284

Continued.

Table 11. Partly radiopaque and partly radiolucent lesions of

Lesion	Usual location	Usual age and sex	Clinical and radiographic features
Ossifying fibroma (fibrous dysplasia)	Either jaw	Adulthood or earlier; either	Solitary radiolucent and radiopaque area; enlargement of jaw; however, no erosion of cortex; teeth may migrate but all vital
Osteogenic sarcoma	Mandible	Under 30 yr; male	Some lesions partly radiolucent and partly radiopaque; rapid growth; pain
Chondrosarcoma	Either jaw	Over 25 yr; either	Rare; radiopacity and radiolucency extend beyond confines of jaw; paresthesia; pain; loosening of teeth
Metastasis from carcinoma of prostate or breast	Either jaw	Old age; either	Rare; solitary or multiple; usually from prostatic carcinoma, less often from breast carcinoma; loosening of teeth; paresthesia; pain
Paget's disease (osteitis deformans)	Either jaw; maxilla slightly more frequently	Over 45 yr; male	Single or multiple areas of irregular cotton wool appearance; in early stages, may have radiolucent and radiopaque appearance; spacing of teeth; systemic symptoms; lesions in other bones; enlarging skull
Condensing osteitis	Mandible	Any age; either	Usually solitary but may be multiple areas of radiopacity and radiolucency; associated with carious teeth, broken roots, or edentulous jaws; asymptomatic or with sporadic symptoms of pain and drainage
Chronic sclerosing osteomyelitis	Mandible	Fourth decade or later; female	Multiple radiopaque areas in jaw; molar and premolar areas; few months to few years in duration; usually asymptomatic; alkaline phosphatase normal

jaws—cont'd

Microscopic features	Treatment	Prognosis	Page ref.
Tumor consists of collagenized tissue with foci of calcification	Local excision	Excellent; lesions may recur but treatment should be conservative	302
Abnormal bone and connective tissue stroma	Wide excision	Fair to poor	316
Cartilage and cartilage-like tissue; atypical chondrocytes	Wide, radical excision	Poor	320
Depend on primary site	Treatment of primary lesions; excision of metastasis	Poor	333
Dense trabecular bone with numerous areas of bone apposition and resorption; fibrous marrow	None	Poor	340
Dense bone; fibrous marrow with infiltration by plasma cells and lymphocytes	Excision; if deep seated and asymptomatic, no treatment necessary	Excellent	350
Dense lamellated bone with many basophilic lines; may resemble Paget's disease; fibrous marrow	None; if secondarily infected, surgical excision	Good	350

Table 12. Swellings of salivary glands

Lesion	Usual location	Usual age and sex	Clinical and radiographic features
Mucocele (mucous retention cyst; retention phenomenon)	Usually lip and tongue but may be anywhere on oral mucosa	Any age; either	Solitary vesicular lesion; compressible, translucent, and sometimes bluish; history of week or more; ruptures and discharges mucoid secretion; recurs
Ranula	Floor of mouth	Adulthood; either	Large compressible enlargement in floor of mouth; may elevate tongue and interfere with speech; associated with submaxillary or sublingual gland
Mumps (infectious parotitis)	Parotid gland	Childhood; either	Unilateral or bilateral diffuse acute enlargement of parotid glands; fever, malaise, anorexia; spontaneous regression within week
Cat-scratch disease	Lymph nodes of any area, including parotid gland	Childhood; either	Painful enlargement of parotid area
Sarcoidosis (Besnier-Boeck-Schaumann disease)	Parotid gland	Adulthood; male	Unilateral or bilateral enlargement of parotid gland; asymptomatic or associated with respiratory symptoms, fever, etc.
Mikulicz's disease (benign lymphoepithelial lesion)	Parotid gland	Over 20 yr; male twice as frequently as female	Nodular or diffuse, unilateral or bilateral enlargement of parotid gland; fluctuates in size; duration, weeks to months; asymptomatic; sometimes spontaneous regression
Sjögren's syndrome (sicca syndrome)	Parotid gland	Old age; female	Same as in Mikulicz's disease; also dryness of conjunctiva, nose, throat, and mouth

Microscopic features	Treatment	Prognosis	Page ref.
Cyst containing mucus and lined by granulation tissue; associated gland may show interstitial inflammation; in some instances, no distinct, well-defined cyst but mucus dispersed in connective tissue	Local excision	Excellent; if associated gland not removed, recurrence most likely	461
Large mucus-containing cyst lined by granulation tissue	Excision or removal of roof of cyst	Excellent	463
Edema of parotid gland with very sparse inflammatory exudate	None	Excellent; similar condition may recur but is caused by other viruses	577
Involves lymph nodes that contain abscesses with necrotic centers and periphery of histiocytes	None	Excellent	577
Circumscribed foci of epithelioid cells and giant cells in gland; no necrosis	None	Fair	580
Circumscribed area of lymphoid tissue or diffuse infiltration of gland by lymphocytes; islands of squamoid and glandular epithelium	None	Usually excellent	582
Same as in Mikulicz's disease	Symptomatic	Fair	585

71

Continued.

Table 12. Swellings of salivary glands—cont'd

Lesion	Usual location	Usual age and sex	Clinical and radiographic features
Fatty infiltration	Parotid gland	Middle age or older; either	Rare condition; unilateral or bilateral diffuse enlargement of parotid gland; long duration; old age, alcoholism, pregnancy, or malnutrition
Hypertrophy	Parotid or minor salivary gland of oral mucosa	Any age; either	Rare; unilateral or bilateral diffuse enlargement of parotid gland; long duration; in minor glands, appears as nodular localized elevation of mucosa
Sialadenitis	Submaxillary or sublingual gland	Middle age or older; male	Diffuse enlargement of involved gland that may increase with eating; pain associated with eating; radiographs may reveal salivary stone in duct
Benign tumor	Parotid gland, palate, submaxillary gland, minor glands of oral mucosa, in that order of frequency	30 yr or older; either	Unilateral solitary nodular swelling of long duration (months to years); overlying skin or mucosa generally normal; absence of neurologic symptoms; tumors usually freely movable
Malignant tumor	Same as for benign tumor of salivary gland	Older age group than for benign tumor; either	Unilateral solitary nodular or diffuse swelling of relatively short duration (weeks to months); rapid growth; fixation to surrounding tissues; ulceration of overlying skin or mucosa common; pain and facial paralysis associated with parotid tumors; palpable cervical nodes may be present; in palatine tumors, radiolucencies and loosening of teeth

Microscopic features	Treatment	Prognosis	Page ref.
Fatty infiltration of involved gland	None	Excellent	585
Normal salivary gland (mucous or serous) tissue	None	Excellent	587
Acute and chronic inflammatory infiltrate of gland, atrophy of acini, and fibrosis	Removal of stone; excision or ligation of duct	Excellent	588
Depends on type	Excision	Good or excellent, depending on type	598
Depends on type	Wide and radical excision	Fair to grave	599

PART II

GENERAL PRINCIPLES OF ORAL PATHOLOGY

CHAPTER 1

Inflammation

Life is a continuous adaptation between an organism and its environment. The mere fact, therefore, that a species or an organism survives implies that it has an inherent ability to adjust to, surmount, or destroy its adversary. All forms of life offer innumerable examples of this phenomenon, and the process of inflammation is only one such example.

The function of inflammation *is to mobilize all the defenses of the body and bring them to the site of battle* with the purpose of overwhelming the source of injury. The latter may be physical or chemical, or it may constitute an attack by some pathogenic microorganism. Regardless of the source of injury, however, the tissue changes in inflammation are essentially the same and have the following purposes:

1. To bring to the area certain phagocytic cells (neutrophilic polymorphonuclear leukocytes, macrophages, histiocytes), which engulf and digest bacteria, dead cells, or other debris
2. To bring antibodies to the site (since antibodies are altered gamma globulins, this is achieved by the escape of fluid and plasma proteins out of the blood vessels and into the tissues)
3. To neutralize and dilute the irritant (by edema)
4. To limit the spread of inflammation (by fibrin formation, fibrosis, or walling off with granulation tissue)
5. To initiate repair

Inflammatory response may be subdivided into four major types:

1. Acute inflammation
2. Subacute inflammation
3. Chronic inflammation
4. Chronic granulomatous inflammation

The four types are not entirely distinct entities. Transitions from one type to another may occur at any time. They are all tissue responses to injury, and the appearance of one or the other depends on the type and intensity of the irritant and the nature of the host (e.g., species, age, nutritional, hormonal, immunologic status).

Acute inflammation. Acute inflammation progresses in the following sequence of events:

1. Arteriolar constriction followed by dilatation
2. Increased blood flow through arterioles, capillaries, and venules
3. Venular and capillary dilatation and increased permeability
4. Exudation of fluid or edema
5. Slowing or stagnation of blood flow
6. Escape of leukocytes from the vessel wall

Immediately after injury there is a transitory arteriolar vasoconstriction that is followed by vasodilatation and increased rate of blood flow through the arterioles, capillaries, and venules.

Under normal circumstances the endothelial lining of capillaries and venules shows "pores" or spaces ranging in size from 90 to 150 Å between adjoining cells. Furthermore, even larger "pores" exist within the cells themselves. In inflammation, first the venules and then the capillaries show an increase in the size of these "pores" (up to five times the normal size) between and within the endothelial cells. As a result of this change, six or seven times the normal amount of water as well as crystalloids and porteins escape into the surrounding tissues. (Of the proteins, the albumin escapes first, followed by globulin and fibrinogen.) The presence of an abnormal amount of fluid in the tissues is called edema.

The increased permeability of the vessel walls is produced not only by the increase in size of the "pores" within and between the endothelial cells but also by the altered filtration pressures. Under normal circumstances the hydrostatic pressure at the arterial end of the capillary is higher than the osmotic pressure in the surrounding tissues, so fluid and nutrients escape from the circulation. At the venous end of the capillary the hydrostatic pressure falls below the osmotic pressure in the surrounding tissues, and the fluid returns to the circulation. This is referred to as *Starling's hypothesis*.

In inflammation the escape of plasma proteins into the tissues causes increased extravascular osmotic pressure and interference with the return of fluid into the venous end of the capillary. This circumstance further leads to edema. The edema fluid in inflammation has a higher specific gravity and a higher protein content than the edema fluid in certain noninflammatory conditions, and it is readily coagulable (because of its fibrinogen content). It is known as *exudate*, whereas that present in some noninflammatory conditions (e.g., heart failure) has a low specific gravity and a low protein content and is referred to as *transudate*.

Although normally the cellular elements of blood move in the center of the stream while the plasma flows at the periphery, with the slowing of blood flow the cellular elements begin to move along the vascular walls. Probably due to altered electrochemical forces, the neutrophils begin to adhere to the capillary wall. This process is referred to as *pavementing* or *margination*. The cells (particularly neutrophilic leukocytes) then leave the blood vessel, enter the surrounding tissues, and move to the injured site by an ameboid motion once believed to be determined by what was called *chemotaxis*. Chemotaxis was defined as positive directional response to a chemical substance at the injured site. This explanation of the movement of leukocytes to the injured area is now regarded as unlikely.

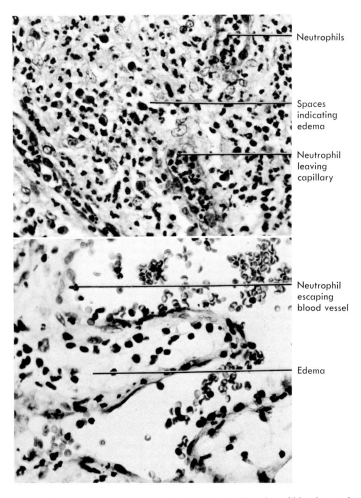

Fig. 1-1. Acute inflammation. Note the edema, the dilatation of blood vessels, and the escape of neutrophils from the blood vessels.

Acute inflammation is thus characterized microscopically by edema and polymorphonuclear leukocytes (Fig. 1-1). Clinically it is characterized by swelling (because of edema), redness, heat (because of hyperemia), and pain. The pain is due to the pressure on, as well as irritation of, the local nerve endings by products of the inflammatory process.

Acute inflammation is often subclassified according to an outstanding feature of the inflammatory process. For example:

serous inflammation Abundant extravascular fluid but few cells and little fibrinogen (e.g., skin blister)

fibrinous inflammation Large amount of fibrin in exudate (e.g., lobar pneumonia)

purulent inflammation Abundant pus in exudate (e.g., abscess)

sanguineous inflammation Exudate containing blood

catarrhal inflammation Acute inflammation of mucous membrane with abundant flow of mucus (e.g., early stage of common cold)

pseudomembranous inflammation Acute inflammation of mucous membrane with associated formation of pseudomembrane, the latter consisting essentially of fibrin, necrotic epithelium, and white cells (e.g., diphtheria)

abscess Acute inflammation localized and associated with tissue destruction and liquefaction as well as formation of pus; the latter consists of dead and dying, as well as viable, neutrophils and products of tissue liquefaction

phlegmonous inflammation Diffuse, spreading acute inflammation of solid tissues (e.g., erysipelas, cellulitis)

When the irritant producing acute inflammation is overcome or eliminated, the inflammatory process resolves. This implies that the edema fluid is gradually drained away from the part via either the lymphatics or the veins, and the cellular elements of blood that had come to the site either reenter the circulation or are locally destroyed and phagocytosed. The tissue thus gradually returns to normal.

Chemical aspects of acute inflammation. It has been observed that, regardless of the type of injury, the tissues respond in a more or less identical manner (e.g., pulpitis caused by trauma is identical to pulpitis caused by bacterial organisms). This is at least partly due to the fact that whenever a cell is injured or destroyed, regardless of the manner of injury, it liberates a number of chemical substances, called chemical media-

tors, which set into motion the process of inflammation. Some
of these substances and their roles are as follows:

H substance Histamine-like substance that supposedly causes erythema due to
vascular dilatation
leukotaxine Produces capillary permeability and also causes emigration of leukocytes (diapedesis)
LPF (leukocytosis-promoting factor) Promotes formation of more leukocytes in
bone marrow
exudin Promotes capillary permeability
necrosin Causes proteolysis or tissue breakdown
pyrexin Causes fever
growth-promoting factors Aid in repair

**Subacute, chronic, and chronic granulomatous inflamma-
tions.** A low-grade, prolonged, and proliferative type of inflammation, *chronic inflammation,* occurs when the irritant is of low
virulence, when resistance of the host is good, or when acute
inflammation is in the late reparative phases. Microscopically it
is characterized by the presence of lymphocytes and plasma
cells and by fibroblastic proliferation (Fig. 1-2). Whereas acute
inflammation lasts from a few days to 2 or 3 weeks, chronic
inflammation extends over a period of months to years.

An inflammatory process having characteristics of both the
acute and the chronic types is called *subacute inflammation;* it
generally extends over a period of weeks or months.

Chronic inflammation may be of such a type that the tissue
response is characterized not only by lymphocytes and plasma
cells but also by a prominent proliferation of histiocytes (macrophages). The latter may form diffuse or circumscribed masses
(Fig. 1-3). This response represents *chronic granulomatous inflammation* and is seen in persons with tuberculosis, syphilis,
sarcoidosis, fungus infections, foreign body reactions, and many
other diseases (p. 673).

Cellular components of inflammation. The cellular elements
that participate in various types of inflammation include neutrophilic polymorphonuclear leukocytes, eosinophilic polymorphonuclear leukocytes, basophilic polymorphonuclear leuko-

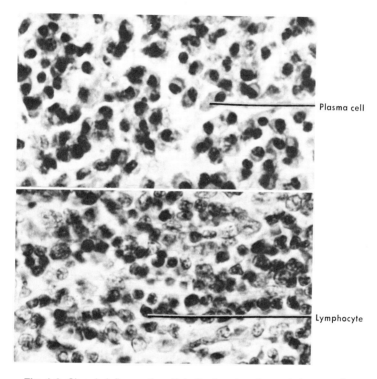

Plasma cell

Lymphocyte

Fig. 1-2. Chronic inflammation. Note the lymphocytes and plasma cells.

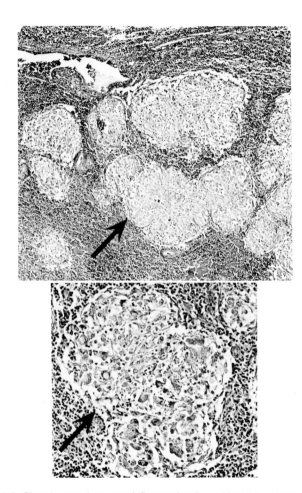

Fig. 1-3. Chronic granulomatous inflammation (sarcoidosis) in a lymph node. Arrows indicate circumscribed foci of histiocytic proliferation.

cytes, lymphocytes, plasma cells, monocytes, and macrophages (histiocytes).

Neutrophilic polymorphonuclear leukocytes. The predominant cell of acute inflammation is the neutrophilic polymorphonuclear leukocyte (Fig. 1-1). These cells have dense, large granules, called the primary granules, and smaller secondary granules. The primary granules have lysozyme, acid phosphatase, peroxidase, and cationic proteins. The latter increases capillary permeability and chemotaxis of mononuclear phagocytes and immobilizes the neutrophils. The secondary granules contain alkaline phosphatase, lysozyme, and lactoferin (antibacterial agent). The life span of a mature polymorphonuclear leukocyte outside the circulation is only about 7 hours, while in circulation the life span is about 120 hours. Its functions are phagocytosis and lysis of bacteria, fibrin, and cellular debris. The intracytoplasmic pH of these cells is remarkably acidic (as low as 3). Also, they contain lytic proteins such as phagocytin and leukin. After phagocytosis the acid environment and the lytic substances of the neutrophils destroy many bacteria. When the neutrophils die, they liberate proteases, peptidases, and lipases, which cause tissue lysis.

Eosinophilic polymorphonuclear leukocytes. Eosinophilic polymorphonuclear leukocytes are seen in patients with hypersensitivity (allergy) and parasitic infections. Their granules have a high content of peroxidase. In addition, they contain ribonuclease, cathepsin, acid, and alkaline phosphatase and plasminogen. Plasminogen is made in the endothelial cells of the capillaries and is the precursor of plasmin, which destroys fibrin. Eosinophils contain histamine but no lysozyme and are not very phagocytic. During cortisone administration their numbers decrease in the peripheral blood but not in the marrow. They are seen in healing tissues.

Mast cells and basophilic polymorphonuclear leukocytes. These cells are very similar or the same. They contain basophil granules, which contain an acid polysaccharide called heparin, histamine, eosinophilic chemotactic factor of anaphylaxis (ECFA), slow-reacting substance of anaphylaxis (SRSA), the platelet activating factor (PAF), and IgE. These cells play an important role in allergy and inflammation.

Lymphocytes and plasma cells. In the fetus the immature lymphocytes develop in the yolk sac, the liver, and the bone marrow. From there they may pass through the thymus and become the T (thymic) lymphocytes or go through the gastrointestinal tract or liver and become the B (bursal, referring to the gastrointestinal tract of a chicken or to bursa) lymphocytes. The T and B lymphocytes populate the lymphoid tissue and circulate in the blood. In the blood 80% of lymphocytes are T cells, 5% to 10% are B cells, and the remainder are unidentified lymphocytes. In the lymphoid tissue the germinal centers contain B cells, while the T cells are located around the follicles. In the medullary part of the lymph node both cells are mixed. When an antigen affects a lymph node, the B cells respond in such a way that they become large, are called *immunoblasts*, and later form plasma cells. Plasma cells are active producers of antibodies and have a prominent, rough endoplasmic reticulum and a Golgi apparatus (which is seen as a perinuclear halo). These cells are therefore responsible for the so-called humoral defense of the body. The antigen alters the T cells immunologically so that they are capable of cell-mediated immunity (suppressive cells, killer cells, helper cells, etc.). Thus the T cells are responsible for the cellular defense of the organism. The exposure to the antigen produces T and B *memory cells* or cells that in a subsequent exposure to the same antigen can quickly multiply to provide cellular and humoral defense.

Monocytes and macrophages (histiocytes). The monocytes of the blood and the macrophages, or histiocytes, of the tissues are closely related cells and are found in patients with all forms of inflammation but particularly those forms with chronic granulomatous processes (Fig. 1-3). These cells move with ease, and their functions are phagocytosis and intracellular digestion by the liberation of proteolytic enzymes. Since they remain active at a pH below 6.8, they persist after the neutrophils have been destroyed by increased acidity of the area. Macrophages also produce antibodies.

Reference

Anderson, W. A. D., and Kissane, J. M.: Pathology, ed. 7, St. Louis, 1977, The C. V. Mosby Co.

CHAPTER 2
Regeneration and repair

As mentioned in the discussion of inflammation, one prerequisite for survival is the ability of an organism to destroy its
adversary. Another prerequisite, the ability of the organism to
repair itself, will now be considered. Some injured single-celled
and multicellular organisms can restitute themselves to their
original form. In more complex animals, the injured tissue may
be replaced either in kind or by a tissue of a different type. The
ability for regeneration and repair, though universal, varies
widely and is dependent on species, tissue, age, nutrition, irritants, local stimuli, blood supply, and mobility of tissues.

1. *Species:* As a rule, the lower and less differentiated animals possess a greater ability for regeneration (e.g., certain amphibians can grow an entire limb, and the earth-
   worm can regenerate a head).
2. *Tissue:* Different tissues in the same animal vary in reparative potential (e.g., the mammalian liver cells can regenerate rapidly, whereas a neuron, once destroyed, is
   incapable of regeneration).
3. *Age:* Young organisms can repair their damage faster than
   older ones.
4. *Nutrition:* Certain nutritional deficiencies, such as protein and vitamin deficiencies (e.g., vitamin C), prolong or
   hinder regeneration and repair.
5. *Irritants:* Whereas mild irritants enhance the reparative
   process, excessive irritants (e.g., persistent infection,
   bone sequestra, lack of rest) inhibit repair and regeneration.

85

6. *Local stimuli:* Local stimuli, such as *trephones* or wound hormones that are liberated by the proteolytic break-down of cellular debris, and certain chemicals (e.g., urea) are believed to stimulate tissue growth. Also, the reduction of local tissue pressures brought about by tissue destruction is a stimulus for cellular growth.
7. *Blood supply:* Tissues with a good vascular supply heal much faster than those in which the blood supply has been diminished due to disease or advanced age.
8. *Mobility of tissues:* Healing in both bone or soft tissues is faster when the injured tissues are immobilized.

REGENERATION

When damaged tissue is replaced by cells that are similar or identical to those destroyed, we speak of regeneration. *Physiologic regeneration* refers to the replacement of cells, such as blood cells and epithelium, that are destroyed under normal circumstances.

In the oral cavity, as elsewhere in the body, the regenerative ability of tissues varies greatly. The oral epithelium is estimated to completely replace itself in about 4 to 6 days. The dorsum of the tongue has the fastest regenerative potential; the cheek, the palate, and the ventral surface of the tongue are next in regenerative speed; and the gingiva is the slowest to regenerate. The connective tissue, bone tissue of the jaws, pulp, odontoblasts, and cementoblasts have good regenerative capacity; but the ameloblasts do not. Wounds of the oral mucous membrane heal rapidly and effectively.

REPAIR

Repair is an all-inclusive term that embraces both regeneration and those processes wherein the damaged tissue is replaced by dissimilar cells. The classic example given in illustrate repair is the healing of wounds. To illustrate this process, five types of oral wounds will be considered:

1. Wounds healing by first intention
2. Wounds healing by second intention
3. Wounds following tooth extraction
4. Transplantation and replantation of teeth
5. Jaw fractures

Wounds healing by first intention. When cut surfaces are approximated or closely sutured, the wound heals without scarring.

The first step in repair is the formation of a clot, which helps to hold the parts together.

Since the area is the site of inflammation, it is edematous and contains polymorphonuclear leukocytes and macrophages. Tissue debris either is lysed by proteolytic enzymes of leukocytes and dead cells or becomes phagocytosed.

With removal of the debris, fibroblasts and capillary loops grow into the clot. The capillary loops are solid at first but soon become canalized, and collagen fibers appear between the fibroblasts. Thus in 3 to 4 days the clot is slowly replaced by tissue consisting of blood vessels, young fibroblasts, and neutrophilic leukocytes. This tissue is called granulation tissue.

The epithelium grows across the wound, and healing is almost completed. In the last stages there is a progressive increase in the amount of collagen, and the number of inflammatory cells decreases.

Wounds healing by second intention. When the opposing edges of a wound (e.g., a large ulcer) are not approximated, the wound fills in from the base (as seen in the healing of a large ulcer) but the healing occurs by essentially the same process. The only distinguishing feature is that all steps are far more exaggerated. Such a process is also called secondary repair.

The inflammatory response and fibroblastic and endothelial proliferation are exuberant, and therefore abundant red granular, easily bleeding granulation tissue can be seen.

When the wound is almost completely filled by granulation tissue, the surface epithelium begins to grow over the vascular-

ized substrate of granulation tissue until the wound is completely epithelialized.

After this, the inflammatory exudate slowly disappears and
the fibroblasts produce collagen so that the wound is replaced
by a scar. However, only rarely do wounds in the oral region
heal with scar formation.

Wounds following tooth extraction. The ensuing discussion
is a brief description of what happens in a wound after a tooth
is extracted.

Immediately after the extraction, bleeding occurs in the
socket and a clot forms.

Within a day the periphery of the clot shows edema and
neutrophilic infiltration. In 2 to 4 days, activity starts at the
periphery of the clot and fibroblasts and endothelial buds enter
it from the surrounding bone marrow spaces. This process is
referred to as *the organization of the clot*.

Simultaneous with acute inflammation and organization of
the clot, the removal of debris takes place. Dead cells, necrotic
tissue, and bone are removed by neutrophils, macrophages, and
osteoclasts.

As soon as the clot is organized (about a week), epithelium
grows over its surface. Instead of being covered by fibrin, the
wound is now epithelialized. The inflammatory component decreases, and collagen fibers in the granulation tissue increase.

In about 10 to 15 days, the periphery of the socket shows
formation of osteoid and immature bone. With time, the
amount of immature bone and osteoid increases from the base
toward the surface of the socket and from the periphery to the
center.

Finally, in about 3 weeks to 6 months, reorganization of the
bone trabeculae in the socket occurs (i.e., immature bone is
removed and replaced by mature bone). The trabeculae are laid
down in a functional pattern—that is, in a manner best suited
to withstand forces that are brought to bear on the alveolar
ridge. It should be recalled here that the immature bone is not
as radiopaque as the mature bone. Consequently a healed

socket containing immature bone is relatively radiolucent. Healing of extraction wounds, therefore, occurs long before anything is apparent on the radiographs.

In some patients, wound healing after extraction is not as uneventful as just described. The usual complication is the so-called *dry socket*, which follows complicated extractions, 95% occurring in the lower premolar and molar areas. The socket is painful, and the patient has foul breath. Examination reveals a socket devoid of a clot, often with the bare bony socket wall visible. Histologic sections reveal the socket wall to be formed by necrotic bone (i.e., containing empty lacunae). The surrounding marrow shows considerable inflammation, and the so-called dry socket represents localized osteitis. Since the necrotic bone must be removed by the osteoclasts before healing can start, dry socket is repaired very slowly.

Although many drugs have been claimed to be beneficial in promoting early healing of extraction wounds, they are of questionable value.

Transplantation and replantation of teeth. Transplantation and replantation of teeth represent two other examples of repair and regeneration in the oral tissue.

Transplantation is the replacement of a lost tooth by another tooth. If the latter is from the same mouth, it is called an *autotransplant;* and if it is from another patient, it is a *homotransplant*. The implantation from one species to another is called a *heterotransplant*. All three procedures are successful, but the degree of success is greatest in autotransplants and least in heterotransplants. Autotransplantation usually implies replacement of a tooth by a developing tooth germ (e.g., a third molar). The transplanted tooth germ may continue to develop normally, establish a new periodontal ligament, and maintain a vital pulp. On the other hand, the tooth germ may undergo resorption and become exfoliated. This procedure is successful in more than 50% of cases.

Replantation is the replacement of a traumatically or otherwise exfoliated tooth in its own socket. This procedure has been used for centuries. The tooth is cleaned, its root canals are filled, and it is inserted back into its socket and splinted. The root surface usually undergoes resorption, and repair follows by bone formation. Thus the tooth is *ankylosed* to the surrounding bone. Although replanted teeth do not have a periodontal ligament in all areas of the root, they may remain serviceable for years. Replantation is successful in about 75% of cases and is always worthy of trial when anterior teeth have been traumatically dislodged.

Jaw fractures. After a jaw fracture, bleeding occurs at the site, a hematoma develops, and a clot forms.

In the first stage—referred to as the *formation of the fibrous or temporary callus* and characterized by inflammation, organization of the clot, and removal of the cellular debris—fibroblasts and endothelial buds from the connective tissue of the periosteum as well as from the bone marrow spaces grow in and organize the clot. Simultaneous with the organization of the clot, edema, neutrophils, leukocytes, plasma cells, and lymphocytes can be seen in the area. Necrotic cells, connective tissue, and bone are removed by phagocytosis, proteolysis, and osteoclasis. Replacement of the clot by granulation tissue takes a few days. Gradually the inflammation decreases, collagen fibers appear, and granulation tissue is transformed into fibrous tissue. The broken ends of the bone are united by collagenous fibers, the fibrous or temporary callus.

In the next stage immature bone trabeculae are formed in the connective tissue of the callus. This stage is referred to as the *formation of the primary bone callus*. The primary callus is composed of immature bone and is therefore radiolucent. Although the fracture at this stage is well on its way toward repair, a radiolucent defect at the fracture site can still be seen. Both the fibrous callus and the primary callus not only bind the broken ends of the bone together but also extend beyond the fracture line in all directions. Thus, as the fracture is repaired by the primary callus, it shows an overabundant amount of immature bone.

In the next stage the immature bone of the primary callus is gradually removed and replaced by mature lamellated bone. This stage is referred to as the *formation of the secondary callus*. The secondary callus is not as exuberant as the primary. Furthermore, it is radiopaque; and on radiographs taken at this stage, the fracture appears healed.

Finally, in the last stage the secondary callus is remodeled (i.e., the excess amount of bone is resorbed and the normal outline of the jaw restored).

REFERENCES

Azaz, B., Zilberman, Y., and Hackak, T.: Clinical and roentgenographic evaluation of thirty-seven autotransplanted impacted maxillary canines, Oral Surg. **45:**8, 1978.

Belinfante, L. S., and others: Incidence of dry socket complication in third molar removal, J. Oral Surg. **31:**106, 1973.

Birn, H., Etiology and pathogenesis of fibrinolytic alveolitis ("dry socket"), Int. J. Oral Surg. **2:**211, 1973.

Cutright, D. E., and Bauer, H.: Cell renewal in the oral mucosa and skin of the rat. I. Turnover time, Oral Surg. **23:**249, 1967.

Jandinski, J. J., Sonis, S., and Doku, H. C.: The incidence of mast cells in selected oral lesions, Oral Surg. **34:**245, 1972.

Lilly, G. E., Osborn, D. B., Rael, E. M., Samuel, H. S., and Jones, J. C.: Alveolar osteitis associated with mandibular third molar extractions, J. Am. Dent. Assoc. **88:**802, 1974.

Natiella, J. R., Armitage, J. E., and Greene, G. W.: The replantation and transplantation of teeth, Oral Surg. **29:**397, 1970.

CHAPTER 3

Immunity and allergy

The fundamental principles and essentials of immunity and allergy are presented in this chapter. Details can be gathered from a number of textbooks on general pathology and immunology.

The following subjects will be discussed:

1. Immunity
2. Allergy
3. Cellular aspects of immunity and allergy

Immunity. The ability of an organism to resist infection is called immunity. Immunity may be divided into two major groups: *innate* or *species immunity*, which is inherent in an entire species (e.g., a rat is immune to syphilis), and *acquired immunity*, which is attained by an individual.

The mechanism of species immunity is unknown and therefore needs no more discussion. Acquired immunity means that an individual (the host) comes in contact with a pathogenic microorganism and this microorganisn stimulates the production of certain specific substances in the body of the host. If, at a subsequent time, the host again comes in contact with the same organism, these newly produced substances (antibodies) will by some means destroy it.

Acquired immunity can be either natural or artificial. The first contact of the host with the organism may be as a result of getting a certain disease, following which the host may resist reinfection with the same organism (*natural immunity*). On the other hand, the first contact may be *artificially* produced in the host by the injection of living or dead organisms or their products, with the resultant immunity called *active immunity*, or by the introduction of antibodies prepared in another host, with the resultant immunity called *passive immunity*.

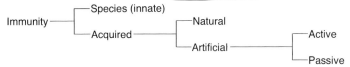

All soluble proteins (e.g., those in bacteria and viruses) introduced into a host stimulate some cells of the host's reticuloendothelial system (lymph nodes, spleen, bone marrow, Kupffer cells of the liver) to produce antibodies. Antibodies are altered serum globulin molecules. When brought in contact with the protein or the microbe that excited their production (i.e., the antigen), they may destroy it by precipitation, lysis, agglutination, neutralization, or promotion of its phagocytosis. Accordingly, these antibodies may be referred to as precipitins, bacteriolysins, agglutinins, neutralizing antibodies, or opsonins. Most likely, plasma cells and reticulum cells produce the antibodies, and plasma cells and lymphocytes carry them.

In addition to the foreign proteins, which are the usual form of antigen, a large carbohydrate-lipid complex may be able to stimulate the formation of antibodies. These foreign proteins and carbohydrate-lipid complexes are referred to as *complete antigens*. A *partial antigen,* or *haptene,* is a simple, nonprotein chemical substance that cannot stimulate antibody production by itself but can attach itself to a protein and thus affect the type of antibody produced.

Allergy. Whereas *immunity* is defined as immunologic reactions that are beneficial to the host, *allergy* may be defined as immunologic reactions that are detrimental to the tissues or physiology of the host.

After antibodies to a particular antigen have been produced by the plasma cells, they are either released into the circulation or become attached to the cells of the host. Thus antibodies are of two types, *circulating* (in the bloodstream) and *fixed* (to cells), and should the host be exposed to the same antigen again, they remain available to react with it.

These antibodies are called immunoglobulins and are made up of five types: IgM, IgG, IgA, IgD, and IgE.

When an individual who has been previously exposed to an antigen is exposed to a second dose of the same antigen, one of two things happens: (1) the antigen may be neutralized or destroyed in the bloodstream by the circulating antibodies, and the person is immune to its untoward effects; or (2) the circulating antibodies are not enough to neutralize or destroy the antigen, and the latter reaches the tissue cells, where it reacts with the fixed antibodies.

When an antigen reacts with fixed antibodies, the reaction either destroys the cell or leads to the release of histamine or histamine-like substances. These substances produce a variety of untoward effects—for example, increased permeability of blood vessel walls (as in angioneurotic edema [Fig. 3-1], skin rash, hay fever, urticaria) or spasm of smooth muscle (asthma). The phenomenon in which a second dose of an antigen reacts with fixed antibodies and produces altered tissue reactions is

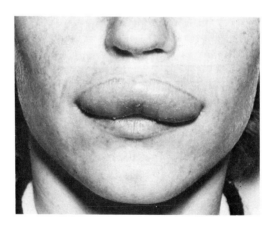

Fig. 3-1. Angioneurotic edema.

called allergy or hypersensitivity. The antigen in this case may be called an allergen, and the individual who has had contact with the allergen and who on second contact shows an allergic response is a *sensitized* individual.

When an allergic response is stimulated artificially—for example, in a laboratory animal or by an accidental injection of a protein into a patient who is sensitive to the protein—it is referred to as an *anaphylactic shock*. If the allergic response is due to a nonbacterial foreign protein, such as strawberries, fish, milk, feathers, hair, or pollen, the process is designated *atopy*. Atopy is believed to be hereditary in nature. Finally, the allergic response may be to a bacterial protein, such as is seen in tuberculosis, and this is referred to as *bacterial allergy*.

In a sensitized patient the second dose may be a mere surface contact with the offending protein. Contact may be on the mucous membrane or the skin and lead to a local allergic reaction called contact allergy. Allergic reactions to lipstick, toothpastes, procaine, etc., are examples of the contact type of allergy. Substances that produce allergic reactions on surface contact may also produce similar reactions when given systemically. It is believed that one attack of contact allergy predisposes an area to additional attacks.

Depending on the speed at which they occur, the allergic reactions are sometimes classified into three types: *immediate* (or anaphylactic) reactions, occurring in 20 to 30 minutes; *accelerated* reactions, occurring in from 1 to 72 hours; and *late* (or delayed) reactions, occurring days or weeks after the administration of the antigen.

Since allergy is usually a result of liberation of histamine, one of the rationales of treatment of allergic responses is the administration of antihistamines. Another rationale is desensitization of the patient by giving small doses of the offending allergen. This increases the level of the circulating antibodies, which prevent the interaction between the allergen and the fixed antibody and thus prevent the allergic response.

Oral lesions of an allergic nature, or that are believed to be so, are stomatitis (also cheilitis, glossitis) medicamentosa (p. 426), stomatitis (also cheilitis, glossitis) venenata (p. 426), erythema multiforme (p. 415), and plasma cell gingivitis (p. 191). Furthermore, delayed allergic reactions may follow injection of local anesthetics (p. 429).

Another tissue reaction related to allergy is represented by the so-called autoimmune responses or diseases. In these conditions the allergen (or the antigen) is not a foreign material but an integral part of the patient's own cells. Thus the patient becomes sensitized, or *allergic,* to his own cells and tissues. Systemic lupus erythematosus, rheumatoid arthritis, and Sjögren's syndrome are examples of autoimmunity.

Cellular aspects of immunity and allergy. A summary of the cellular basis of both immunity and allergy are as follows: Two types of small sensitized lymphocytes populate the lymph nodes throughout the body—the T and the B lymphocytes.

A *T lymphocyte* is any small lymphocyte that, after its formation by a stem cell in the bone marrow, is released into the circulation. It passes through the thymus gland, and at this time it is sensitized by the thymus; it then continues on the partially populate a lymph node. From here it will produce cells responsible for fixed (cellular) immunity and delayed hypersensitivity (e.g., organ transplant rejection, tuberculin reaction).

A *B lymphocyte* also arises in a nonspecific manner from the bone marrow stem cell. It follows a different course in the circulation, however, and dictated only by chance finds its way into an area thought to be located in the gastrointestinal tract and in the liver. At this time it is sensitized, and it proceeds to help populate the same lymph nodes as do the T cells. B lymphocytes, in response to the proper stimulus, form plasma cells, which are the chief source of antibody formation. These antibodies are the mediators of humoral immunity and allergy (hypersensitivity).

For an individual (host) to be immunologically competent, two cell types in addition to the T and B lymphocytes must be present: the macrophage and the polymorphonuclear leukocyte (PML).

The *macrophage* attacks and engulfs the antigen. During this procedure the antigen is "processed" or somehow altered so that it will trigger a response by the T and/or B lymphocytes. Without processing, no lymphocyte response can occur.

The function of the *PML* appears to be to phagocytose and destroy the antigen-antibody complex. This function is markedly enhanced by the serum complement system, which actively participates in the destruction of foreign cells. The complement system of nine functioning interrelated components, while not completely defined at the present time, may be the most important component of the immune system.

REFERENCES

Anderson, W. A. D., and Kissane, J. M.: Pathology, ed. 7, St. Louis, 1977, The C. V. Mosby Co.

Chue, P. W. Y.: Acute angioneurotic edema of the lips and tongue due to emotional stress, Oral Surg. **41:**734, 1976.

Donlon, W. C.: Immunology in dentistry, J. Am. Dent. Assoc. **100:**220, 1980.

Giunta, J., and Zablotsky, N.: Allergic stomatitis caused by self-polymerizing resin, Oral Surg. **41:**631, 1976.

La Via, M. F., and Hill, R. B., Jr.: Principles of pathology, New York, 1975, Oxford University, Press, Inc.

Lopez, M., and Carvel, R. I.: Clinical immunology with reference to the oral cavity, J. Oral Med. **28:**90, 1973.

Uhr, J. W.: Delayed hypersensitivity, Physiol. Rev. **46:**359, 1966.

PART III

PATHOLOGY OF TEETH AND JAWS

CHAPTER 4

Developmental disturbances of jaws, dentition, and individual teeth

The jaws, dentition, and individual teeth may be involved in a number of disturbances in such a manner that the shape, form, or number of these structures is altered. Some of these conditions are hereditary or familial (i.e., mutations or genetic disturbances), whereas others are caused by local abnormalities.

The following classification is based on the severity of the disturbance—whether it affects the skull, jaws, and teeth or the jaws only or is limited to a single tooth or groups of teeth. This is not a rigid, inflexible grouping but merely a convenient way to remember the different types of abnormalities.

Developmental disturbances affecting skull, jaws, and teeth

1. Cleidocranial dysostosis (Sainton's disease)
2. Craniofacial dysostosis (Crouzon's disease; maladie de Crouzon)
3. Mandibulofacial dysostosis (Treacher-Collins syndrome; Franceschetti's syndrome)

Developmental disturbances affecting jaws

1. Macrognathia
2. Micrognathia
3. Agnathia
4. Cleft palate
5. Pierre Robin syndrome
6. Cleft mandible

Developmental disturbances affecting teeth

Disturbances during initiation of tooth germs
1. Ectodermal dysplasia
2. Anodontia
3. Accessory and supernumerary teeth

4. Prediciduous dentition

5. Postpermanent dentition

Disturbances during morphodifferentiation of tooth germs
1. Hutchinson's incisors
2. Mulberry molar
3. Pflüger molar
4. Peg-shaped lateral incisors
5. Macrodontia
6. Microdontia
7. Dens in dente (dens invaginatus)
8. Dens evaginatus (evaginated odontoma)
9. Gemination
10. Fusion
11. Dilaceration
12. Taurodontism

Disturbances during apposition of hard dental tissues
1. Enamel hypoplasia
2. Amelogenesis imperfecta
3. Dentinogenesis imperfecta (opalescent dentin)
4. Dentinal dysplasia
5. Shell teeth
6. Odontodysplasia
7. Pigmentation of enamel and dentin
8. Cemental hypoplasia

Disturbances during calcification of hard dental tissues
1. Enamel hypocalcification
2. Interglobular dentin

Disturbances during eruption of teeth
1. Malocclusion
2. Concrescence
3. Retarded eruption
4. Shortened and submerged teeth
5. Supraeruption

DEVELOPMENTAL DISTURBANCES AFFECTING SKULL, JAWS, AND TEETH

Cleidocranial dysostosis (Sainton's disease). Cleidocranial dysostosis is characterized by delayed closure of the fontanelles and cranial sutures and the presence of wormian bones (small, irregular bones within the sutures of the skull) (Fig. 4-1, *A*), underdevelopment of the upper face (particularly the maxilla), underdevelopment of paranasal sinuses, a high and narrow palate, and prognathism or a relative prominence of the mandible (Fig. 4-1, *B*). In addition, there is a delayed eruption of teeth, malocclusion, and the presence of numerous supernumerary teeth and impacted teeth, some of which may be associated with follicular cysts. There is an absence or hypoplasia of the clavicles, so the patient can approximate the shoulders with ease (Fig. 4-1, *C*).

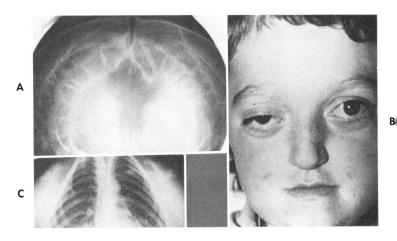

Fig. 4-1. Cleidocranial dysostosis ("Sainton's disease"). **A,** Delayed closure of the fontanelles and cranial sutures and presence of wormian bones. **B,** Underdevelopment of the upper face. **C,** Absence of the clavicles.

Craniofacial dysostosis (Crouzon's disease; maladie de Crouzon). Craniofacial dysostosis is essentially the same condition as cleidocranial dysostosis except that the clavicles are normal and the disturbance is limited to the skull, the upper face, and the dentition. It would appear to be a variant of the same mutation that causes cleidocranial dysostosis.

Mandibulofacial dysostosis (Treacher-Collins syndrome; Franceschetti's syndrome). In its classic form, mandibulofacial dysostosis is characterized by hypoplasia of the facial bones (especially the zygomatics), anomalies of the external ear and lower eyelids, and marked hypoplasia of the mandibular body—all of which gives the patient a bird-face or fish-face appearance (Fig. 4-2). The teeth are crowded and malposed.

DEVELOPMENTAL DISTURBANCES AFFECTING JAWS

Macrognathia. Macrognathia refers to a large jaw. This condition is rare.

Micrognathia. Micrognathia is a small jaw. This condition is extremely rare.

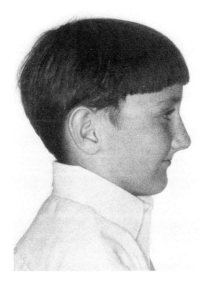

Fig. 4-2. Mandibulofacial dysostosis. Note the hypoplasia of the mandible. No ear defect is present.

Agnathia. Failure of developmental of a jaw is referred to as agnathia. This condition is extremely rare. When it is seen, it is often associated with other developmental disturbances and is usually incompatible with life.

Cleft palate. Cleft palate is a result of lack of fusion of the two palatal processes with each other or with the frontonasal process (primitive palate), varying in severity from the so-called bifid uvula (i.e., cleft of the uvula) to a cleft that involves the uvula, soft palate, hard palate, alveolar ridge, and upper lip (Fig. 4-3). Cleft lip is more common that cleft palate and may be unilateral or bilateral (Fig. 4-4). It is represented by a defect in the upper lateral incisor and canine areas. It occurs more commonly in males than in females and far more commonly on the left side than on the right.

The cause of cleft palate or cleft lip is unknown, but there is a high incidence in the offspring of parents who have these de-

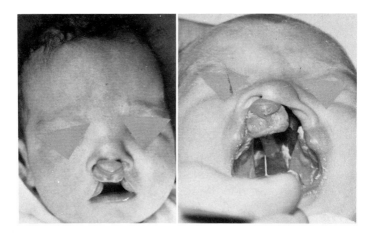

Fig. 4-3. Bilateral cleft lip and cleft palate.

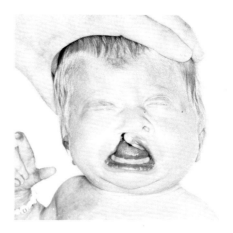

Fig. 4-4. Unilateral cleft lip.

fects. Heredity, therefore, is an important factor. Experimental work in animals has shown that vitamin A and B deficiencies and trauma, if instituted prior to palatal closure, produce clefts in a high percentage of cases. Roughly 1 out of 1,000 newborn infants has a cleft lip or cleft palate.

Clinically cleft palate presents as a defect in the oral roof. When the median nasal septum meets and fuses with one of the palatal processes, the defect is unilateral. Otherwise it is bilateral. In the anterior part of the palate, the cleft deviates to the right or left (or both) to extend between the lateral incisors and the canines. Due to communication between the oral and nasal cavities, the patient has difficulty in speech and deglutition. Treatment of cleft palate is surgical and/or mechanical (obturators, etc.) closure.

Pierre Robin syndrome. The Pierre Robin syndrome is characterized by micrognathia (Fig. 4-5), glossoptosis (dropping of the tongue), and cleft palate. The small jaw leads to downward

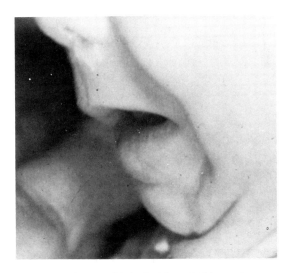

Fig. 4-5. Micrognathia in the Pierre Robin syndrome.

and backward displacement of the tongue, which obstructs the epiglottis and interferes with breathing. In addition to these deformities, other abnormalities such as mongolism, atresia of ears, and absence of the temporomandibular joint may be present.

Cleft mandible. Cleft mandible is an extremely rare condition in which a failure of fusion between the right and left mandibular processes leads to a defect in the midline of the mandible.

DEVELOPMENTAL DISTURBANCES AFFECTING TEETH

Development of the teeth is usually subdivided into *initiation, morphodifferentiation, apposition, calcification,* and *eruption*. The developmental anomalies may be grouped correspondingly.

Disturbances during initiation of tooth germs

Ectodermal dysplasia. Ectodermal dysplasia is a hereditary disease that involves all structures derived from the ectoderm. It is a recessive mutation, and males are much more frequently involved than females. General and oral manifestations include absence or reduction in amount of hair (hypotrichosis), absence of sweat glands (anhidrosis) and sebaceous glands (asteatosis), temperature elevation (because of anhidrosis), dry skin, depressed bridge of the nose, protrusion of the lips, defective mental development, and complete or partial anodontia of both the deciduous and the permanent dentitions, with malformation of any teeth that may be present (Fig. 4-6).

Anodontia. True anodontia implies the absence of teeth. It may be total and involve both the deciduous and the permanent dentitions, as in some patients with ectodermal dysplasia, or it may be partial (hypodontia) and limited to a single tooth or group of teeth (Fig. 4-7). The tooth germs may fail to initiate, or initiation may occur but further development of the tooth germ will be aborted.

False anodontia is the clinical absence of a tooth. Impacted

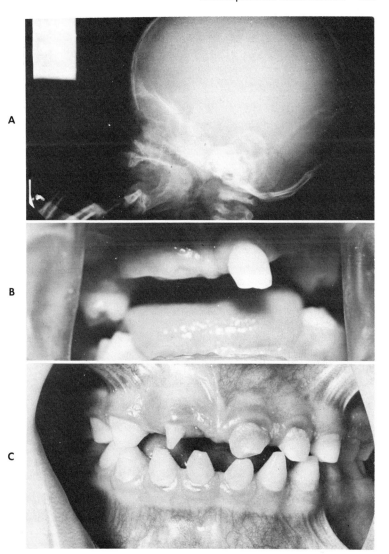

Fig. 4-6. Ectodermal dysplasia. **A,** Complete absence of teeth. **B,** Partial absence of teeth. **C,** Presence of malformed teeth.

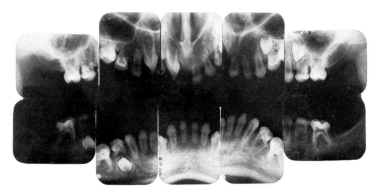

Fig. 4-7. Partial anodontia. Note the absence of much of the permanent dentition.

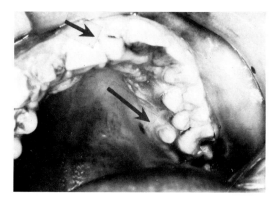

Fig. 4-8. Mesiodens (upper arrow) and paramolar (lower arrow).

or ankylosed teeth (or tooth) that fail to erupt leave vacant places in the dental arch and represent false anodontia. Obviously, this condition is never complete. An example of false anodontia is seen in patients with cleidocranial dysotosis, in whom numerous teeth are present in the jaws but do not erupt.

Accessory and supernumerary teeth. Teeth in excess of the normal complement are referred to as accessory or supernumerary. The term *accessory* is sometimes used for teeth that do not

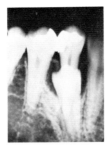

Fig. 4-9. "Third dentition." Note the unerupted third premolar.

resemble the normal form, whereas *supernumerary* is used for teeth that mimic the normal shape.

An accessory tooth between the maxillary central incisors is called a *mesiodens* (Fig. 4-8), whereas one located buccal to the arch is a *peridens*. An accessory tooth distal to the third molar is a *distomolar,* and one located buccal or lingual to the molars a *paramolar* (Fig. 4-8).

Accessory and supernumerary teeth are far more common in the maxilla than in the mandible (9:1), and the most frequent sites are between the maxillary central incisors and distal to the molars.

Predeciduous dentition. Predeciduous dentition is an extremely rare condition that implies the presence of teeth preceding the deciduous dentition. Such teeth are generally present at birth or may erupt soon after birth (natal and neonatal teeth, respectively). These are usually aborted structures and consist only of caps of enamel or enamel and dentin. If loose, they may be accidentally aspirated and therefore should be removed. Occasionally a normal member of the deciduous dentition will erupt prematurely. This should be distinguished from a predeciduous tooth and not be extracted.

Postpermanent dentition. On extremely rare occasion, teeth may erupt after the loss of permanent dentition. Usually these are impacted accessory teeth (Fig. 4-9) that erupt after the insertion of dentures.

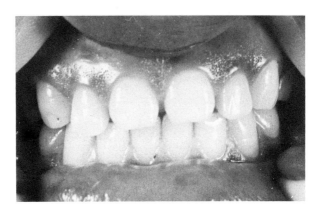

Fig. 4-10. Hutchinson's incisors (maxillary central).

Disturbances during morphodifferentiation of tooth germs

Hutchinson's incisors. The shape of the central incisors is altered in 10% to 30% of children with congenital syphilis. These teeth may resemble a screwdriver (incisal edges narrower than the middle part of the crown) or may show notching of the incisal edges (Fig. 4-10). Although the maxillary central incisors are the most frequently involved, the maxillary lateral incisors and the mandibular incisors may also be affected. Deciduous dentition is not altered. In about 1% of patients with congenital syphilis, Hutchinson's incisors are associated with interstitial keratitis (inflammation and scarring of the cornea) and deafness. This symptom complex is referred to as *Hutchinson's triad*. The ateration in the shape of the teeth is due to the changes in the tooth germ during the stage of morphodifferentiation—changes consisting of inflammation in and around the tooth germ and hyperplasia of the epithelium of the enamel organ.

Mulberry and Pflüger molars. The shape of the permanent first molars is altered in 10% to 30% of patients with congenital syphilis. The occlusal surfaces are much narrower than normal and give the crown a pinched appearance. The teeth also show

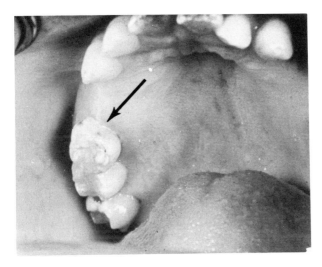

Fig. 4-11. Mulberry molars (arrow). The occlusal surface is narrow, and there is enamel hypoplasia.

hypoplasia of the enamel and are called mulberry molars (Fig. 4-11). Pflüger molars are identical to mulberry molars except that hypoplasia is not present.

Peg-shaped lateral incisors. The peg-shaped lateral incisor is an example of a disturbance during morphodifferentiation.

Macrodontia. Macrodontia refers to a large tooth.

Microdontia. Microdontia refers to a small tooth.

Dens in dente (dens invaginatus). As the term indicates, dens in dente is a "tooth within a tooth." There are two types of dens invaginatus: the coronal, which is by far the most common, and the radicular, which is very rare.

The *coronal* type (Fig. 4-12) is caused by an invagination of all layers of the enamel organ into the dental papilla. As the hard tissues are formed, the invaginated enamel organ produces a small "tooth" within the future pulp chamber. The stages in its development are shown in Fig. 4-13. It occurs in about 2% of the population and can be diagnosed best by radiographic

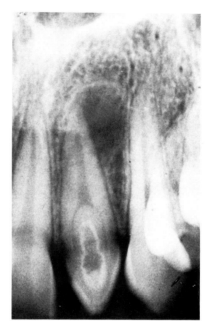

Fig. 4-12. Coronal type of dens in dente (dens invaginatus). Note the apical radiolucency.

examination. The maxillary lateral incisor is most frequently involved. The pulp is usually exposed and therefore necrotic or inflamed. Not infrequently a periapical lesion is associated with this condition. The pulp canals of the teeth should be cleaned and filled.

In the *radicular* type of dens invaginatus (Fig. 4-14), there is a folding of Hertwig's sheath into the developing root. This invaginated epithelial organ then produces enamel and dentin within the root much like what occurs in the coronal type of malformation. These teeth often contain pulp necrosis and apical lesions.

Dens evaginatus (evaginated odontoma). This condition oc-

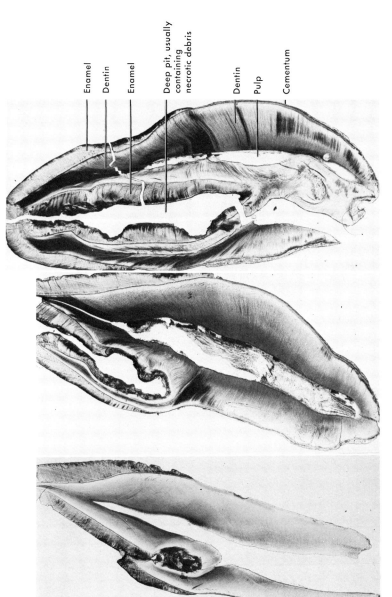

Enamel

Dentin

Enamel

Deep pit, usually containing necrotic debris

Dentin

Pulp

Cementum

Fig. 4-13. Three cases of dens in dente demonstrating the stages in the development of this anomaly.

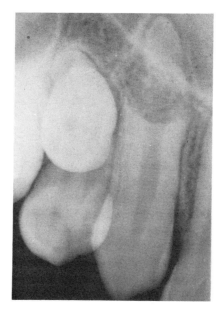

Fig. 4-14. Dens in dente (radicular type).

curs primarily in the mongoloid races (about 2% of the population), but cases have been described among whites. It is a hereditary trait (probably autosomal dominant) and has been reported in successive generations. It is the antithesis of dens invaginatus and consists of the presence of a tuberclelike or nipplelike protuberance on the occlusal surface of premolars (Fig. 4-15). Very rarely, however, canines and molars may also be affected.

There are two types of dens evaginatus: in one the tubercle arises from the lingual ridge of the buccal cusp, and in the other it is located in the center of the occlusal surface. Attrition or fracture of the tubercle leads to exposure of the dentin and a pinpoint depression on the occlusal surface. The pulp extends into this protuberance and often undergoes necrosis. Dens evaginatus is believed to be caused by the abnormal develop-

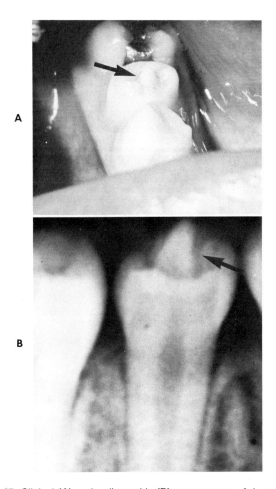

Fig. 4-15. Clinical **(A)** and radiographic **(B)** appearances of dens evaginatus (arrows). (Courtesy John Nelson, D.D.S., Washington, D.C.)

ment of the inner enamel epithelium into stellate reticulum. Since dens evaginatus is not a neoplasm, the term *evaginated odontoma* is not entirely appropriate for this malformation.

Gemination. When a single tooth germ splits or attempts to split to form two completely or partially separated crowns, the process is called gemination (twinning). There is usually a single root canal with a single root (Fig. 4-16).

Fusion. When two adjoining tooth germs join to form a single large crown, the process is called fusion (Fig. 4-17). It is usually seen in the incisor area. The single crown may have two roots or a grooved root, but there are usually two root canals. It is often difficult to distinguish between gemination and fusion.

Dilaceration. Twisting. bending, or other distortion of the root is referred to as dilaceration (Fig. 4-18).

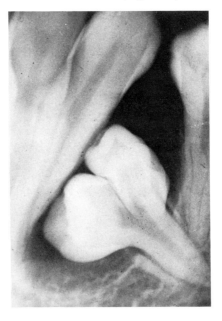

Fig. 4-16. Gemination. Note the presence of two crowns but a single root and root canal.

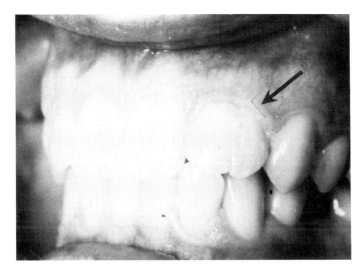

Fig. 4-17. Fusion of a lateral incisor and a supernumerary tooth has produced a large tooth (arrow). Such teeth have two root canals.

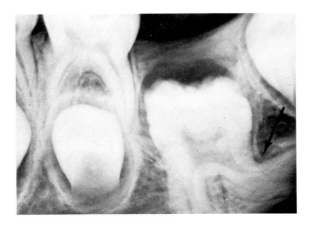

Fig. 4-18. Dilaceration of the distal root of a first molar.

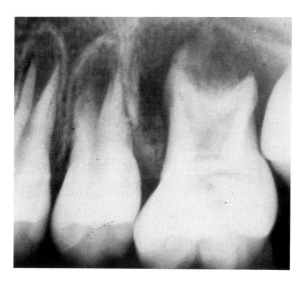

Fig. 4-19. Taurodontism or taurodontia. The pulp chamber is large, and the roots are short and pointed.

Taurodontism. In a hereditary disturbance the pulp chambers of teeth may be unusually large and extend into the root area (Fig. 4-19). Since these teeth remotely resemble those seen in the ungulates, the condition is called taurodontism or taurodontia (*taurus,* bull). It can occur in deciduous or permanent dentitions but is more common in the latter. First molars are least affected, and third molars are most severely affected. Taurodontism is often associated with other anomalies. In roentgenograms, teeth show a long, rectangular body with short roots. The pulp chamber is elongated in an apico-occlusal direction and lacks constriction at the cervix.

Disturbances during apposition of hard dental tissues

Enamel hypoplasia. The term enamel hypoplasia implies a reduction in the amount (thickness) of enamel formed and does not refer to the quality of calcification (Fig. 4-20). Enamel hypoplasia may be due to local, systemic, or hereditary factors.

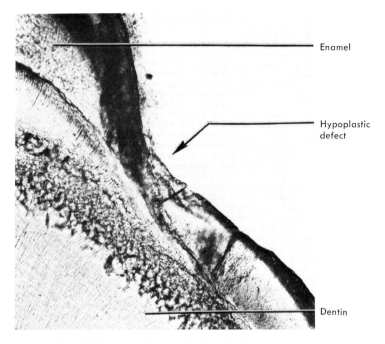

Fig. 4-20. Enamel hypoplasia. Note the hypoplastic defect.

Local enamel hypoplasia affects a tooth or a part of a tooth and is due to a local cause—for example, periapical infections or trauma associated with a deciduous tooth may affect the amount of enamel formed on the underlying permanent tooth.

In systemic enamel hypoplasia (Fig. 4-21) the abnormality is caused by a generalized disease (e.g., rickets, smallpox, German measles). It involves all teeth that are developing at this time, and the defect is seen in areas of the crowns in which amelogenesis was in progress at the time of disturbance.

Hereditary enamel hypoplasia (Fig. 4-22) involves not only all teeth but also their entire crowns. Both permanent and deciduous dentitions are involved. Since the enamel thickness is reduced, the crowns may appear yellow. The condition is also

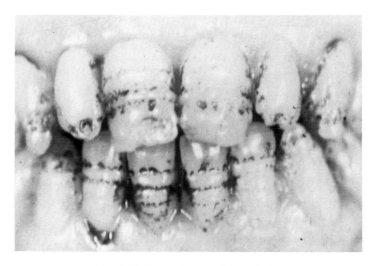

Fig. 4-21. Systemic enamel hypoplasia.

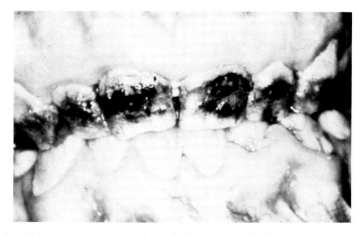

Fig. 4-22. Hereditary enamel hypoplasia. The enamel of the entire crown of each tooth is defective.

called *hereditary brown teeth.* Soon after eruption of the teeth, the thin enamel wears or chips off, and the teeth appear as if they had been prepared for porcelain jacket crowns. The condition is transmitted as a dominant mendelian character.

Amelogenesis imperfecta. This is an ill-defined term used to denote hereditary enamel hypoplasia, aplasia, or hypocalcification.

Dentinogenesis imperfecta (opalescent dentin). Dentinogenesis imperfecta is a hereditary disturbance that affects the development of dentin and may be accompanied by a similar disturbance in the bones (osteogenesis imperfecta).

Clinically both deciduous and permanent dentitions are affected. All teeth are involved and may appear opalescent or gray (Fig. 4-23). Attrition is rapid and marked, carious lesions are not uncommon, the enamel is normal but chips off easily, and the crowns are bulbous (Fig. 4-24).

Radiographs show that the roots are short and conical, and that the pulp chambers are wide in the early stages but narrowed or completely obliterated later (Fig. 4-24).

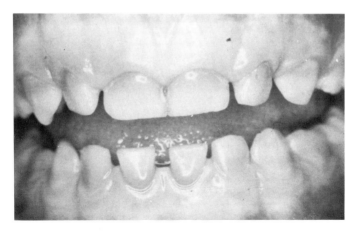

Fig. 4-23. Dentinogenesis imperfecta. The teeth appear gray or opalescent.

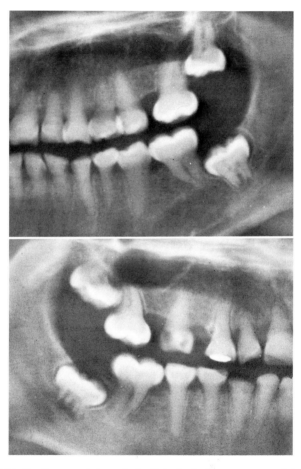

Fig. 4-24. Dentinogenesis imperfecta. Note the bulbous crowns and the obliteration of pulp canals and pulp chambers.

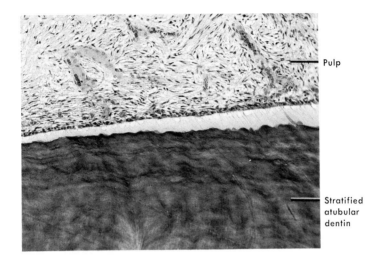

Fig. 4-25. Dentinogenesis imperfecta. Note that the dentin is atubular and stratified and that the odontoblasts are not columnar.

Microscopically the dentin just below the dentinoenamel junction (mantle dentin) is normal. The remainder of the dentin shows reduction of tubules, cellular inclusion, and numerous resting lines—giving the appearance of stratification (Fig. 4-25). The pulp chambers and canals are wide in the early stages but become progressively obliterated and replaced by atypical dentin.

Dentinogenesis imperfecta may be associated with other developmental anomalies (e.g., albinism, cardiac malformation, osteogenesis imperfecta, blue sclerae). Briefly, osteogenesis imperfecta is characterized by atypical bone tissue, so that bones fracture easily (p. 346).

Dentinal dysplasia. This rare disturbance is probably related to dentinogenesis imperfecta. It is a hereditary disease transmitted as an autosomal dominant characteristic.

Both the deciduous and the permanent dentitions are affected. The teeth appear clinically normal but are lost prema-

turely. Radiographs show short pointed roots, periapical radiolucencies, and obliteration of pulp chambers and root canals
(Fig. 4-26). The obliteration occurs much faster than in dentinogenesis imperfecta.

Microscopic sections of teeth show normal coronal dentin.

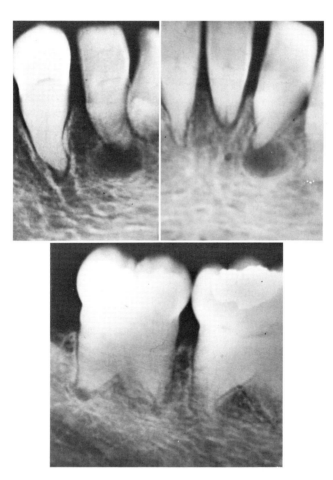

Fig. 4-26. Dentinal dysplasia. Note the obliteration of pulp canals and pulp
chambers, the short pointed roots, and the apical radiolucencies.

The remainder of the dentin, however, has a whorllike, globular, disorganized pattern. There is no treatment for dentinal dysplasia.

Shell teeth. The term shell teeth refers to a modification of dentinogenesis imperfecta. The roots fail to form, the pulp

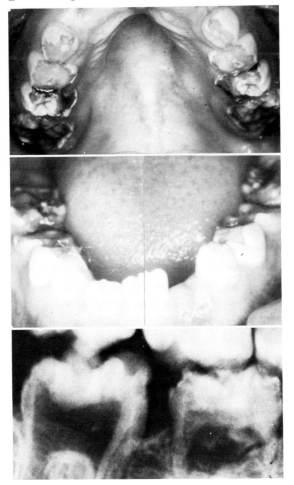

Fig. 4-27. Odontodysplasia. Clinically and radiographically the crowns of teeth have a moth-eaten appearance. The pulp chambers are wide and irregular.

chambers are very wide (therefore "shell teeth"), and the dentin is of the type seen in the teeth of persons with dentinogenesis imperfecta. The enamel is normal.

Odontodysplasia. Also called odontogenic dysplasia, ghost teeth, odontogenesis imperfecta, and regional odontodysplasia, this developmental disorder affects both the ectodermal and mesodermal dental components. Any tooth may be affected, but usually one or more quadrants are involved. The disorder is characterized by defective dentin and enamel formation and discolored, hypoplastic, and hypocalcified teeth with short roots (Fig. 4-27). These teeth usually fail to erupt, and radiolucent areas may be seen around their crowns. They have wide pulp chambers.

Odontodysplasia is usually seen in the deciduous or early mixed dentitions, and females are more often affected than males. Although usually restricted to single quadrants, the disorder may be bilateral as well as involve teeth in both jaws. The

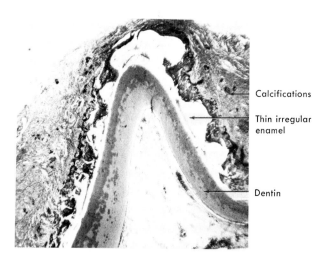

Calcifications

Thin irregular
enamel

Dentin

Fig. 4-28. Odontodysplasia. Microscopic features consist of interglobular dentin, an irregular thin layer of enamel, calcifications around the enamel organ, and a wide pulp chamber.

maxilla is affected twice as often as the mandible. When deciduous teeth are involved, the disorder also affects the permanent teeth.

Microscopically there is distortion of enamel matrix, absence of enamel rods, and focal calcifications in the connective tissue around the crown (Fig. 4-28). Electron microscopic studies have shown that the calcifications represent cementum (Fig. 4-29). The dentin is almost entirely of the interglobular type and may show cellular inclusions and clefts. Coronal dentin in severe cases shows amorphous areas, which in ultrastructural studies are found to be free of collagen. The pulp contains calcifications.

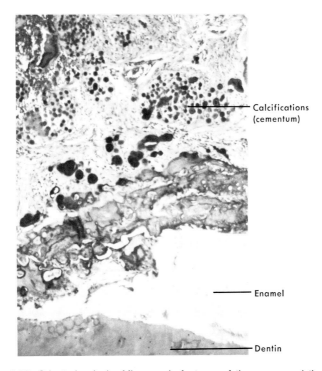

Calcifications
(cementum)

Enamel

Dentin

Fig. 4-29. Odontodysplasia. Microscopic features of the crown and tissues around the crown. The calcified foci represent cementum.

This disturbance does not affect the entire dentition, and its cause is unknown. However, it involves all the tooth structures and has therefore been called odontodysplasia.

Pigmentation of enamel and dentin. Vital pigmentation of dentin and enamel is rare. However, it is seen in patients with erythroblastosis fetalis (Fig. 4-30; also p. 653) and in those with congenital hematoporphyrinuria. In recent years an increasing number of children have been observed with gray or brown pigmentation of the teeth. This pigmentation is caused by administration of tetracyclines during the period of crown development. It has been reported in children with cystic fibrosis (because of tetracycline administration) and ochronosis. Discoloration of teeth is due to deposition of the tetracycline in the dentin. Deposition in the enamel is minimal. The extent of discoloration therefore depends on how close to the dentinoenamel junction the deposits occur, and this in turn depends on the stage of odontogenesis at which the drug is given. Since the enamel is thinnest in the cervical part of the tooth, the discoloration is first observed in that area.

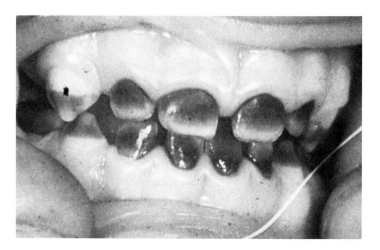

Fig. 4-30. Pigmentation of the teeth in erythroblastosis fetalis.

Discoloration of enamel can be eliminated or improved by applying gauze soaked in 30% hydrogen peroxide and heated to about 88° F. with a hand-held heat source for 30 minutes. Treatments can be repeated to get the desired coloration.

Cemental hypoplasia. This rare condition affects the deciduous and permanent dentitions and is characterized by marked reduction in the amount and rate of cementum formation. Clinically these teeth are lost prematurely and appear to be shed without apparent cause.

In a hereditary metabolic disease called hypophosphatasia, there is hypoplasia of the cementum and the deciduous teeth are prematurely lost without root resorption. In the severe form, impaired calcification of bone, reduced tissue and plasma alkaline phosphatase, and ricketslike changes in the skeleton are seen.

Disturbances during calcification of hard dental tissues

Enamel hypocalcification. Enamel hypocalcification is a condition in which the calcification of enamel is subnormal but the amount of enamel is not changed. Like hypoplasia of enamel, hypocalcification may be local, systemic, or hereditary.

Local hypocalcification is due to local causes and affects only part of a tooth. Clinically it appears as a white opaque area on the crown.

Systemic hypocalcification is caused by some general disturbance. It affects a number of teeth and areas of teeth that are in the process of development at the time of the disturbance. Mottled enamel is the best-known example of systemic enamel hypocalcification.

Hereditary enamel hypocalcification affects the entire crown of all teeth.

Interglobular dentin. Interglobular dentin is seen as areas of uncalcified dentin. Normally after dentin matrix is formed, globules of calcospherites are deposited in it until the entire area is calcified. If calcification is defective, the dentin shows areas of calcification with interspersed irregular zones of uncal-

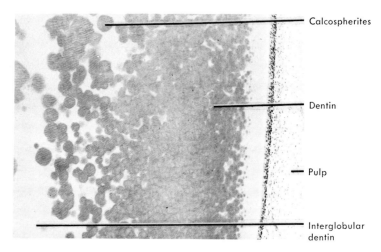

Fig. 4-31. Interglobular dentin. Microscopic features consist of irregular areas of uncalcified dentin matrix.

cified dentin matrix (Fig. 4-31). This is called interglobular dentin. It is seen in patients with numerous conditions (e.g., physical or bacterial trauma to a developing tooth, rickets, chickenpox or any other exanthematous fevers).

Disturbances during eruption of teeth

Malocclusion. This is common and is caused by numerous factors. The details of its etiology can be found in any textbook on orthodontics.

Concrescence. When two independently formed teeth become fused, the phenomenon is called concrescence (Fig. 4-32). Microscopically the teeth are found to have separate pulp canals and roots, but the latter are fused to each other by cementum or bone. Both teeth may be erupted or embedded, or one tooth may be embedded and the other erupted.

Retarded eruption. Teeth may be slow in eruption. This may be due to endocrine disturbances (hypopituitarism or hypothy-

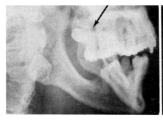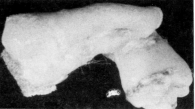

Fig. 4-32. Concrescence (arrow). Two independent teeth have become fused by cementum.

roidism), vitamin deficiencies (rickets), or local causes (lack of space, dentigerous cysts, eruption cysts, malposition, etc.).

Shortened and submerged teeth. Both the permanent and the deciduous teeth may "enter" the oral cavity, but their eruptions subsequently cease. Since the adjoining teeth continue to erupt, these teeth appear to be shortened or submerged. Microscopically they show fusion of the root to the surrounding bone (ankylosis).

Supraeruption. When an antagonist to a tooth is lost, the tooth may erupt beyond the occlusal plane. This is called supraeruption.

REFERENCES

Alexander, W. N., and Allen, H. J.: Hereditary ectodermal dysplasia in three brothers, Oral Surg. **20:**802, 1965.

Alexander, W. N., and Ferguson, R. L.: Beta thalassemia minor and cleidocranial dysplasia: a rare combination of genetic abnormalities in one family, Oral Surg. **49:**413, 1980.

Alexander, W. N., Lilly, G. E., and Irby, W. B.: Odontodysplasia, Oral Surg. **22:**814, 1966.

Arens, D. E., Rich, J. J., and Healey, H. J.: A practical method of bleaching tetracycline-stained teeth, Oral Surg. **34:**812, 1972.

Augsburger, R. A., and Brandebura, J., Jr.: Bilateral dens invaginatus with associated radicular cysts, Oral Surg. **46:**260, 1978.

Bartlett, R. C., Eversole, L. R., and Adkins, R. S.: Autosomal recessive hypohidrotic ectodermal dysplasia, Oral Surg. **33:**736, 1972.

Beumer, J., Trowbridge, H. O., Silverman, S., and Eisenberg, E.: Childhood hypophosphatasia and the premature loss of teeth, Oral Surg. **35:**631, 1973.

Bhatt, A. P., and Dholakia, H. M.: Radicular variety of double dens invaginatus, Oral Surg. **39**:284, 1975.

Bouschor, C. F., and Dorman, H. L.: Bleaching fluoride stained teeth, Tex. Dent. J. **91**:6, 1973.

Bradlaw, R. V.: The dental stigmata of prenatal syphilis, Oral Surg. **6**:147, 1953.

Casamassimo, P. S., Nowak, A. J., Ettinger, R. L., and Schlenker, D. J.: An unusual triad: microdontia, taurodontia, and dens invaginatus, Oral Surg. **45**:107, 1978.

Chabora, A. J., and Horowitz, S. L.: Cleft lip and cleft palate: one genetic system, Oral Surg. **38**:181, 1974.

Chandra, S., and Chawla, T. N.: Clinical evaluation of the sandpaper disk method for removing fluorosis stains from teeth, J. Am. Dent. Assoc. **90**:1273, 1975.

Chaudhry, A. P., Wittich, H. C., Stickel, F. R., and Holland, M. R.: Odontogenesis imperfecta: report of a case, Oral Surg. **14**:1099, 1961.

Chosack, A., Eidelman, E., Wisotski, I., and Cohen, T.: Amelogenesis imperfecta among Israeli Jews and the description of a new type of local hypoplastic autosomal recessive amelogenesis imperfecta, Oral Surg. **47**:148, 1979.

Chow, M. H.: Natal and neonatal teeth, J. Am. Dent. Assoc. **100**:215, 1980.

Ciola, B., Bahn, S. L., and Goviea, G. L.: Radiographic manifestations of an unusual combination Type I and Type II dentin dysplasia, Oral Surg. **45**:317, 1978.

Congleton, J., and Burkes, E. J., Jr.: Amelogenesis imperfecta with taurodontism, Oral Surg. **48**:540, 1979.

Conklin, W. W.: Double bilateral dens invaginatus in the maxillary incisor region, Oral Surg. **39**:949, 1975.

Conklin, W. W.: Bilateral dens invaginatus in the mandibular incisor region, Oral Surg. **45**:905, 1978.

Curzon, M. E. J., and others: Evaginated odontomes in the Keewatin Eskimo, Br. Dent. J. **129**:324, 1970.

Druck, J. S.: Amelogenesis imperfecta, Oral Surg. **39**:502, 1975.

Durr, D. P., Campos, C. A., and Ayers, C. S.: Clinical significance of taurodontism, J. Am. Dent. Assoc. **100**:378, 1980.

Eastman, J. R., Melnick, M., and Goldblatt, L. I.: Focal odontoblastic dysplasia: dentin dysplasia Type III? Oral Surg. **44**:909, 1977.

Elzay, R. P., and Robinson, C. T.: Dentinal dysplasia, Oral Surg. **23**:338, 1967.

Elzay, R. P., and van Sickels, J. E.: Oromandibular-limb hypogenesis syndrome: Type II C, hypoglossia-hypodactylomelia, Oral Surg. **48**:146, 1979.

Fraser, F. C.: The genetics of cleft lip and cleft palate, Am. J. Hum. Genet. **22**:336, 1970.

Gardner, D. G.: The dentinal changes in regional odontodysplasia, Oral Surg. **38**:887, 1974.

Gardner, D. G., and Girgis, S. S.: Taurodontism, short roots, and external resorption, associated with short stature and a small head, Oral Surg. **44:**271, 1977.

Gardner, D. G., and Sapp, J. P.: Regional odontodysplasia, Oral Surg. **35:**351, 1973.

Gardner, D. G., and Sapp, J. P.: Ultrastructural, electron-probe, and microhardness studies of the controversial amorphous areas in the dentin of regional odontodysplasia, Oral Surg. **44:**549, 1977.

Gertzman, G. B., Gaston, G., and Quinn, I.: Amelogenesis imperfecta: local hypoplastic type with pulpal calcification, J. Am. Dent. Assoc. **99:**637, 1979.

Giansanti, J. S.: A kindred showing hypocalcified amelogenesis imperfecta, J. Am. Dent. Assoc. **86:**675, 1973.

Giansanti, J. S., and Allen, J. D.: Dentin dysplasia, type II, or dentin dysplasia, coronal type, Oral Surg. **38:**911, 1974.

Giansanti, J. S., and Budnick, S. D.: Six generations of hereditary opalescent dentin: report of a case, J. Am. Dent. Assoc. **90:**439, 1975.

Gibbard, P. D., Lee, K. W., and Winter, G. B.: Odontodysplasia, Br. Dent. J. **135:**525, 1973.

Gotoh, T., Kawahara, K., Imai, K., Kishi, K., and Fujiki, Y.: Clinical and radiographic study of dens invaginatus, Oral Surg. **48:**88, 1979.

Guggenheimer, J., Nowak, A. J., and Michaels, R. H.: Dental manifestations of the rubella syndrome, Oral Surg. **32:**30, 1971.

Gyenes, V., de Grosz, I., and Toth, I.: Some observations concerning mandibulofacial dysostosis (Franceschetti's syndrome), Oral Surg. **16:**68, 1963.

Herman, N. G., and Moss, S. J.: Odontodysplasia: report of case, J. Dent. Child. **44:**52, 1977.

Hintz, C. S., and Peters, R. A.: Odontodysplasia, Oral Surg. **34:**744, 1972.

Houpt, M. I., Kenny, F. M., and Listgarten, M.: Hypophosphatasia: case reports, J. Dent. Child. **37:**127, 1970.

Jedrychowski, R., Jr., and Duperon, D.: Childhood hypophospatasia with oral manifestations, J. Oral. Med. **34:**18, 1979.

Johnson, D. C.: Prevalence of delayed emergence of permanent teeth as a result of local factors, J. Am. Dent. Assoc. **94:**100, 1977.

Kalliala, E., and Taskinen, P. J.: Cleidocranial dysostosis, Oral Surg. **15:**808, 1962.

Kelln, E. E., Chaudhry, A. P., and Gorlin, R. F.: Oral manifestations of Crouzon's disease, Oral Surg. **13:**1245, 1960.

Kramer, R. M., and Williams, A. C.: The incidence of impacted teeth: a survey at Harlem Hospital, Oral Surg. **29:**237, 1970.

Kutscher, A. H., Zegarelli, E. V., Fahn, B. S., Denning, C. R., and Dougles, R. N.: Tetracycline discoloration of teeth: diagnosis by long-wave and short-wave ultraviolet light, Oral Surg. **23:**91, 1967.

Lunin, M., and Devore, D.: The etiology of regional odontodysplasia, J. Dent. Res., **55**:B 109, Abstr. 192, 1976.

Lustmann, J., Klein, H., and Ulmansky, M.: Odontodysplasia, Oral Surg. **39**:781, 1975.

Lustmann, J., and Ulmansky, M.: Structural changes in odontodysplasia, Oral Surg. **41**:193, 1976.

Mader, C. L.: Fusion of teeth, J. Am. Dent. Assoc. **98**:62, 1979.

McLarty, E. L., Giansanti, J. S., and Hibbard, E. D.: X-linked hypomaturation type of amelogenesis imperfecta exhibiting lyonization in affected females, Oral Surg. **36**:678, 1973.

Melnick, M., Eastman, J. R., Goldblatt, L. I., Michaud, M., and Bixler, D.: Dentin dysplasia, Type II: a rare autosomal dominant disorder, Oral Surg. **44**:592, 1977.

Mena, C. A.: Taurodontism, Oral Surg. **32**:812, 1971.

Metro, P. S.: Mandibulofacial dysostosis (Treacher-Collins syndrome), Oral Surg. **20**:583, 1965.

Michaels, R. H., and Kenny, F. M.: Postnatal growth retardation in congenital rubella, Pediatrics **43**:251, 1969.

Miller, W. A., and Seymour, R. H.: Odontodysplasia, Br. Dent. J. **125**:56, 1968.

Miller, W. A., Winkler, S., Rosenberg, J. J., Mastracola, R., Fischman, S. L., and Wolfe, R. J.: Dentinogenesis imperfecta traceable through five generations of a part American Indian family, Oral Surg. **35**:180, 1973.

Moffitt, J., Cooley, R. O., Olsen, N. H., and Hefferren, J. J.: Prediction of tetracycline-induced tooth discoloration, J. Am. Dent. Assoc. **88**:547, 1974.

Orlowski, R. M., and Reeve, C. M.: Uninherited dentinogenesis imperfecta, Oral Surg. **9**:742, 1975.

Palmer, M. E.: Case reports of evaginated odontomes in Caucasians, Oral Surg. **35**:772, 1973.

Perl, T., and Farman, A. G.: Radicular (Type I) dentin dysplasia, Oral Surg. **43**:746, 1977.

Pimstone, B., Eisenberg, E., and Silverman, S.: Hypophosphatasia: genetic and detal studies, Ann. Intern. Med. **65**:722, 1966.

Pruhs, R. J., Simonsen, C. R., Sharma, P. S., and Fodor, B.: Odontodysplasia, J. Am. Dent. Assoc. **91**:1057, 1975.

Reichart, P., and Tantiniran, D.: Dens evaginatus in the Thai, Oral Surg. **39**:615, 1975.

Rosenblum, F. N.: Odontodysplasia: report of a case, J. Dent. Child. **38**:327, 1971.

Rushton, M. A.: Anomalies of human dentin, Br. Dent. J. **98**:431, 1955.

Sapp, J. P., and Gardner, D. G.: Regional odontodysplasia: an ultrastructural and histochemical study of the soft-tissue calcifications, Oral Surg. **36**:383, 1973.

Sarnat, B. G., and Shaw, N. G.: Dental development in congenital syphilis, Am. J. Dis. Child. **64**:771, 1942.

Sauk, J. J., Jr., Vickers, R. A., Copeland, J. S., and Lyon, H. W.: The surface of genetically determined hypoplastic enamel in human teeth, Oral Surg. **34**:60, 1972.

Spyropoulos, N. D., Patsakas, A. J., and Angelopoulos, A. P.: Simultaneous presence of partial anodontia and supernumerary teeth, Oral Surg. **48**:53, 1979.

Stark, R. B.: Development of the face, Surg. Gynecol. Obstet. **137**:403, 1973.

Stenvik, A., Zachrisson, B. U., and Svatun, B.: Taurodontism and concomitant hypodontia in siblings, Oral Surg. **33**:841, 1972.

Stewart, R. E., Dixon, G. H., and Graber, R. B.: Dens evaginatus (tuberculated cusps): genetic and treatment considerations, Oral Surg. **46**:831, 1978.

Taylor, G. N., and McDaniel, R. K.: Extraradicular communicating dens invaginatus, Oral Surg. **4**:931, 1977.

Thomas, J. G.: A study of dens in dente, Oral Surg. **38**:653, 1974.

Turvey, T. A., Long, R. E., and Hall, D. J.: Multidisciplinary management of Crouzon syndrome, J. Am. Dent. Assoc. **99**:205, 1979.

Ulmansky, M., and Hermal, J.: Double dens in dente in a single tooth, Oral Surg. **17**:92, 1964.

Vogel, R. I., and Austin, G.: Tetracycline-induced extrinsic discoloration of the dentition, Oral Surg. **44**:50, 1977.

Walker, R. V., and Maloney, J. A.: Pierre Robin syndrome: report of six cases, J. Oral Surg. **21**:140, 1963.

Walton, J. L., Witkop, C. J., Jr., and Walker, P. O.: Odontodysplasia, Oral Surg. **46**:676, 1978.

Weinmann, J. P., Svoboda, J. F., and Woods, R. W.: Hereditary disturbances of enamel formation and calcification, J. Am. Dent. Assoc. **32**:397, 1945.

Wesley, R. K., Wysocki, G. P., Mintz, S. M., and Jackson, J.: Dentin dysplasia, type I, Oral Surg. **41**:516, 1976.

Witkop, C. J., Brearley, L. J., and Gentry, W. C.: Hypoplastic enamel, onycholysis, and hypohidrosis inherited as an autosomal dominant trait, Oral Surg. **39**:71, 1975.

Yip, W.: The prevalence of dens evaginatus, Oral Surg. **38**:80, 1974.

Zegarelli, E. V., Kutscher, A. H., Applebaum, E., and Archard, H. O.: Odontodysplasia, Oral Surg. **16**:187, 1963.

CHAPTER 5

Lesions of hard dental tissues

The following lesions of hard dental tissues are discussed in this chapter:

1. Caries
   a. Radiation
2. Erosion
3. Abrasion
4. Attrition
5. Secondary dentin
6. Irregular dentin
7. Hypercementosis
8. Root resorption

Caries. Dental caries, the most common disease of man, is characterized by decalcification and disintegration of the hard dental tissues. It affects persons of all races, countries, and economic strata and can occur at any age and in either sex. Its predisposing factors, mechanism of development, control, microscope appearance, and clinical aspects are well known.

Predisposing factors. There are numerous factors that predispose an animal or a person to develop caries.

Certain *species* are more susceptible to caries than others. However, this is probably due to the shape and structure of teeth and to food habits. *Civilization* is believed to be a predisposing factor. It has been shown that *heredity* influences somewhat the susceptibility and immunity to caries. A strain of caries-immune or caries-susceptible rats can be produced by selective breeding. Also, parents with a low caries index can pass relative immunity on to their children. Some *races* (e.g., the Australian aborigines) are less predisposed to caries.

The type of *diet* has considerable bearing on caries susceptibility. A diet rich in fermentable carbohydrates promotes caries, whereas a diet consisting of raw, coarse foods tends to reduce the incidence of caries. *Ingestion of fluorides* in the water reduces susceptibility. Increased concentrations of boron, strontium, lithium, molybdenum, titanium, and vanadium in the drinking water are believed to reduce tooth decay. The *composition of teeth* also has some bearing on incidence. Caries-immune teeth have been shown to possess a higher fluoride content than caries-susceptible teeth.

The *physical form* of teeth may determine susceptibility (e.g., areas with deep pits and fissures are especially predisposed). Poor *oral hygiene* is known to be a predisposing factor. Finally, the *saliva* contains an immunoglobulin called the secretory immunoglobulin A (IgA). Its main function is to protect against viruses that invade the respiratory or intestinal tract. This antibody is known to coat some plaque bacteria and make them liable to phagocytosis by oral neutrophils. The saliva of caries-immune individuals, therefore, may contain bacteriolytic factors. Also, the viscosity and amount of saliva can affect the incidence of decay.

Mechanism of development. Caries is initiated by demineralization of the enamel by organic acids that are produced locally by bacteria. In addition to demineralization, bacteria destroy the protein content of teeth (especially dentin). Caries is therefore a bacterial disease and is transmitted from one to other members of the species.

In the development of caries, certain oral bacteria colonize the surfaces of teeth in the form of a sticky gelatinous film that besides the bacteria contains mucus, desquamated cells, and food debris. It is called dental plaque (Fig. 5-1; for additional discussion of plaque see p. 177). The bacteria that are primarily concerned with dental decay in man are the *Streptococcus mutans*. These organisms proliferate in the supragingival dental plaque; they are seen in mouths with natural or artificial teeth; and their numbers are markedly lower before teeth erupt or after teeth are lost. In addition to *Streptococcus mutans*, *Lactobacillus acidophilus* probably also play a minor role in acid production in the plaque.

The stickiness of the plaque is caused by *dextran* which is

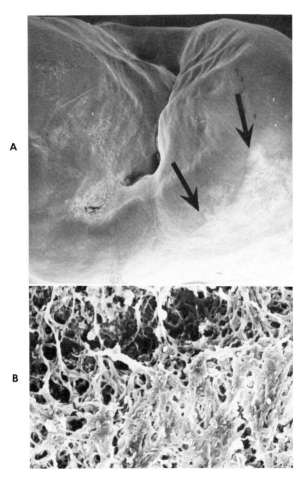

Fig. 5-1. A, Mesio-occlusal view of a premolar. Arrows point to plaque. **B** and **C,** Scanning electron micrographs (×600 and ×1,500) of the plaque. Note the honeycomb-like mass. The three round bodies in **C** are erythrocytes.

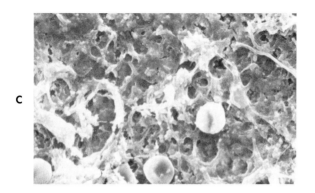

C

Fig. 5-1, cont'd. For legend see opposite page.

produced by the fermenting of dietary sucrose by *Streptococcus mutans*. Dextran forms about 10% of the weight and 33% of the volume of the plaque, and it traps in it all types of oral organisms. The plaque bacteria, particularly *Streptococcus mutans*, act upon dietary fructose to produce lactic acid, which causes enamel decalcification (at or below about 5.5 pH). When carbohydrates are abundant in the oral environment, the plaque bacteria can store intracellular polysaccharides (amylopectin); and during periods of carbohydrate deficiency, they can act on this store to continue producing lactic acid. Thus the plaque and dietary carbohydrates are important in the initiation of enamel caries.

Finally, the rate of caries initiation and extension depends on the *susceptibility* of *enamel*.

To get a carious lesion, therefore, all three conditions must be present: the plaque, the diet, and the susceptibility of enamel.

In addition to acid production, some of the plaque bacteria produce proteolytic enzymes that break down the organic portions of the enamel and dentin. This mechanism plays an important role in dentin decay, which has considerable organic components. However, even in enamel caries proteolytic breakdown is important in the progression of decay through enamel lamellae and other protein-filled defects.

Control. Since caries is a result of the interplay between bacteria (plaque), diet, and enamel—its control can be accomplished by a variety of means:

1. Incorporation of fluorides in enamel, particularly in the outer layers. This can be done by fluoridating water or by topical application of various fluoride compounds.
2. Elimination of sucrose from the diet. There is some evidence that addition of inorganic and organic phosphates to diets high in sucrose may render such diets harmless to teeth.
3. Use of antibiotics and antiseptics as mouthwashes. Since only a suppression of plaque bacteria is necessary to reduce dental decay, this need not be done daily. The bacteria in plaque grow at a rate of about 2 or 3 cell divisions rather than 40 to 50 a day as elsewhere. Therefore, recovery from the use of an antimicrobial agent would be very slow (estimated at half a day or longer).
4. Careful daily removal of the plaque from all tooth surfaces.

Microscopic appearance. In caries of enamel, decalcification of the interprismatic substance occurs first, followed by decalcification of the interglobular material. This leads to an accentuation of the bands of Retzius and to a prominence of the rods themselves. The decalcification is followed by breakage and loss of enamel rods so that broken rods and voids are seen in histologic sections. As the process of decalcification progresses to the dentinoenamel junction, it spreads laterally along the junction and the caries of dentin is initiated.

Under low power, a carious lesion appears triangular, with the apex of the cone pointed toward the dentin. The exception to this is the carious lesion in occlusal fissures, in which the apex is directed occlusally. These patterns are determined by the direction of the enamel rods in different areas of the tooth.

Sections through a carious lesion in dentin show four zones.

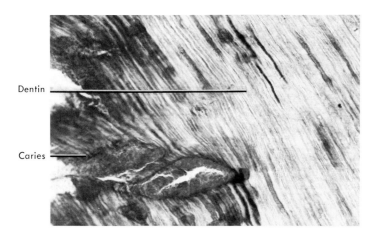

Fig. 5-2. Caries of dentin. Note the clefts and dilated tubules.

The deepest zone is that of *fatty degeneration* of the dentinal tubules. Next is a zone of *sclerosis*, in which the dentin appears transparent as a result of calcification of the dentinal tubules (sclerosis)—also called the transparent zone. Coronal to the zone of sclerosis is a zone that shows *decalcification* and invasion of the tubules by microorganisms. In this area, longitudinal and horizontal clefts and dilatation of tubules are present (Fig. 5-2). The most superficial zone of the lesion consists of completely *necrotic dentin*, whose morphologic details are erased. The necrotic zone and the decalcified zone contain numerous saprophytic organisms that digest and remove necrotic dentin. The pupal end of the carious dentin shows formation of secondary dentin (p. 143). Depending on the severity of the lesion, the underlying pulpal tissue may show edema or infiltration by neutrophils, plasma cells, or lymphocytes.

Clinical aspects. The clinical appearance of caries, from its inception as a chalky white area on enamel to a far-progressed, deep lesion, is well known.

When lesions progress rapidly, as they sometimes do in children, the term *acute caries* is used (Fig. 5-3, *A*). Slowly progressing carious lesions in older patients are *chronic caries* (Fig. 5-3, *B*). In acute caries, pulp involvement occurs rapidly. In chronic caries the pulp responds by forming secondary dentin and is exposed only in the late stages of the disease.

A lesion may cease to progress, in which instance it is referred to as *arrested caries*. This usually occurs on the occlusal surfaces where, due to the breakage of the enamel walls, a large

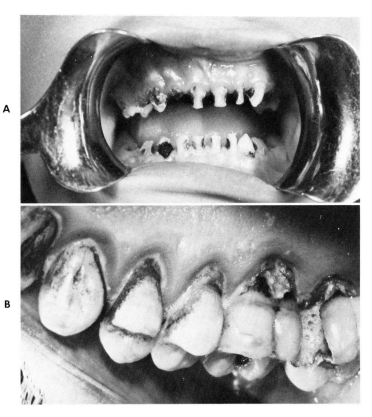

A

B

Fig. 5-3. A, Extensive acute caries. **B,** Chronic caries.

carious lesion becomes exposed to the cleansing action of tooth-brushing, saliva, and mastication. The soft dentin is then worn off, leaving a hard, eburnated layer of brown or black dentin.

The term *recurrent caries* is used for carious lesions that begin around the margins of defective restorations.

Although no tooth is immune to caries, it has been shown that the maxillary teeth are involved slightly more frequently than the mandibular teeth. Involvement of individual teeth occurs in the following order of frequency: first molars, second molars, second premolars, first premolars, maxillary canines and incisors, and mandibular canines and incisors. Tooth surfaces are involved in the following order of frequency: occlusal, mesial, distal, buccal, and lingual.

Radiation caries. In patients receiving large doses of radiation for treatment of malignant lesions around the head and neck, a specific form of carious lesion is often observed.

These lesions begin a few weeks to a few months after radiation and consist of what looks like a decalcification process around the cervical area of teeth. Radiation caries can surround the entire crown and cause its amputation. The mechanism of this disease is not known. Radiographs show what look like carious lesions.

Erosion. The term erosion refers to the idiopathic loss of hard dental tissues along the gingival margins of the teeth. The lesions are shaped like a dish, wedge, or crescent; they occur usually on the buccal surfaces, have sharp margins, and present a hard, polished, shiny base.

The cause of erosion is obscure. There are many theories, most of them speculative. The manner in which the teeth are brushed may play a role in the causation or spread of the lesion. Neurologic disturbances, hyperthyroidism, abnormal secretion from mucosal glands, and discharge from gingival pockets are other factors that have been mentioned. The process of erosion may cease spontaneously or be progressive. Even restorations in the area do not hinder its spread. There is no known treatment for erosion.

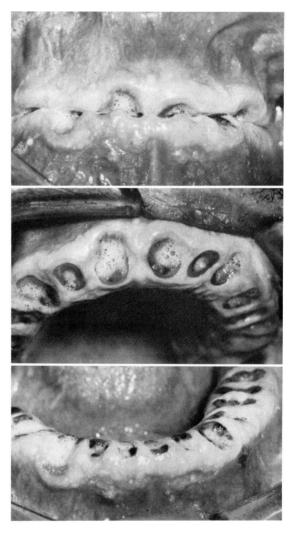

Fig. 5-4. Advanced case of attrition and caries.

Abrasion. Loss of tooth structure due to mechanical wear (e.g., by clasps, toothbrushing) is called abrasion. It is seen in patients who use a large amount of dentifrice and a hard toothbrush. These patients usually have low plaque scores but more gingival recession than normal. Teeth most commonly showing abrasion are the maxillary first molars, maxillary premolars, and mandibular premolars.

Attrition. Loss of tooth structure when related to mastication is called attrition (Fig. 5-4). Obviously, it occurs on the occlusal surfaces of the teeth; and it is usually more pronounced in peoples whose diet consists mainly of coarse foods (e.g., Eskimos).

Loss of tooth structure, which superficially resembles attrition, is seen in patients who regurgitate or who habitually suck on lemons or other acidic foods. These lesions are most often seen on the lingual aspect of maxillary teeth.

•   •   •

Histologic features in erosion, abrasion, and attribution are identical. Microscopic sections in all these conditions show only loss of tooth structure and apposition of irregular or secondary dentin in the pulp.

Secondary and irregular dentin. Sometimes the terms secondary dentin and irregular dentin are used synonymously. However, secondary dentin is atypical and formed in the pulp as a result of progressive crowding of the odontoblasts whereas irregular dentin is formed in response to injury.

As the odontoblasts recede from the dentinoenamel junction, the surface area progressively narrows (except on the pulpal floor, where it gets wider) and some odontoblasts are destroyed. The subsequently formed dentin, which has fewer dentinal tubules, is called secondary dentin.

Whenever dentinal tubules are cut, irritated, or injured (in caries, abrasion, or cavity preparation), the odontoblasts at the pulpal ends of these tubules form new dentin that has fewer tubules and may be atubular, has cellular inclusions, and shows irregular pulpal borders. Such dentin is called irregular dentin

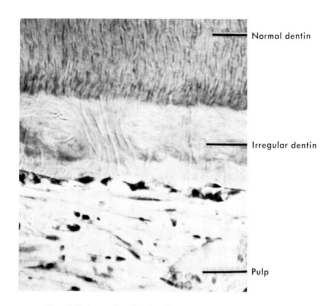

Normal dentin

Irregular dentin

Pulp

Fig. 5-5. Irregular dentin. There are very few tubules.

(Fig. 5-5). On rare occasion, it may even resemble bone tissue (osteodentin).

Teeth with irregular or secondary dentin in their pulp chambers (i.e., having undergone attrition, abrasion, or other irritational exposure) show a greater amount of collagen in their pulp tissue—implying that the response of dentin to irritation is not only a new layer of dentin formation but also pulpal fibrosis.

Hypercementosis. Excessive deposition of cementum on the root surface is called hypercementosis. It may be confined to one area of a root or to a single tooth, or it may involve the entire dentition. Its cause will not always be apparent, but it may be associated with periapical granulomas, Paget's disease, acromegaly, gigantism, or local injury such as occlusal trauma.

Microscopically the tooth shows cellular and acellular cementum that is excessive in quantity but normal in structure.

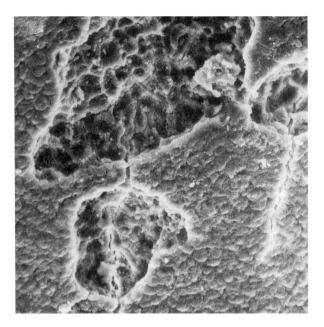

Fig. 5-6. Scanning electron micrograph of the root surface of a tooth showing three areas of resorption. (×800). (Courtesy John Brady, D.D.S., Washington, D.C.)

Root resorption. Microscopic areas of root resorption from the side of the periodontal membrane (external resorption) are common in old age (Fig. 5-6).

Serial sections through the jaws of elderly persons show a number of small foci in which cementum or cementum and dentin are undergoing resorption and being replaced by connective tissue. In some instances these foci are repaired by cementum. Microscopic root resorption is of no clinical significance; it is asymptomatic and cannot be seen radiographically.

Clinically apparent external resorption of the root can be seen in excessive occlusal trauma, orthodontic tooth movement, and some cysts and central tumors of the jaw. It may also be

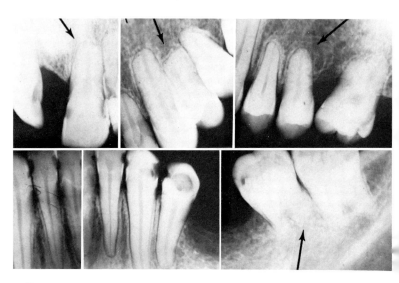

Fig. 5-7. Idiopathic root resorption. Arrows point to some of the many areas of root resorption.

observed after radiation therapy, or it may be idiopathic (Fig. 5-7). The microscopic features of resorption in these conditions are the same as those described previously except that repair usually is not prominent. In cases of cysts and tumors, the defect in the root is usually filled by the offending lesion.

Internal resorption of teeth is discussed with the diseases of the pulp (Chapter 6).

REFERENCES

Berman, D. S., and Slack, G. L.: Susceptibility of tooth surfaces to carious attack: a longitudinal study, Br. Dent. J. **134:**135, 1973.

Bibby, B. G.: The cariogenicity of snack foods and confections, J. Am. Dent. Assoc. **90:**121, 1975.

Bowen, W. H.: A vaccine against dental caries: a pilot experiment in monkeys (Macacca irus), Br. Dent. J. **126:**159, 1969.

Bowen, W. H., and Cornick, D. E.: The microbiology of gingival-dental plaque, Int. Dent. J. **20:**382, 1970.

Brady, J. M., and Woody, R. D.: Scanning microscopy of cervical erosion, J. Am. Dent. Assoc. **94:**726, 1977.

Briner, W. W.: Plaque in relation to dental caries and periodontal disease, Int. Dent. J. **1**:293, 1971.

Edgar, W. M., Bibby, B. G., Mundorff, S., and Rowley, J.: Acid production in plaques after eating snacks: modifying factors in foods, J. Am. Dent. Assoc. **90**:418, 1975.

Jordan, H. V.: A systematic approach to antibiotic control of dental caries, J. Can. Dent. Assoc. **39**:703, 1973.

Karmiol, M., and Walsh, R. F.: Dental caries after radiotherapy of the oral regions, J. Am. Dent. Assoc. **91**:838, 1975.

Kleinberg, I.: Regulation of the acid-base metabolism of the sentogingival plaque and its relation to dental caries and periodontal disease, Int. Dent. J. **20**:451, 1970.

Lehner, T., Wilton, J. M. A., and Ward, R. G.: Serum antibodies in dental caries in man, Arch. Oral Biol. **15**:481, 1970.

Levin, M. P., Yearwood, L. L., and Carpenter, W. N.: The desensitizing effect of calcium hydroxide and magnesium hydroxide and hypersensitive dentin, Oral Surg. **35**:741, 1973.

Marciani, R. D., and Plezia, R. A.: Management of teeth in the irradiated patient, J. Am. Dent. Assoc. **88**:1021, 1974.

Scherp, H. W.: Dental caries, prospect for prevention, Science **173**:199, 1971.

Sims, W.: The concept of immunity in dental caries, Oral Surg. **34**:69, 1972.

Sognnaes, R. F., Wolcott, R. B., and Xhonga, F. A.: Dental erosion. I. Erosion-like patterns occurring in association with other dental conditions, J. Am. Dent. Assoc. **84**:571, 1972.

Stein, J. J., James, A. G., and King, E. R: The management of the teeth, bone, and soft tissues in patients receiving treatment for oral cancer, Am. J. Roentgenol. **108**:257, 1970.

Volpe, A. R., Kupczak, L. J., Brant, J. H., King, W. J., Kestenbaum, R. C., and Schlissel, H. J.: Antimicrobial control of bacterial plaque and calculus and the effects of these agents on oral flora, J. Dent. Res. (suppl.) **48**:832, 1969.

White, D. K., Hayes, R. C., and Benjamin, R. N.: Loss of tooth structure associated with chronic regurgitation and vomiting, J. Am. Dent. Assoc. **97**:833, 1978.

Xhonga, F. A., Wolcott, R. B., and Sognnaes, R. F.: Dental erosion. II. Clinical measurements of dental erosion progress, J. Am. Dent. Assoc. **84**:577, 1972.

Zipkin, I., and McClure, F. G.: Salivary citrate and dental erosion. II. Clinical measurements of dental erosion progress, J. Am. Dent. Assoc. **84**:577, 1972.

CHAPTER 6

Diseases of pulp

The pulp is composed of connective tissue that, with slight modifications, is identical to connective tissue present elsewhere in the body. It consists of fibroblasts, blood vessels, undifferentiated mesenchymal cells, nerves, reticular and collagen fibers, and odontoblasts. However, it differs from connective tissue elsewhere in the body insofar as its intercellular ground substance is denser than that in loose connective tissue and it is encased in a hard, unresilient shell of dentin.

The following diseases of the pulp are discussed in this chapter:

1. Pulpitis
   a. Acute pulpitis and hyperemia
   b. Chronic pulpitis
   c. Hyperplastic pulpitis (pulp polyp)
2. Anachoresis
3. Aerodontalgia
4. Necrosis
5. Reticular atrophy
6. Calcifications
7. Internal resorption
8. Metaplasia

Pulpitis. Pulpitis may be acute, chronic, or hyperplastic.

Acute pulpitis and hyperemia. Acute pulpitis results from (1) physical agents such as heat and cold (these conditions may be associated with deep or extensive fillings, sudden severe physical trauma, or careless cavity preparation with excessive associated heat production and dehydration), (2) chemical injury such as the application of irritants to exposed dentin, and (3) bacterial invasion such as that seen in deep carious lesions. In extremely rare instances, inflammation of the pulp may follow the hematogenous route (e.g., in persons with bacteremias and septicemias).

Clinically acute pulpitis is characterized by severe pain that varies from a continuous throbbing type to less severe and intermittent attacks. The severity of pain increases while the patient is lying down and with changes in temperature. The extreme pain associated with inflammation of the pulp as compared to pain experienced with inflammation elsewhere in the body is due to the fact that in pulp the edema is confined in a rigid chamber of dentin and the pressure is greater than in loose connective tissue. This pressure, as well as the products of inflammation, acts upon the nerve endings to produce pain.

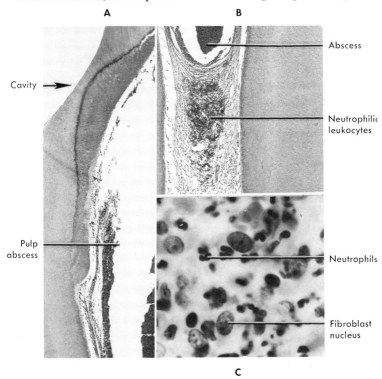

Fig. 6-1. A and **B,** Acute pulpitis with pulp abscess, a response to cavity preparation. **C,** High-power view of an area from **B** showing numerous neutrophilic leukocytes.

With an electric vitality tester, the tooth reacts at a far lower threshold than normal.

Microscopically acute pulpitis is characterized by edema, moderate to dense infiltration by neutrophils (Fig. 6-1), and disorganization of the odontoblastic layer. In some cases, there is a dense localized accumulation of neutrophils. Such an area is associated with tissue liquefaction and is called pulp abscess (Fig. 6-1). If the liquefied material (pus) is lost in slide preparation, the area appears as a space surrounded by neutrophils. The inflammatory changes just mentioned may involve the entire pulp *(total acute pulpitis)* or only a part of the pulp *(partial acute pulpitis)*. Special stains may reveal microorganisms in the pulp.

The term *pulp hyperemia* is a clinical designation; the condition does not exist as a separate clinicopathologic entity. Clinicians use the term for what microscopically are early stages of partial acute pulpitis. The tooth is sensitive to heat and especially sensitive to cold.

Treatment of acute pulpitis consists of removal of the cause, pulp capping, or root canal treatment, depending on the clinical evaluation of the extent of pulp involvement.

The cracked tooth syndrome is a condition in which pulpitis results from a crack in the tooth. Patients compalin of ill-defined pain. Although clinically usually invisible, the crack in the crown extends into the pulp; and the saliva and organisms produce pulp inflammation. In clinical practice, therefore, when tooth pain cannot be explained by any other cause, the possibility of a cracked tooth should be considered. Since it is often difficult to detect, drying of the tooth and/or application of a dye are used in making the diagnosis. Treatment depends on the location of the crack and consists of a full crown (with or without endodontic therapy) or extraction.

Chronic pulpitis. The cause of chronic pulpitis is the same as that of acute pulpitis except the irritant is of low virulence and therefore the response is milder and more protracted.

Clinically the tooth may exhibit intermittent dull aching.

Sensitivity to heat and cold is less striking than that present in acute pulpitis, and with the electric pulp tester the tooth responds at higher levels than does the normal tooth. Microscopically infiltration of the pulp by plasma cells and lymphocytes and a mild degree of fibrosis (i.e., formation of collagen fibers) are found.

Treatment of chronic pulpitis is the same as for acute pulpitis.

Hyperplastic pulpitis (pulp polyp). In teeth, particularly the deciduous molars, with extensive carious lesions leading to wide exposures of the pulp tissue, the inflammatory changes are characteristic and terminate in what is called a pulp polyp. The clinical features of a pulp polyp are as follows: it is generally seen in children, the tooth involved has a large cavity that is usually on the occlusal surface, a red fleshy mass of tissue lies in the cavity or projects beyond the occlusal surface, the growth is not painful, the tooth remains vital, and the most frequently involved teeth are the deciduous molars and the first permanent molars (Fig. 6-2).

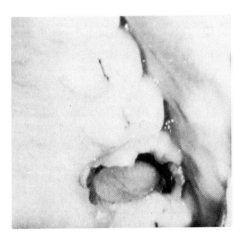

Fig. 6-2. Pulp polyp in the maxillary molar.

The following sequence of events leads to the production of a pulp polyp: Caries produces acute pulpitis; however, because of the wide exposure, acute pulpitis does not lead to pulp necrosis but gradually to chronic pulpitis, which is characterized by the formation of abundant granulation tissue (the latter protrudes out of the exposure into the cavity); then the desquamated cells from the oral mucosa, many of which are viable, become implanted on the granulation tissue and by rapid proliferation and migration cover the surface.

Microscopic sections of a pulp polyp show vital pulp tissue

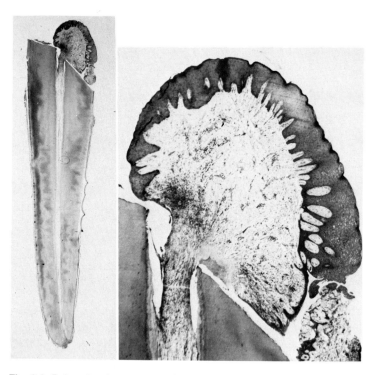

Fig. 6-3. Pulp polyp, low-power and high-power views. Note that the polyp is attached to the vital pulp.

with chronic inflammatory cells (plasma cells and lymphocytes) and young vascular connective tissue (granulation tissue) that projects from the pulp into the carious lesion (Fig. 6-3). It also shows infiltration by plasma cells, lymphocytes, and neutrophils. The entire lesion is covered by stratified squamous epithelium (Fig. 6-3).

Treatment consists of surgical excision of the polyp from the floor of the pulp chamber and pulp capping. In successful cases this is followed by the formation of a dentin bridge at the junction of the excised area and the pulp-capping material (Fig. 6-4).

Anachoresis. If the bacteria circulating in the bloodstream settle in areas of inflammation or of lowered resistance in the pulp and produce pulpitis, abscess, or necrosis, the phenomenon is referred to as anachoresis.

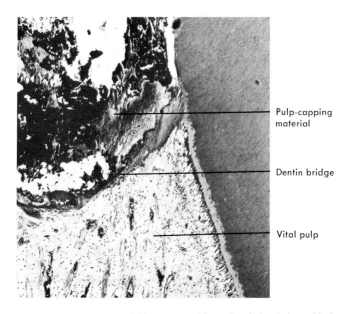

Pulp-capping material

Dentin bridge

Vital pulp

Fig. 6-4. Pulp-capping material is separated from the vital pulp by a thin layer of dentin.

Aerodontalgia. In some persons, high-altitude flights produce pain in teeth that at ground level are asymptomatic. The pain, called aerodontalgia, begins during flight or starts a few hours or days later. This condition occurs only in teeth with subclinical pulpitis.

Necrosis. Untreated pulpitis may lead to death of the pulp. The inflammatory exudate compressed within a hard shell of dentin brings about compression of blood vessels, particularly the apical, which causes infarction and necrosis.

Clinically necrosis is characterized by cessation of all symptoms. Microscopic sections through such a tooth show either an empty pulp chamber and canals or isolated areas of necrotic structureless masses.

Reticular atrophy. Reticular atrophy is really an artifact but at one time was believed to be a regressive change of the pulp. Microscopic sections show numerous spaces and intertwining bundles of fibers (reticular pattern) in the pulp (Fig. 6-5). It is not a change seen in old age.

Calcifications. The pulp may be the site of calcifications. The

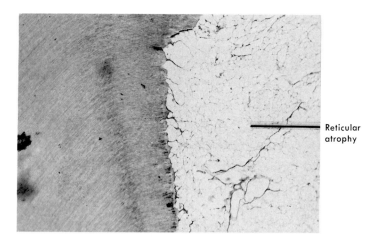

Reticular atrophy

Fig. 6-5. Reticular atrophy of the pulp. In reality, this is an artifact and does not represent a pathologic state.

cause of these is not known. They are usually asymptomatic, and, unless large, cannot be identified radiographically. It has been estimated that only about 10% of the pulp calcification can be seen by radiographic observation.

Calcification may be *diffuse* or *nodular* (pulp stones) (Fig. 6-6).

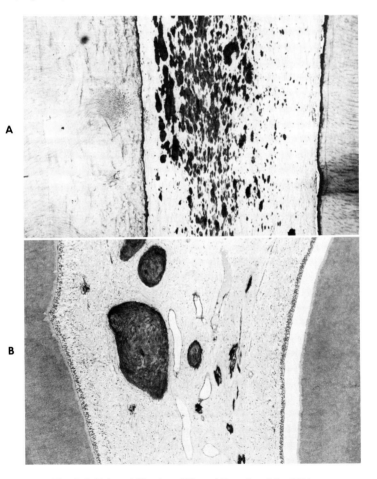

Fig. 6-6. Pulp calcification. Diffuse **(A)** and nodular **(B)** types.

The diffuse type is characterized by dispersed or scattered calcifications in the pulp chamber and/or pulp canal. On microscopic examination it appears as a conglomerate or multitude of small, deeply basophilic granules. This type of calcification is probably preceded by local tissue necrosis.

The nodular type of calcification is called a pulp stone and usually is seen in the pulp chamber. Pulp stones may be composed of dentin (true denticles) or may be amorphous (false denticles).

Nodular calcifications are called *free, attached,* or *embedded*—depending on whether they are free in the pulp, attached to the pulp wall, or embedded in the dentin. As observed through a microscope, a nodular calcification either is made up of dentin or appears as a deeply basophilic, laminated mass.

Internal resorption. When resorption of teeth occurs from

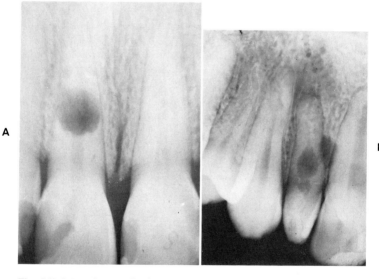

Fig. 6-7. Internal resorption in a central incisor **(A)** and a dens in dente **(B).**

within the pulp cavity, it is referred to as internal or idiopathic resorption (Fig. 6-7).

The cause of this condition is not known, but trauma is believed to be a contributory factor. If the resorption occurs in the crown of the tooth, the dentin may be destroyed and vascular tissue of the pulp can be seen through the enamel as a pink spot (pink tooth). Internal resorption may be progressive and lead to perforation or fracture of a tooth, or it may cease spontaneously.

Microscopic examination reveals few or numerous irregular areas of resorption of the pulpal surface of dentin (Fig. 6-8), giant cells adjacent to certain areas of resorption, repair of some resorbed areas by atypical dentin or bone (Fig. 6-8), and extension of other resorbed areas to enamel or cementum. In the root, resorption may extend into the periodontal ligament.

Although the cause of internal resorption is obscure, the

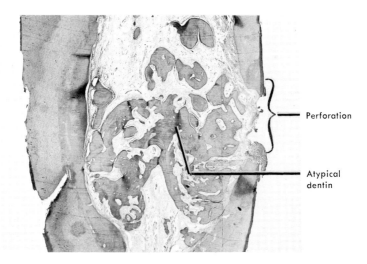

Perforation

Atypical
dentin

Fig. 6-8. Internal resorption with perforation. Resorption has occurred along the entire pulpal wall, and some areas have been repaired. Atypical dentin has been laid down in the pulp cavity.

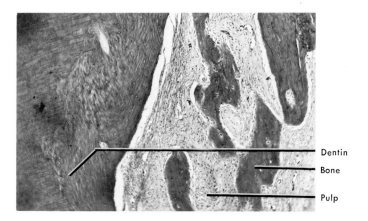

Dentin

Bone

Pulp

Fig. 6-9. Metaplasia of the pulp. Note the deposition of bone trabeculae in the pulp tissue.

most likely possibility is that the following sequence of events takes place: some sudden trauma to the tooth produces intrapulpal hemorrhage; the hemorrhage organizes (i.e., is replaced by granulation tissue); then proliferating granulation tissue compresses the dentin walls, predentin formation ceases, odontoclasts differentiate from the connective tissue, and resorption begins.

Internal resorption is best treated by prompt root canal therapy and the removal of the offending tissue.

Metaplasia. Deposition of bone tissue in the pulp is referred to as metaplasia of the pulp (Fig. 6-9).

INTERRELATIONSHIPS OF PULP DISEASES

Possible interrelationships in diseases of the pulp are summarized in the accompanying diagram.

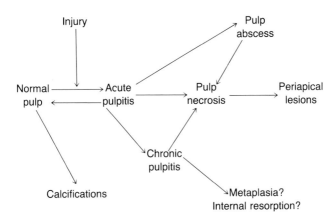

REFERENCES

Bender, I. B., and Seltzer, S.: The effect of periodontal disease on the pulp, Oral Surg. **33**:458, 1972.

Cotton, W. R.: Dental pulp histology observed by scanning electron microscopy, Oral Surg. **39**:136, 1975.

Cutright, D. E., and Bhaskar, S. N.: Pulpal vasculature as demonstrated by a new method, Oral Surg. **27**:678, 1969.

Garrington, G. E., and Crump, M. C.: Pulp death in a patient with lepromatous leprosy, Oral Surg. **25**:427, 1968.

Haskell, E. W., Stanley, H. R., Chellemi, J., and Stringfellow, H.: Direct pulp capping treatment: a long-term follow up, J. Am. Dent. Assoc. **97**:607, 1978.

Hayes, R. L.: Idiopathic internal resorption of teeth, Oral Surg. **13**:723, 1960.

Hodges, F. R.: Barodontalgia at 12,000 feet, J. Am. Dent. Assoc. **97**:66, 1978.

Holcomb, J. B., and Gregory, W. B., Jr.: Calcific metamorphosis of the pulp: its incidence and treatment, Oral Surg. **24**:825, 1967.

Kakehashi, S., Stanley, H. W., and Fitzgerald, R. J.: The effects of surgical exposures on dental pulps in germ-free and conventional laboratory rats, Oral Surg. **20**:340, 1965.

Langeland, K., and Langeland, L. K.: Cutting procedures with minimized trauma, J. Am. Dent. Assoc. **76**:991, 1968.

Mjor, I. A., and Tronstad, L.: The healing of experimentally induced pulpitis, Oral Surg. **38**:115, 1974.

Mount, G. J.: Idiopathic internal resorption, Oral Surg. **33**:801, 1972.

Naidorf, I. J.: Inflammation and infection of pulp and periapical tissues, Oral Surg. **34**:486, 1972.

Ostby, B. N., and Schilder, H.: Inflammation and infection of the pulp and periapical tissues: a synthesis, Oral Surg. **34**:498, 1972.

Rabinowitch, B. Z.: Internal resorption, Oral Surg. **33**:263, 1972.

Saunders, I. D. F.: Idiopathic internal resorption, Br. Dent. J. **135**:498, 1973.

Seltzer, S., and Bender, I. B.: The dental pulp, Philadelphia, 1965, J. B. Lippincott Co.

Shiller, W. R.: Aerodontalgia under hyperbaric conditions, Oral Surg. **20**:694, 1965.

Snyder, D. E.: The cracked-tooth syndrome and fractured posterior cusp, Oral Surg. **41**:698, 1976.

Southam, J. C., and Hodson, J. J.: Neurohistology of human dental pulp polyps, Arch. Oral Biol. **18**:1255, 1973.

Southam, J. C., and Hodson, J. J.: The growth of epithelium, melanocytes, and Langerhans cells on human and experimental dental pulp polyps, Oral Surg. **37**:546, 1974.

Stanley, H. R.: The effect of systemic diseases on the human pulp, Oral Surg. **33**:606, 1972.

Sundell, J. R., Stanley, H. R., and White, C. L.: The relationship of coronal pulp stone formation to experimental operative procedures, Oral Surg. **25**:579, 1968.

Tronstad, L., and Mjor, I. A.: Capping of the inflamed pulp, Oral Surg. **34**:477, 1972.

Witkop, C. J., Jr.: Manifestations of genetic diseases in the human pulp, Oral Surg. **32**:278, 1971.

CHAPTER 7

Periapical lesions

About 23% of all biopsies examined by an oral pathologist are periapical diseases. This group of lesions therefore comprises the largest number of tissue specimens removed in a dental office (Table 17, p. 474). The following are discussed in the present chapter:

1. Dental granuloma
2. Radicular cyst
3. Residual cyst
4. Periapical (dentoalveolar) abscess
5. Apical scar
6. Cholesteatoma

Dental granuloma. This lesion represents the apical extension of a pulp inflammation. Clinically the tooth is either asymptomatic or slightly painful on percussion. The patient may give a history of severe pain that later subsides and disappears. The tooth associated with a dental granuloma is usually nonvital, but it may respond poorly to vitality tests.

According to one study the dental granuloma constitutes about 48% of all periapical lesions. Other estimates range from 65% to 90%. In any case, the lesion is more common in the maxilla than in the mandible and usually occurs in the third decade of life.

A dental granuloma appears as an area of radiolucency that may be either a slight widening of the periapical periodontal ligament or a circumscribed lesion of varying size (Fig. 7-1).

Microscopically the pulp of the associated tooth is necrotic or it shows dense to moderate infiltration with plasma cells and lymphocytes. The alveolar bone proper and the periodontal ligament in the periapical area are replaced by granulation tissue

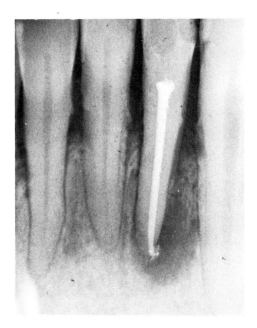

Fig. 7-1. Dental granuloma. From the radiograph alone, it is impossible to distinguish between a granuloma and a radicular cyst.

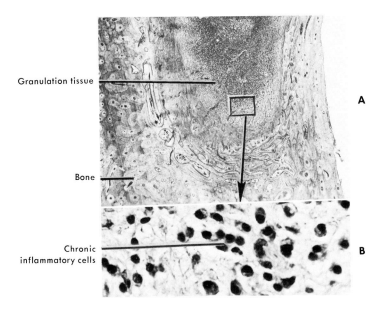

Granulation tissue

Bone

Chronic
inflammatory cells

A

B

Fig. 7-2. Dental granuloma. **A,** Apical tissue. **B,** High-power view of an area
from **A** (inset) showing plasma cells and lymphocytes.

(Fig. 7-2)—the latter consisting of fibroblasts, blood vessels,
plasma cells, and lymphocytes and a varying amount of collagen. In some dental granulomas, islands of epithelium can be
seen (Fig. 7-3). Other granulomas show foam cells (pseudoxanthoma cells) and cholesterol clefts (Fig. 7-4). Foam cells are
macrophages that contain lipoid material, the product of fatty
degeneration in the area. Bone tissue on the periphery of the
granulation tissue shows resorption, and osteoclasts may be
seen lining its surface. Cementoblasts adjacent to the lesion
may have increased activity, and there may be hypercementosis
of the root surface.

Bacteriologic studies show that organisms cannot be cultured from the majority of dental granulomas.

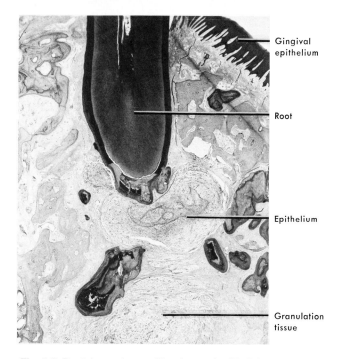

Gingival
epithelium

Root

Epithelium

Granulation
tissue

Fig. 7-3. Dental granuloma with a focus of epithelial proliferation.

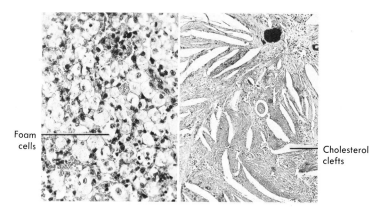

Foam
cells

Cholesterol
clefts

Fig. 7-4. Dental granuloma. High-power views showing foam cells (pseudo-xanthoma cells) and cholesterol clefts.

The mechanism of formation of a dental granuloma is as follows: In the beginning there is pulpitis from which the tooth fails to recover; this either leads to necrosis or progresses from the pulp chamber to the root canal and then toward the apex; in either case, chronic inflammation extends into the periapical periodontal ligament; the chronic inflammation is associated with the formation of granulation tissue (i.e., fibroblasts, blood vessels, infiltration by plasma cells and lymphocytes); granulation tissue therefore replaces the apical periodontal ligament; the bone surrounding the granulation tissue undergoes resorption due to the pressure of the growing granulation tissue.

As soon as some of the periapical bone is destroyed and replaced by granulation tissue, the lesion becomes visible radiographically.

Dental granuloma is treated by either extraction or root canal therapy (i.e., by the removal of the irritant that evoked the change).

Radicular cyst. A radicular cyst is usually asymptomatic. Occasionally, however, the associated tooth is sensitive to percussion. Rarely the lesion may be associated with a fistula. The tooth is nonvital and may show a deep carious lesion or a restoration. The patient often gives a history of pain and subsequent relief in the tooth. Radicular cysts do not produce gross deformity of the involved jaw. They constitute a little more than 11% of all tissue specimens removed in a dental practice. According to a number of studies, they comprise about 43% of all periapical radiolucencies; but other estimates range as low as 10%. The radicular cyst is far more common in the maxilla than in the mandible and occurs most often in the third decade of life.

A radicular cyst characteristically appears as a more or less clearly demarcated radiolucency associated with the apical area of the affected tooth (Fig. 7-5). The lesion varies in size considerably. It is usually larger than a dental granuloma and may extend over the area of two or more teeth. Rarely a radicular cyst involving almost an entire quadrant of the jaw may be seen.

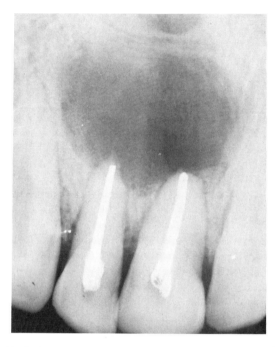

Fig. 7-5. Radicular cyst. Unless the lesion is more than 200 mm^2 in size, apical radiolucencies of dental granuloma, radicular cyst, and periapical abscess are indistinguishable.

On radiographs a distinction cannot be made between a radicular cyst, a dental granuloma, and other cystic lesions in the area. The presence of a devitalized tooth with a periapical radiolucency, however, indicates that the lesion is a radicular cyst, a dental granuloma, or an apical abscess. It has been suggested that if an apical radiolucency is more than 200 mm^2, it is almost always a radicular cyst.

When the cyst is removed in toto, the gross specimen has a saclike appearance. When sectioned, the cyst either contains necrotic debris or exudes fluid. The inner surface is smooth.

Microscopically the cyst cavity contains structureless ne-

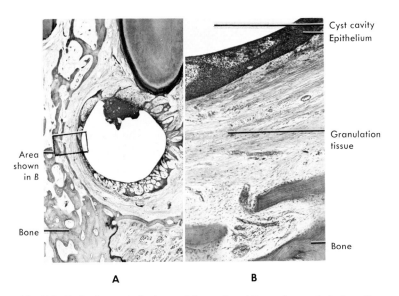

Cyst cavity
Epithelium

Granulation
tissue

Area
shown
in B

Bone

Bone

A   B

Fig. 7-6. Radicular cyst. A, Apex of the root and the entire cystic lesion. B, The cyst cavity is lined by epithelium and surrounded by a wide zone of granulation tissue.

crotic debris or homogeneous eosinophilic material. In addition, the cyst contents consist of cholesterol crystals (seen as clefts because the alcohol used in the preparation of a histologic section dissolves the cholesterol crystals, leaving empty spaces) and some viable cells. If the contents are lost during surgical procedures or the preparation of sections, the cyst cavity will be empty. The cyst is lined by stratified squamous epithelium (Fig. 7-6). On rare occasion, however, respiratory or other forms of epithelium may be seen. Connective tissue of varying density surrounds the epithelial lining. The connective tissue is almost always infiltrated by plasma cells and lymphocytes and shows edema. Cholesterol clefts surrounded by giant cells, hemosiderin, and large pale macrophages (foam cells or pseudoxanthoma cells) may also be seen in the connective tissue (Fig.

7-4). Within or surrounding the connective tissue, bone trabeculae are sometimes present.

The mechanism of formation of a radicular cyst is the same as that of a dental granuloma (p. 165). However, subsequent to the formation of a circumscribed lesion that consists of granulation tissue and is located at the apex of the tooth, the following changes occur:

As a result of inflammation, the epithelium in the periapical area (epithelial rests of Malassez) proliferates and by continuous proliferation forms a large mass of cells (Fig. 7-7, *A*); since the epithelium has no blood vessels of its own, its blood supply must come from the surrounding connective tissue; and since the central cells in the epithelial mass are farthest away from the blood supply, they degenerate and form a small cavity lined by epithelium (Fig. 7-7, *B*). This is the beginning of the radicular cyst.

Once begun, the cystic cavity increases in size by three mechanisms. The epithelial cells are shed into the cavity; and since these cells consist of protein material, the osmotic pres-

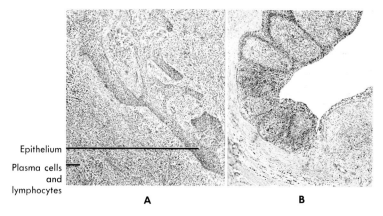

Epithelium

Plasma cells
and
lymphocytes

A **B**

Fig. 7-7. A, Epithelial island in a dental granuloma. **B,** Formation of a cystic cavity. The cyst results from degeneration of the central cells of the epithelial island.

sure within the cyst progressively becomes greater than that in the surrounding tissues. Tissue fluids and edema fluid are therefore gradually imbibed by the cavity. This, in turn, compresses the surrounding tissue and bone. The bone is resorbed, and the radiolucency becomes larger. Secondly, the granulation tissue of the cyst wall also continues to proliferate, destroying bone and thus enlarging the bone defect.

Finally, the third mechanism in the growth of a radicular cyst consists of what may be called sequestration of the connective tissue wall. The epithelial lining extends into the connective tissue of the cyst wall and incorporates parts of this tissue into the cystic cavity.

A radicular cyst may be treated by one of several methods: extraction of the tooth and apical curettage, root canal filling and apical curettage, or root canal filling alone. It was previously believed that all radicular cysts required surgical removal; but more recently it has been shown that secondary infection and/or hemorrhage during endodontic therapy may destroy the epithelial lining and promote healing of a cyst. In these cases, which are the majority, surgical intervention is not necessary. In a few instances, however, if it is not removed surgically, a radicular cyst will persist in the jaw and radiographs taken years later will show a cystic lesion in an edentulous space.

A radicular or primordial cyst that develops along the lateral side of a root is called a *lateral periodontal cyst* (Fig. 7-8). The distinction between the two can sometimes be made by the presence or absence of vitality in the associated tooth, but a definitive diagnosis is possible only by histologic examination.

Residual cyst. If a tooth associated with a radicular cyst is extracted but the cyst is left undisturbed, it may persist within the jaw (Fig. 7-9). Such a lesion is called a residual cyst.

The microscopic features of a residual cyst are the same as those of a radicular cyst. Residual cysts constitute about 3.5% of all periapical lesions. They occur in the maxilla more often than in the mandible, and the majority of patients are in the fourth decade of life. Treatment consists of surgical enucleation.

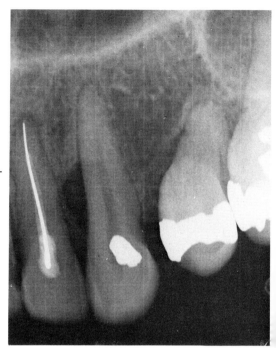

Fig. 7-8. Lateral periodontal cyst.

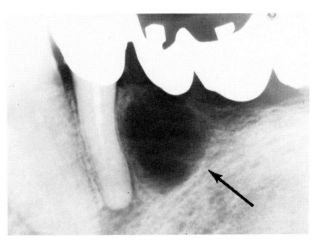

Fig. 7-9. Residual cyst (arrow). The lesion represents a radicular cyst that was associated with a tooth that has been extracted.

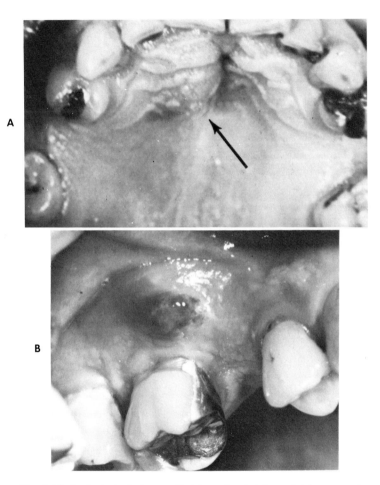

Fig. 7-10. A, Periapical abscess that has elevated the palatal mucosa (arrow). **B,** Periapical abcess presenting as a gumboil.

Periapical (dentoalveolar) abscess. A periapical abscess is associated with an acute onset, swelling, pain, reddening of the overlying skin, elevation of the tooth in the socket, extreme sensitivity on percussion, and (when severe) elevation of temperature. It may, however, be insidious and present none of the above symptoms. The involved tooth usually has a deep carious lesion, a restoration, or an inadequate root canal filling; but it may be intact. Depending on its duration and location, the abscess may "point" intraorally or extraorally. When it "points" intraorally, it may do so on the buccal or lingual surface (Fig. 7-10, *A*). Sometimes a periapical abscess may appear as a parulis, or gumboil (Fig. 7-10, *B*). In these instances it must be distinguished from a peridontal abscess (p. 201).

Radiographs can present either a normal picture or a diffuse area of radiolucency not always restricted to a single tooth. Lesions that originate in a preexisting dental granuloma or cyst, however, show a well-demarcated boundary.

A periapical abscess is characterized by a necrotic pulp or a pulp densely infiltrated by neutrophils. The periapical tissues show dense, almost solid masses of neutrophils (pus) and clefts or spaces (indicating areas out of which pus has been lost during histologic preparation). From the central area toward the periphery, there is a gradual reduction in the intensity of polymorphonuclear infiltration. Bone trabeculae in the periapical area may show empty lacunae (i.e., death of osteocytes). Such trabeculae represent dead bone or sequestra. Since bone marrow spaces are infiltrated by polymorphonuclear leukocytes, they represent acute inflammation of marrow (acute osteitis or osteomyelitis).

Initial treatment of a periapical abscess consists of drainage, which can be established through the pulp chamber or from the periapical area. After acute symptoms subside, root canal therapy is instituted. In some instances, extraction is the only choice.

Apical scar. This lesion comprises about 3% of all periapical radiolucencies. It occurs in the maxilla more often than in the mandible, and the patients are usually in their fifth decade of life. The anterior maxilla is the preferred site.

Clinically the tooth is asymptomatic, and the radiolucency is discovered on routine examination. There is a history of a periapical lesion and root canal filling, or of a root canal filling and apical curettage. An apical scar is characterized by a circumscribed radiolucency (Fig. 7-11).

Microscopically an apical scar shows dense collagen bundles,

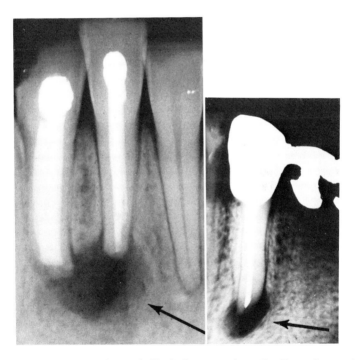

Fig. 7-11. Apical scar (arrows). The lesion occurs in teeth with previous root canal fillings and produces no symptoms.

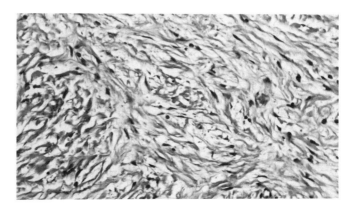

Fig. 7-12. Apical scar. Note the dense hyalinized collagen bundles. There are no inflammatory cells.

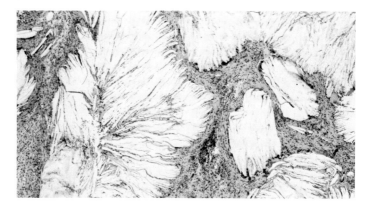

Fig. 7-13. Cholesteatoma. Note the numerous cholesterol clefts.

many of which are hyalinized (Fig. 7-12). Fibroblasts are few in number and spindle shaped. The lesion represents an area where the healing process has terminated in the formation of dense collagen rather than bone. However, this condition is not pathologic. It remains asymptomatic and requires no treatment.

Cholesteatoma. Less than 1% of periapical radiolucencies are cholesteatomas. Except for the microscopic features, this lesion has all the characteristics of a dental granuloma.

Microscopically a cholesteatoma consists of dense masses of cholesterol crystals that appear as clefts (Fig. 7-13). In addition to cholesterol, it contains foam cells, plasma cells, and lymphocytes. It represents a dental granuloma in which a great deal of fatty degeneration has led to the formation of abundant cholesterol.

Treatment of a cholesteatoma consists of root canal filling and apical curettage.

REFERENCES

Bender, I.: A commentary on General Bhaskar's hypothesis, Oral Surg. **34:**469, 1972.

Bhaskar, S. N.: Periapical lesions—types, incidence, and clinical features, Oral Surg. **21:**657, 1966.

Bhaskar, S. N.: Bone lesions of endodontic origin, Dent. Clin. North Am., p. 521, November, 1967.

Bhaskar, S. N.: Oral pathology in the dental office: survey of 20,575 biopsy specimens, J. Am. Dent. Assoc. **76:**761, 1968.

Bhaskar, S. N.: Nonsurgical resolution of radicular cysts, Oral Surg. **34:**458, 1972.

Bhaskar, S. N., and Rappaport, H. M.: Dental vitality tests and pulp status, J. Am. Dent. Assoc. **86:**409, 1973.

Bozzo, L., Valdrighi, L., and Vizioli, M. R.: Lipid components of human dental periapical lesions, Oral Surg. **34:**166, 1972.

Chilton, N. W.: Periodontic-endodontic relationships, a synthesis, Oral Surg. **34:**327, 1972.

Kirkham, D. B.: The location and incidence of accessory pulpal canals in periodontal pockets, J. Am. Dent. Assoc. **91:**353, 1975.

Lalonde, E. R.: A new rationale for the management of periapical granulomas and cysts; an evaluation of histopathological and radiographic findings, J. Am. Dent. Assoc. **80:**1056, 1970.

Lalonde, E. R., and Leubke, R. G.: The frequency and distribution of periapical cysts and granulomas, Oral Surg. **25:**861, 1968.

Leonard, E. P., Lunin, M., and Provenza, D. V.: On the occurrence and morphology of Russell bodies in the dental granuloma, Oral Surg. **38:**584, 1974.

Patterson, S. S., and Hillis, P. D.: Scar tissue associated with the apices of pulpless teeth prior to endodontic therapy, Oral Surg. **33:**450, 1972.

Reeve, C. M., and Wentz, F. M.: The prevalence, morphology, and distribution of epithelial rests in the human periodontal ligament, Oral Surg. **15:**785, 1962.

Stallard, R. E.: Periodontic-endodontic relationships, Oral Surg. **34:**314, 1972.

Torabinejad, M., and Kiger, R. D.: Experimentally induced alterations in periapical tissues of the cat, J. Dent. Res. **59:**87, 1980.

Torneck, C. D.: Pedodontic-endodontic practices: a synthesis, Oral Surg. **34:**310, 1972.

CHAPTER 8

Periodontal diseases

Periodontal diseases include conditions that primarily involve the periodontal tissues. The latter consist of the gingiva, periodontal ligament, and alveolar bone. There are numerous and diverse classifications of periodontal diseases, but the following is most satisfactory:

1. Gingivitis
   a. Chronic
   b. Hyperplastic (elephantiasis gingivae; fibromatosis gingivae)
   c. Hormonal
   d. Desquamative
   e. Necrotizing
   f. Acute recurrent
   g. Allergic (plasma cell gingivitis, plasma cell gingivostomatitis; idiopathic gingivostomatitis)
   h. Miscellaneous lesions

2. Periodontitis
   a. Periodontal pocket
   b. Periodontal abscess (parulis)
3. Juvenile periodontitis (periodontosis)
4. Occlusal trauma

With few exceptions, periodontal disease begins in the marginal and interdental gingivae and progresses apically. One exception is the lesion of occlusal trauma, in which the abnormal changes begin in the deep structures. Gingivitis and periodontitis are initiated and sustained by a bacterial mass on the tooth surface called *plaque* (p. 178). The portion of the plaque that lies in the vicinity of the gingival sulcus produces gingival lesions. Since plaque also produces caries, its removal is a critical step in the management and control of both periodontal diseases and caries. Once removed, plaque begins to form within

2 hours and is well established in 24 hours. Therefore its frequent removal is essential to clinical success.

Within a few seconds a recently cleaned tooth surface exposed to saliva absorbs glycoproteins and mucoproteins (from the saliva), which deposit on it in the form of a *pellicle*. It has extensions into the enamel surface, and this part of the pellicle is called the *dendritic pellicle*. Soon after its formation, gram-positive aerobic organisms, especially *Streptococcus sangius*, begin to stick to the pellicle and *plaque* formation begins. Once bacteria stick, they proliferate along the tooth surface and at right angles to it. After *S. sanguis*, *Actinomyces*, especially *A. naeslundii* and *A. viscosus*, begin to join the plaque. With time, more and more bacteria attach to the plaque and those already in the plaque multiply. In about 36 hours gram-negative bacteria begin to attach to the plaque, and at about this time the plaque is well attached to the tooth surface. In a healthy mouth with no gingival inflammation the plaque is about 20 cells thick, while in early gingivitis it is about 300 cells thick. If the supragingival plaque is not removed, both the plaque and the accompanying inflammation progress apically along the tooth surface.

A great deal of new information about plaque has recently been accumulated. The plaque that produces caries is basically different in its microbiologic inhabitants from the plaque that produces periodontal disease. The plaque associated with healthy gingiva and teeth is different from that associated with disease. The nature of plaque may vary from tooth to tooth, patient to patient, and from time to time in the same patient. With regard to periodontal disease, the plaque that forms along the gingival margin of the tooth surface and that which forms below the gingival margin is of the greatest significance. The plaque in these areas is thus classified into *supragingival plaque* and *subgingival plaque*. The supragingival plaque is mostly attached to the tooth surface and is composed mainly of gram-positive aerobic organisms such as *Streptococcus sangius*, *S. mutans*, *S. salivarius*, and *Actinomyces*. In patients with very poor oral hygiene the supragingival attached plaque may be covered with a layer of loosely attached plaque. The supragingival plaque, therefore, has an *attached* component and may have a *loosely attached* component. The subgingival plaque also has an *attached* and loosely attached or *unattached* component. The subgingival attached plaque does not extend to the bottom of the pocket (or crevis) and is composed predominantly of gram-negative anaerobic rods and cocci. It is estimated that there is no attached plaque in the bottom 0.1 mm of the pocket. The subgingival *unattached* plaque lies between the attached plaque and the lining of the pocket and also extends to the bottom of the pocket. Because of its location and composition, this plaque is the most pathogenic of all forms of plaque. It consists primarily of gram-negative cocci and of rods and spirochetes. Toxic substances, enzymes, and antigens produced by these organisms are the major factor in producing and sustaining advanced periodontal disease. Whereas the attached plaque is responsible for caries and calculus formation, the unattached plaque is the primary cause of periodontal disease.

Periodontal disease is almost universal, is usually bilateral (except occlusal trauma), is primarily interdental, and is episodic in its progression. This latter characteristic means that it does not begin and progress at a constant rate, rather, it has periods of fast progression that are interspersed with long periods of relative stability or inactivity.

Gingivitis. As the name implies, gingivitis is inflammation of the gingiva. Based on the proved or suspected causes of gingivitis, various types, such as chronic, acute, hyperplastic, hormonal, etc., are recognized.

Chronic gingivitis. The most common form of gingival disease, chronic gingivitis. is universal in distribution. It is caused by plaque or poor restorations and occurs in two forms: the *edematous* and the *fibrous* types. The two types are not clear-cut entities; rather they represent extremes of a common process.

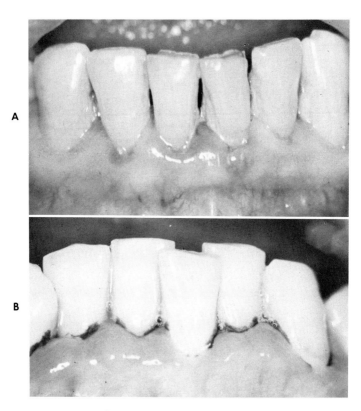

Fig. 8-1. Edematous **(A)** and fibrous **(B)** types of chronic gingivitis.

In the *edematous* type the gingiva is enlarged and glossy, loses its stippling, and bleeds easily (Fig. 8-1). Microscopic sections reveal that the keratinized stratified squamous epithelium, which normally covers the gingiva, either is unaltered or shows absence of a keratin layer. The connective tissue under the epithelium shows edema and infiltration by plasma cells, lymphocytes, and neutrophilic leukocytes (Fig. 8-2, *A*). The cellular infiltrate is particularly marked on the side of the gingival sulcus (i.e., toward the side of the irritant). Inflammation extends nei-

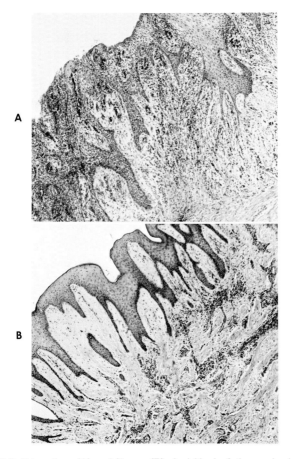

Fig. 8-2. Edematous **(A)** and fibrous **(B)** gingivitis. In **A** the predominant features consist of inflammatory cells and edema. In **B** inflammatory cells and increased fibrous tissue can be seen.

ther into the periodontal ligament space nor into the marrow of
the underlying bone. There is no resorption of the alveolar
crest. The epithelial attachment is normal, without pocket formation. Treatment consists of removal of the local cause by
hand instruments or ultrasonic devices, following which recovery is rapid.

The *fibrous* type of chronic gingivitis is the later stage of the
edematous type and is characterized by enlarged, firm gingiva
that may bleed during toothbrushing (Fig. 8-1). Microscopically
the predominant feature is the formation of fibrous tissue, but
plasma cells and lymphocytes are present in varying amounts
(Fig. 8-2, *B*). This type of chronic gingivitis improves after ultrasonic and hand scaling; but gingivectomy may be necessary
in advanced disease.

**Hyperplastic gingivitis (elephantiasis gingivae; fibromatosis
gingivae).** Exuberant fibrous growth of the gingiva is known to
occur under certain conditions—following the administration of
drugs (Dilantin), in certain genetic anomalies (hereditary fibro-

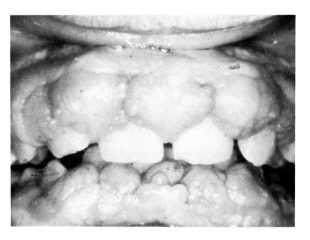

Fig. 8-3. Dilantin hyperplasia. Note the generalized fibrous enlargement of
the gingiva.

matosis gingivae, tuberous sclerosis), without any known cause (idiopathic), or in association with severe mouth-breathing problems. In all patients the gingiva is firm and fibrous and covers varying amounts of the crowns of teeth. In severe cases the teeth may be completely covered and tooth migration may occur. Since the gingiva is enlarged, it leads to the formation of a deep sulcus, or a *pseudopocket*. The term pseudopocket is used to distinguish this "pocket" from the *true pocket*, which is associated with the loss of bone and periodontitis. Microscopically the gingiva shows a covering of stratified squamous epithelium, but the major bulk of the enlarged gingiva is made up of dense collagen bundles. The inflammatory cells are minimal in number.

From 10% to 30% of patients who receive phenytoin (Dilantin) for control of epilepsy have a generalized enlargement of the gingiva, with the labial gingiva of the maxillary and mandibular teeth most frequently involved (Fig. 8-3). Some enlarge-

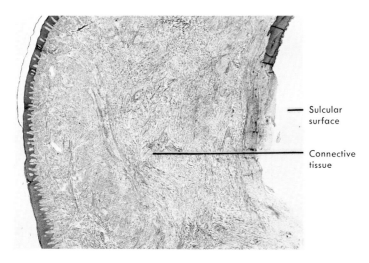

Sulcular surface

Connective tissue

Fig. 8-4. Dilantin hyperplasia of the gingiva. Note the marked increase in connective tissue.

ment of the gingiva has been reported in as many as 78% of
patients receiving the drug. The mechanism of this hyperplasia
is unknown. The microscopic features are essentially the same
as those observed in other forms of hyperplastic gingivitis except that the collagen formation is far more pronounced and the
epithelial covering shows long, thin ridges that extend deep into
the connective tissue (Fig. 8-4). Although other drugs, such as
mephenytoin (Mesantoin), have been used in the control of epilepsy, Dilantin is much more effective. For this reason, fibromatosis gingivae is often unavoidable.

Another type of hyperplasia of the gingiva is the so-called
hereditary gingival hyperplasia (hereditary fibromatosis gingivae). The condition resembles Dilantin hyperplasia both clinically and microscopically but differs from the latter in being hereditary and sometimes associated with other developmental
defects such as mental deficiency and hypertrichosis.

Gingival hyperplasia without known cause is called *idiopathic fibromatosis* and is essentially identical to that just described. Gingival hyperplasia may also occur in mouth breathers
and is usually limited to the anterior teeth.

Treatment of all types of hyperplastic gingivitis is gingivectomy followed by periodic checkups. If the condition recurs,
reexcision is necessary.

Hormonal gingivitis. Hormonal gingivitis is the term given to
gingivitis occurring during phases of life that are associated with
an alteration or adjustment of sex hormones, such as adolescence, pregnancy, and menstruation. Also, the use of oral contraceptives may produce this type of gingivitis.

Clinically the gingiva is enlarged, red or bluish red, and
edematous and puffy; and it bleeds easily (Fig. 8-5). Enlargement of the gingiva produces pseudopockets. The lesions usually begin in the interdental papillae and later affect the marginal gingiva. This type of gingivitis may involve a few teeth or
a single arch, or it may be generalized. The most frequent and
earliest site of involvement, however, is the anterior segment of
the mouth.

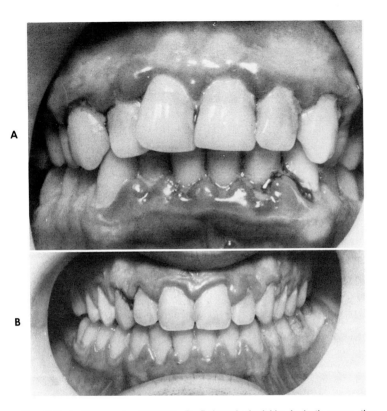

Fig. 8-5. A, Pregnancy gingivitis. **B,** Pubertal gingivitis. In both cases the gingiva is swollen and red and bleeds easily.

Gingivitis occurring during puberty is *pubertal gingivitis* (Fig. 8-5, *B*), whereas that occurring during pregnancy is *pregnancy gingivitis* (Fig. 8-5, *A*). The latter is seen in more than 50% of pregnant women. Both pubertal gingivitis and pregnancy gingivitis commonly are precipitated by poor oral hygiene. However, when the patient is past these physiologic states, spontaneous regression of the gingival lesions may occur. Nevertheless, local treatment consisting of hand or ultrasonic scaling is always beneficial. Patients who take oral contracep-

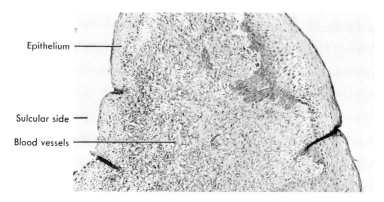

Fig. 8-6. Pregnancy gingivitis. Note the numerous capillaries, edema, and extravascular inflammatory cells.

tives often show gingival lesions that are comparable to those seen in pregnancy. The gingiva is red and bleeds easily, and it responds poorly to treatment. The incidence of periodontitis in such patients is greater than in the average population.

Microscopically pubertal, pregnancy, and oral contraceptive gingivitis shows a thin epithelial covering of the gingiva, areas of ulceration on the side of the pseudopocket, infiltration of the subepithelial connective tissue by neutrophils, plasma cells, and lymphocytes, edema, and the presence of numerous capillaries in the subepithelial tissue (Fig. 8-6). Changes are far more pronounced in patients with pregnancy gingivitis than in those with the other two forms. Treatment of hormonal gingivitis consists of ultrasonic scaling and improved home care procedures.

Desquamative gingivitis. This is a disease of unknown etiology that is characterized by desquamation of the epithelium and the subsequent presence of raw patches on the attached gingiva and alveolar mucosa. (Fig. 8-7). It affects females three to six times more frequently than males and may occur at any age past puberty, but usually the patients are young and middle-aged women. It can affect edentulous patients or patients with natural dentition. Sometimes lesions start as vesicles that later rup-

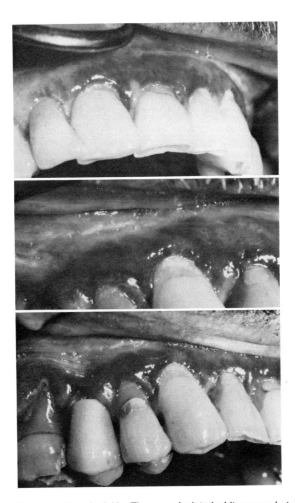

Fig. 8-7. Desquamative gingivitis. There are isolated white areas, but most of the attached gingiva shows desquamation of epithelium. (This patient was 52 years old and male.)

ture, leaving raw surfaces. Desquamative gingivitis may be the gingival manifestation of a variety of systemic diseases. Although it has not been proved, it is believed that this disease has an immunopathologic basis.

Clinically desquamative gingivitis resembles erosive lichen planus or the oral manifestations of pemphigus, pemphigoid (pp. 389, 418, 421) and erythema multiforme (p. 415). However, it can be distinguished from these conditions by the fact that the lesions are limited to the gingiva, with neither the skin nor any other area of the oral mucosa involved. In many cases gingival epithelium can be separated from the underlying tissue by a moderate amount of finger pressure (Nikolsky's sign).

Microscopic sections show areas in which the epithelial covering is elevated or missing and the connective tissue is exposed (ulcer) (Fig. 8-8). The ulcer is covered by fibrin, and the connective tissue shows polymorphonuclear infiltration. The inflammatory exudate corresponds to the extent of the secondary infection.

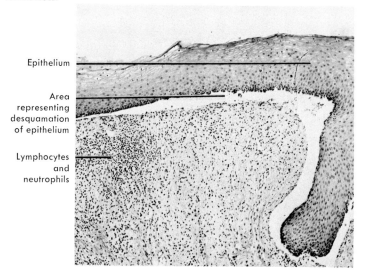

Epithelium

Area
representing
desquamation
of epithelium

Lymphocytes
and
neutrophils

Fig. 8-8. Desquamative gingivitis. Note the clean separation between the epithelium and the underlying connective tissue.

Treatment consists of improving oral hygiene and symptomatic therapy. Local and systemic administration of corticoids has been tried, with questionable success. In very painful conditions mouthwashes containing diphenhydramine and lidocaine prior to meals may be of value.

Necrotizing gingivitis. Necrotizing gingivitis is also referred to as acute necrotizing ulcerative gingivitis, ulceromembranous gingivitis, Vincent's gingivitis, fusospirochetal gingivitis, and oral fusospirochetosis (with stomatitis). The causative organism or organisms are not known, but a vibrio, *Bacillus fusiformis*, *Bacteroides melaninogenicus*, *Borrelia vincentii* (or *Spirochaeta plauti-vincentii*) have all been assumed to be the causative agents. However, spirochetes are present in large numbers in lesions of necrotizing gingivitis. This disease has a strong correlation with stress, smoking, and poor oral hygiene; and it is more common in winter months.

The clinical features of oral fusospirochetosis are striking. The patient has fever; cervical lymphadenopathy; malaise; a swollen, red, painful, bleeding gingiva; and necrosis of the interdental papillae (Fig. 8-9). Because of necrosis and sloughing,

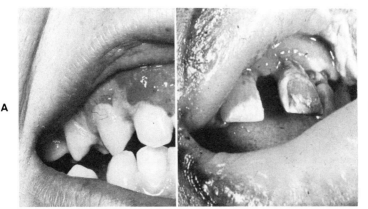

A

B

Fig. 8-9. Necrotizing (Vincent's) gingivitis. **A,** Early stage with beginning necrosis of the interdental papilla. **B,** Late stage with marked destruction of the tissues.

the papillae become inverted. The ulcerated areas are covered by a pseudomembrane. Because of necrotic tissue, the patient has fetid breath. Radiographic findings are normal.

Microscopic sections prepared from a lesion are not pathognomic. They show an ulcer covered by fibrin and necrotic debris. The underlying connective tissue is edematous and infiltrated by neutrophils (Fig. 8-10). Electron microscopic studies have shown that lesions of necrotizing gingivitis have four main zones. A superficial zone characterized by many bacteria, a second zone consisting predominantly of neutrophils, a third zone of necrotic cells, and a fourth layer of viable tissue with many spirochetes of the intermediate and large type.

Treatment of necrotizing gingivitis consists of rest, fluids, aspirin, and debridement of the area with hand scalers or an ultrasonic device. After debridement the ulcer is covered with a periodontal dressing or a mildly anesthetic solution, such as a mixture containing equal parts of kaolin and pectin (Kaopectate) and elixir of diphenhydramine (Benadryl).

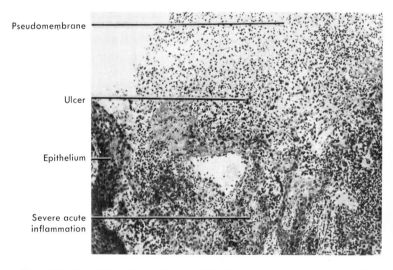

Pseudomembrane
Ulcer
Epithelium
Severe acute inflammation

Fig. 8-10. Necrotizing (Vincent's) gingivitis. Note the necrotic tissue and the dense neutrophilic infiltrate. These make up the pseudomembrane.

Acute recurrent gingivitis. This is a rare type of gingivitis that is characterized by a self-limiting, recurrent, painful gingivitis that involves the interdental papilla. Regional lymphadenopathy is present, and the lesion spreads to adjacent marginal and papillary areas. Ulceration is absent, and there is no pseudomembrane formation or interdental cratering. Oral hygiene is generally good, and lesions resolve in about 10 days. The cause of this disease is not known; but like necrotizing ulcerative gingivitis, it is related to stress.

Allergic gingivitis (plasma cell gingivitis; plasma cell gingivostomatitis; idiopathic gingivostomatitis). Allergic gingivitis, also called plasma cell gingivitis (because microscopically the lesions show dense plasma cell aggregates), plasma cell gingivostomatitis, and idiopathic gingivostomatitis, is a lesion of the marginal and attached gingivae. Most cases are an allergic response to chewing gum, but reactions to animal epithelium (dog

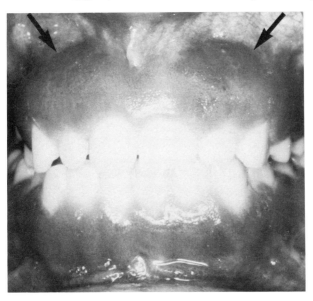

Fig. 8-11. Plasma cell (allergic) gingivitis. Note that the lesion stops at the mucogingival junction (arrows).

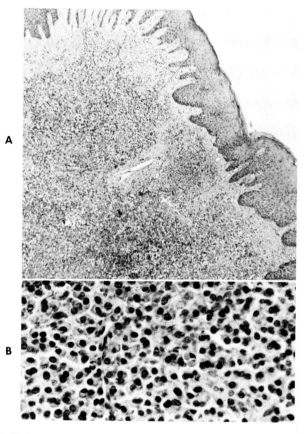

Fig. 8-12. Low-power **(A)** and high-power **(B)** views of plasma cell gingivitis. Note the dense plasma cell aggregations.

or cat dander) have been observed. The majority of cases involve only the marginal and the attached facial gingivae of both the maxilla and the mandible, and the lesion abruptly ends at the mucogingival junction (Fig. 8-11). However, it may also involve the palatal, lip, and tongue mucosa. The involved mucosa is red, swollen, and sometimes granular. Although patients may complain of a burning sensation or pain, the discomfort is far less than the clinical appearance would indicate. In some cases the lesion is restricted to a few isolated areas of the gingiva, whereas in others loss of periodontal bone is seen.

Microscopically the gingiva is covered by keratinized or parakeratotic stratified squamous epithelium. Ulceration is rare, and the gingiva is infiltrated by a dense mass of plasma cells arranged in solid sheets or in a lobular pattern (Fig. 8-12). Treatment consists of removal of the cause and improved oral hygiene.

Miscellaneous lesions. A papillomatous, cobblestone appearance of attached gingiva has been reported in Cowden's syndrome (multiple hamartoma and neoplasia syndrome).

•　　•　　•

It is apparent from the preceding discussion that the diagnosis of various forms of gingivitis is made primarily on clinical features.

Periodontitis. When an inflammatory process, whatever its cause, extends from the gingiva into the underlying bone, the lesion is referred to as periodontitis. As will be pointed out in the subsequent description, such a spread of inflammation is inevitably accompanied by *bone destruction* and *pocket formation*, which are therefore the two most important clinical features of the disease. Periodontitis is associated with the subgingival plaque. The unattached component of this plaque, which consists of anaerobic gram-negative cocci and rods and spirochetes, is the most important factor in the development and progress of this disease. Endotoxins, peptidoglycans, hyaluronidase, collagenase, and cytotoxic substances such as ammonia, proteases, indole, hydrogen sulfide, toxic amines, and organic acids produced by the plaque cause the destructive changes that are seen in periodontitis.

Clinically periodontitis is characterized by changes in gingival color, loss of stippling, edema, hyperplasia or recession, formation of clefts, presence of true pockets (which may exude pus on pressure), and tooth mobility (Fig. 8-13). Radiographs show evidence of bone destruction (Fig. 8-14), seen as a reduction in the height of the interdental and interradicular septa. Loss of the lamina dura on the alveolar crest gives the crest a concave (cupped) or shaggy appearance. In the interdental areas there may be a vertical resorption of bone and narrowing of the bony septa.

Periodontal pocket. The following events lead to the development of periodontitis and the formation and progression of a periodontal pocket: The supragingival plaque leads to inflammation of the gingiva (gingivitis). This inflammation persists as long as the cause persists and is associated with degeneration of the gingival fibers of the periodontal ligament immediately under the sulcus (Figs. 8-15 to 8-17). The cementoblasts in this area become necrotic, and cementum formation ceases; the epithelial attachment (also called *junctional epithelium*) now grows along the surface of the denuded cementum. As the epithelial attachment grows in depth, its coronal portion separates from the tooth surface, the sulcus deepens, and the periodontal "pocket" is initiated.

As the sulcus deepens, more plaque and debris accumulate, inflammation progresses further downward, more gingival fibers are destroyed, and an additional area of cementum becomes denuded. Furthermore, the apically progressing inflammation reaches the alveolar crest, and bone resorption begins. The resorption of bone is caused by endotoxins of the plaque and by a number of other substances, prominent among which is the osteoclast activating factor (OAF), which acts upon the osteoclasts. This peptide is produced by the lymphocytes in the area

Text continued on p. 200.

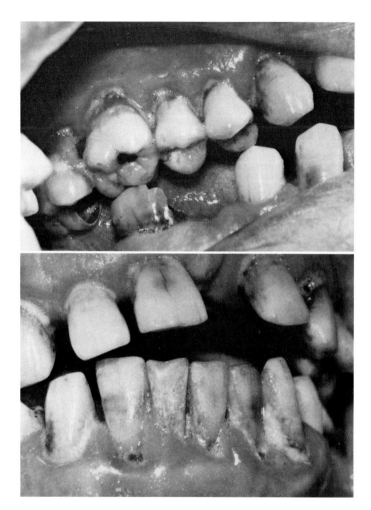

Fig. 8-13. Advanced periodontitis. Note loss of normal architecture of gingiva, blunting of papillae, diastemas, extensive supragingival plaque and suppuration.

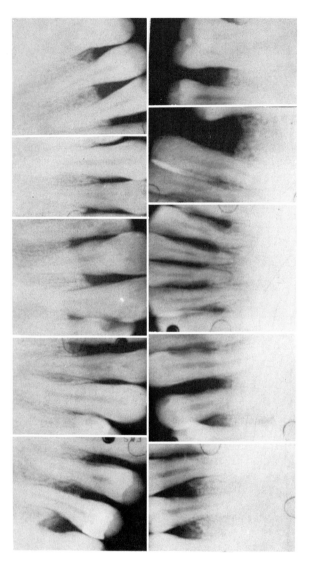

Fig. 8-14. Advanced periodontitis. Note the bone destruction in almost all segments of the jaws.

Calculus
and plaque

Pocket

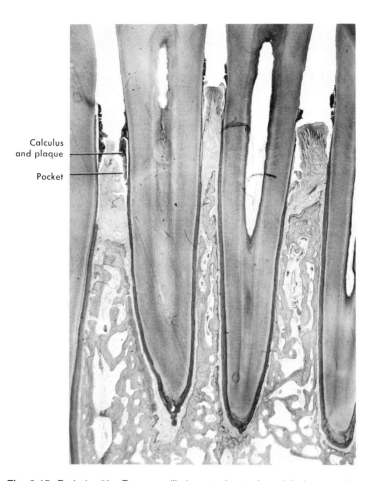

Fig. 8-15. Periodontitis. Four mandibular anterior teeth and their supporting bone show periodontitis. Note the plaque and calculus, the pockets, and the alveolar crest resorption.

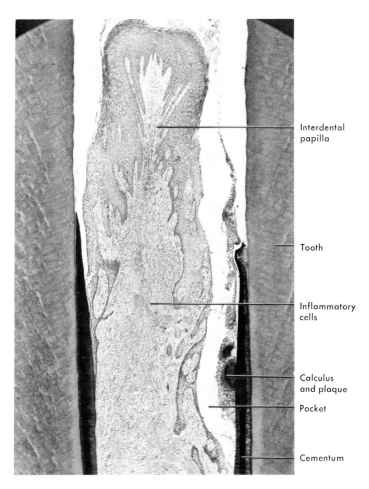

Interdental
papilla

Tooth

Inflammatory
cells

Calculus
and plaque

Pocket

Cementum

Fig. 8-16. Periodontal pocket in periodontitis. The tooth on the right has a deep pocket that contains calculus and plaque. The gingiva is densely infiltrated by inflammatory cells.

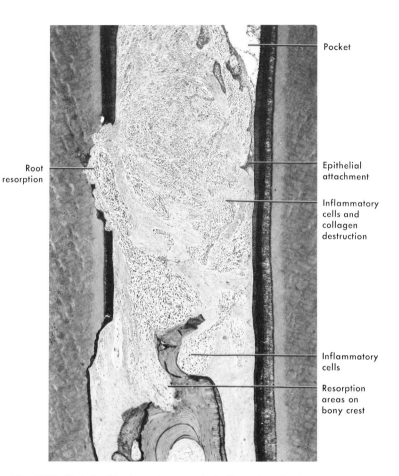

Fig. 8-17. Periodontitis (suprabony pocket). Note that the bottom of the pocket is coronal to the alveolar crest.

and is not seen in lymphocytes elsewhere in the body. The apical end of the epithelial attachment continues to grow along the denuded cementum while the coronal end progressively separates from the tooth surface, and the cycle continues.

In summary, the essential steps in the development of periodontitis are gingivitis, degeneration of collagen bundles of the periodontal ligament, cessation of cementum formation, downward growth of the epithelial attachment (junctional epithelium) with separation of the coronal part of the epithelial attachment from the surface of the tooth, pocket formation, the presence of OAF in the lymphocytes of the area, and a progressive destruction of the alveolar crest.

Because of the local anatomic features, two types of periodontal pocket are recognized: suprabony and intrabony, or infrabony. The *suprabony* pocket (Fig. 8-17) was described in the preceding discussion. In this type, the bottom of the pocket is coronal to the alveolar crest. A suprabony pocket is most commonly seen in anterior teeth. An *intrabony,* or *infrabony,*

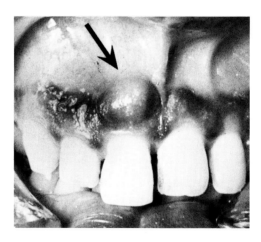

Fig. 8-18. Parulis (arrow).

pocket, in which the bottom of the pocket is apical to the alveolar crest, occurs most frequently in the interproximal areas of the premolars and molars or on the buccal and lingual areas of molars.

Periodontitis is treated by scaling and surgical elimination of the soft tissue and osseous defects.

Periodontal abscess (parulis). Deep periodontal pockets are sometimes associated with abscess formation—the so-called gumboil, or parulis. Clinically this lesion appears as a small, circumscribed boil on the gingiva of the affected tooth (Fig. 8-18). It is not painful, but the patient is aware of it and may give a history of numerous such lesions, each of which terminated in rupture and discharge of pus. A chronic apical abscess may appear as a gumboil (Fig. 7-9, *B*). It can be distinguished from the periodontal abscess by the presence of a nonvital tooth. Furthermore, in a periapical abscess a deep periodontal pocket is usually absent.

Microscopic sections show a dense, solid aggregation of neutrophils in the gingiva and the periodontal pocket (Fig. 8-19). In the histogenesis—or mechanism of formation—of a parulis, the coronal opening of a periodontal pocket closes due to the swelling of the gingiva. As a result the pocket becomes an ideal incubating chamber. Bacteria proliferate, and an abscess forms. Following the line of least resistance, the abscess "points" on the gingival soft tissues. Recent microbiologic studies have shown that the organisms that colonize the periodontal abscess are primarily gram-negative anaerobic rods. One of the most consistent organisms found in these lesions is the *Bacteroides melaninogenicus*.

Periodontal abscess is treated by incision, drainage, and surgical elimination of the pocket.

Juvenile periodontitis (periodontosis). Juvenile periodontitis is characterized by a rapid loss of alveolar bone about more than one tooth of the permanent dentition with small accumulation of plaque and little or no evidence of clinical inflammation (Fig.

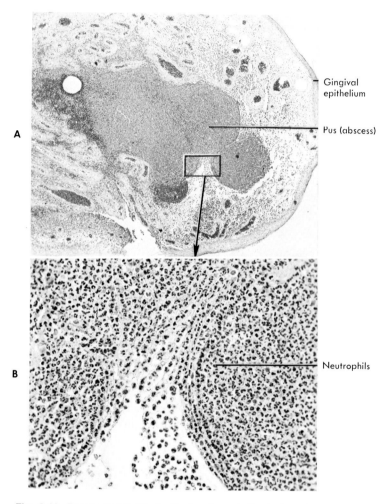

A

Gingival
epithelium

Pus (abscess)

B

Neutrophils

Fig. 8-19. Parulis (gumboil). **A,** Section through the lesion. **B,** High-power
view of an area from **A** (inset).

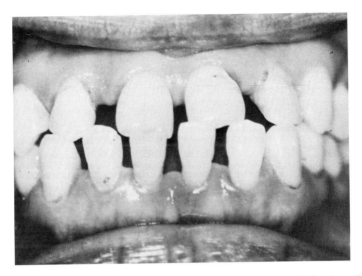

Fig. 8-20. Clinical features of juvenile periodontitis consist of migration of teeth, diastema formation, extrusion, pocket formation, and development of malocclusion.

8-20). Patients are healthy adolescents, and in the classical form the only teeth affected are the first molars and incisors. Sometimes regional lymph nodes are involved, and bone loss progresses at three or four times the rate seen in typical periodontitis. Females are affected more frequently than males, and there is a familial tendency for this disease. Patients with juvenile periodontosis show increased concentrations of IgG, IgM, and IgA; and their polymorphonuclear leukocytes have an intrinsic defect in chemotaxis. Microbiologic studies have shown that the lesions are primarily associated with gram-negative anaerobic rods (Figs. 8-21 and 8-22). Clinically bone destruction begins at about 11 to 13 years of age and in early stages is not associated with inflammation. As the disease progresses, however, there is rapid development of deep pockets, inflammation, suppuration, tooth mobility, tooth migration, and diastema

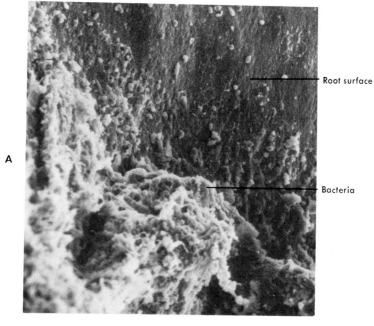

A

Root surface

Bacteria

Fig. 8-21. Scanning electron micrographs (**A,** ×300; **B,** ×3,200) from the bottom of a juvenile periodontitis pocket. The root (cemental) surface is covered by short rod-shaped bacteria and erythrocytes. (Courtesy John Brady, D.D.S., Washington, D.C.)

B

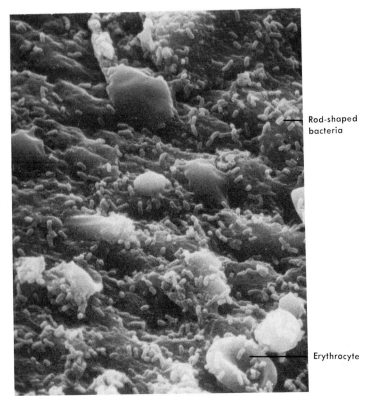

Rod-shaped
bacteria

Erythrocyte

Fig. 8-21, cont'd. For legend see opposite page.

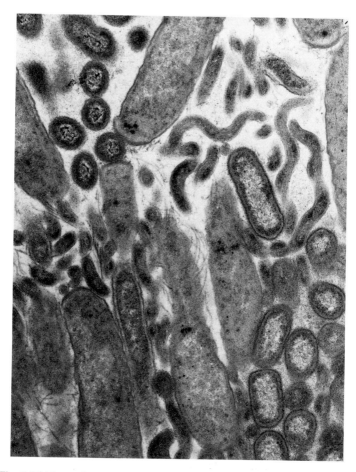

Fig. 8-22. Transmission electron micrograph (× 18,000) of bacterial flora from a juvenile periodontitis pocket. Note the rods, cocci, flagellated rods, and spirochetal forms. (Courtesy John Brady, D.D.S., Washington, D.C.)

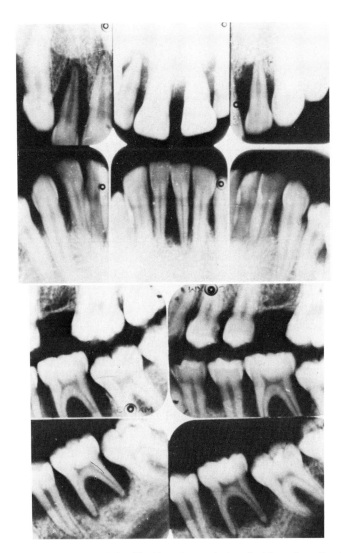

Fig. 8-23. Juvenile periodontitis. Note the marked vertical bone loss, the diastemas, and the erratic bone destruction.

formation. Classically the maxillary incisors show distolabial migration and diastema formation, while the lower incisors migrate less frequently. Roentgenographic findings include extensive vertical bone loss that is usually bilateral. Often there is an arc-shaped bone loss extending from the distal surface of the second bicuspid to the mesial surface of the second molar (Fig. 8-23).

If left untreated, the disease progresses until the affected teeth are lost. In a few cases, when patients reach the mid or late twenties without tooth loss, the disease shows a slowing down of bone destruction and a "burnout" phenomenon.

Radiographs show widening of the periodontal space and marked vertical bone resorption (Fig. 8-23).

The treatment of juvenile periodontitis is local and symptomatic and consists of elimination of the irritant (scaling), surgical removal of the periodontal pocket, splinting of the loose teeth, and elimination of any existing occlusal trauma.

Because of the recent evidence concerning its infective nature, some patients have been treated with antibiotics. The results of this therapy are encouraging.

Periodontosis-like lesions are an important feature of the *Papillon-Lefevre syndrome*, which includes hyperkeratosis of the palms and soles. A genetic disturbance, this disease is sometimes referred to as *generalized juvenile periodontitis*. The palmar and plantar keratosis may be worse in the winter months. The teeth show a sparcity of cementum on the middle and coronal thirds of the roots. The treatment of oral lesions is symptomatic. It is doubtful that the oral lesions in this disease are of infective origin.

Occlusal trauma. When the teeth are exposed to excessive occlusal forces, the resultant changes in the supporting tissues are referred to as traumatism or occlusal trauma.

The causes of occlusal trauma are essentially twofold: (1) because of malocclusion or bruxism, there may be an absolute increase in the occlusal force; (2) because of some pathology of the supporting tissues, such as periodontitis, the normal occlusal

forces may become abnormally intense for the reduced supporting tissues. Although in the past fifty years numerous conditions
such as erosion, caries, gingivitis, periodontitis, gingival recession, and trigeminal neuralgia have been ascribed to occlusal
trauma, it has been repeatedly shown that occlusal trauma can
produce only migration or loosening of teeth.

When a tooth is subjected to occlusal trauma, the forces that
are most damaging are those that act in a lateral direction. Thus
the periodontal ligament of the affected tooth has areas of pressure and tension, as shown in Fig. 8-24.

Microscopic changes in the areas of pressure are narrowing
of the periodontal space and compression and necrosis of collagen fibers (Fig. 8-25, *A*), thrombosis of the blood vessels of the
periodontal ligament (Fig. 8-25, *B*), and differentiation of osteo-

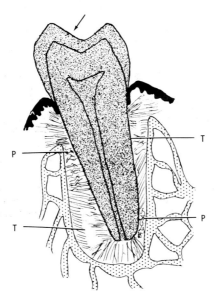

Fig. 8-24. Occlusal trauma (arrow). *P,* Area of pressure; *T,* area of tension.

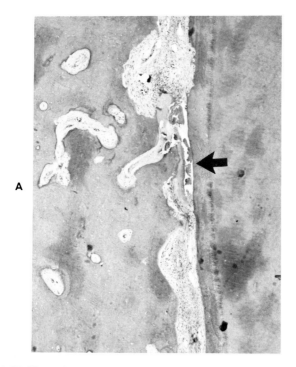

Fig. 8-25. Photomicrographs of the periodontal ligament on the pressure side. Tooth is shown on the right, and bone on the left. **A,** Note the narrowing of the ligament and the necrotic area (arrow). **B,** Thrombosis of vessels and bone resorption.

B

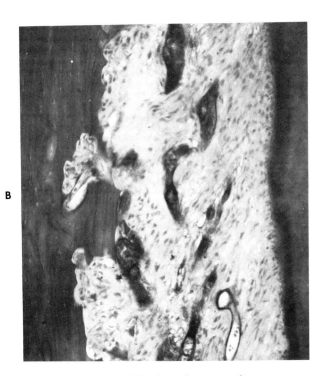

Fig. 8-25, cont'd. For legend see opposite page.

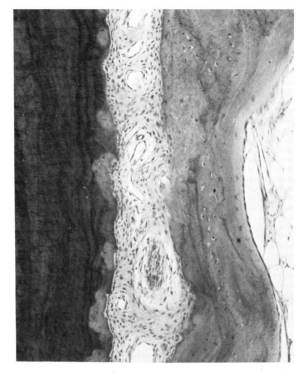

Fig. 8-26. Photomicrograph of a periodontal ligament that was previously under occlusal trauma but has now undergone repair. Note the repaired areas on the bone (right) and the cemental surface (left).

clasts on the bone surface and resorption of bone (Fig. 8-25, *B*). Bone resorption continues until pressure is relieved, and then a small amount of new bone is formed to re-embed the fibers of the periodontal ligament (Fig. 8-26).

Microscopic changes in areas of tension consist of widening of the periodontal ligament, stretching of periodontal fibers, differentiation of osteoblasts, and formation of new bone on the wall of the socket. In cases of extreme tension, thrombosis of blood vessels can sometimes be seen.

The final result of these changes is that the tooth moves out of the area of occlusal trauma.

If a tooth is exposed to lateral movements that act in two directions (i.e., jiggling movements), all parts of the periodontal ligament become areas of pressure, bone resorption occurs everywhere, the periodontal ligament widens, and the tooth becomes loose. Radiographs of such teeth show a periodontal ligament that may be three times normal width.

Excessive occlusal forces acting in one or two directions therefore do not produce gingivitis, or periodontitis. However, a tooth with periodontal disease may, by migration, come under an unfavorable occlusal relationship and occlusal trauma. Furthermore, due to the loss of supporting bone around a tooth with periodontal disease, even the normal occlusal forces may become traumatic. Occlusal trauma facilitates the spread of inflammation from the area of the periodontal pocket into the underlying tissues. Whereas normally the inflammatory process extends from the pocket to the interdental bone, in teeth under occlusal trauma the inflammation may reach into both the bone and the periodontal ligament. Therefore, in the treatment of periodontal disease, not only should the pocket be eliminated but also any occlusal trauma present should be alleviated.

REFERENCES

Acevedo, A., and Buhler, J. E.: Plasma-cell granuloma of the gingiva, Oral Surg. **43**:196, 1977.

Albjerg, L. E.: Idiopathic gingival hyperplasia, Oral Surg. **23**:823, 1967.

Angelopoulos, A. P., and Goaz, P. W.: Incidence of diphenylhydantoin gingival hyperplasia, Oral Surg. **34**:898, 1972.

Baer, P. N.: The case for periodontosis as a clinical entity, J. Periodontol. **42**:516, 1971.

Barnes, G. P., Bowles, W. F., III, and Carter, H. G.: Acute necrotizing ulcerative gingivitis: a survey of 218 cases, J. Periodontol. **44**:35, 1975.

Becker, W., Collings, C. K., Zimmerman, E. R., De La Rosa, M., and Singdahlsen, D.: Hereditary gingival fibromatosis, Oral Surg. **24**:313, 1967.

Bhaskar, S. N., and Frisch, J.: Occlusion and periodontal disease, Int. Dent. J. **17**:251, 1967.

Bowen, W. H., and Cornick, D. E.: The microbiology of gingival-dental plaque, Int. Dent. J. **20**:382, 1970.

Brady, J. M., Gray, W. A., and Bhaskar, S. N.: Electron microscopic study of the effect of water jet lavage devices on dental plaque, J. Dent. Res. **52**:1310, 1973.

Briner, W. W.: Plaque in relation to dental caries and periodontal disease, Int. Dent. J. **21**:293, 1971.

Brownstein, M. H., and Skolnik, P.: Papillon-Lefevre syndrome, Arch. Dermatol. **106**:533, 1972.

Brusati, R., and Bracchetti, A.: Electron microscopic study of chronic desquamative gingivitis, J. Periodontol. **40**:388, 1969.

Carranza, F. A.: Glickman's clinical periodontology, Philadelphia, W. B. Saunders Co., 1979.

Carvel, R. I.: Palmo-plantar hyperkeratosis and premature periodontal destruction, J. Oral Med. **24**:73, 1969.

Das, A. K., Bhowmick, S., and Dutta, A.: Oral contraceptives and periodontal disease. II. Prevalence and severity, J. Indiana Dent. Assoc. **43**:155, 1971.

Eastcott, A. D., and Stallard, R. E.: Sequential changes in developing human dental plaque as visualized by scanning electron microscopy, J. Periodontol. **44**:218, 1973.

El-Ashiry, G. M., El-Kafrawy, A. H., Nasr, M. F., and Younis, N.: Comparative study of the influence of pregnancy and oral contraceptives on the gingivae, Oral Surg. **30**:472, 1970.

Emerson, T. G.: Hereditary gingival hyperplasia, Oral Surg. **19**:1, 1965.

Eversole, L. R.: Allergic stomatitides, J. Oral Med. **34**:93, 1979.

Fournel, J.: Periodontosis, juvenile periodontosis or Gottlieb Syndrome? Report of 4 cases, J. Periodontol. **45**:234, 1974.

Giansanti, J. S., Hrabak, R. P., and Waldron, C. A.: Palmer-plantar hyperkeratosis and concomitant periodontal destruction (Papillon-Lefevre syndrome), Oral Surg. **36**:40, 1973.

Gilmore, E. L., and Bhaskar, S. N.: Effect of tongue brushing on bacteria and plaque formed in vitro, J. Periodontol. **43**:418, 1972.

Gilmore, E. L., Gross, A., and Whitley, R.: Effect of tongue brushing on plaque bacteria, Oral Surg. **36**:201, 1973.

Hall, W. B.: Mast cells in desquamative gingivitis, lichen planus, and pemphigoid, Oral Surg. **28**:646, 1969.

Hamner, J. E., and Croft, L. K.: Clinical, endocrinological, and histopathological findings in allergic gingivostomatitis, J. Periodont. Res. **8**:192, 1973.

Han, S. S., Hwang, P. J., and Lee, O. H.: A study of the histopathology of gingival hyperplasia in mental patients receiving sodium diphenylhydantoinate, Oral Surg. **23**:774, 1967.

Henefer, E. P., and Kay, L. A.: Congenital idiopathic gingival fibromatosis in the deciduous dentition, Oral Surg. **24**:65, 1967.

International Conference on Dental Plaque, American Dental Association, New York, 1969.

Kaslick, R. S., Chasens, A. I., Tuckman, M. A., and Kaufman, B.: Investigation of periodontosis with periodontitis: literature survey and findings based on ABO blood groups, J. Periodontol. **42:**420, 1971.

Kaufman, A. Y.: An oral contraceptive as an etiologic factor in producing hyperplastic gingivitis and a neoplasm of the pregnancy tumor type, Oral Surg. **28:**666, 1969.

Kelstrup, J., and Gibbons, R. J.: Induction of dental caries and alveolar bone loss by a human isolate resembling Streptococcus salivarius, Caries Res. **4:**360, 1970.

Kerr, D. A., McClatchey, K. D., and Regezi, J. A.: Idiopathic gingivostomatitis (cheilitis, glossitis, gingivitis syndrome, atypical gingivostomatitis, plasmacell gingivitis, plasmacytosis of gingiva), Oral Surg. **32:**402, 1971.

Klar, L. A.: Gingival hyperplasia during Dilantin therapy; a survey of 312 patients, J. Public Health Dent. **33:**180, 1973.

Langeland, K., Rodrigues, H., and Dowden, W.: Periodontal disease, bacteria, and pulpal histopathology, Oral Surg. **37:**257, 1974.

Listgarten, M.: Electron microscopic observations on bacterial flora of acute necrotizing ulcerative gingivitis, J. Periodontal. **36:**328, 1965.

Listgarten, M.: Structure of the microbial flora associated with periodontal health and disease in man, J. Periodontal. **47:**1, 1976.

Listgarten, M., and Lewis, D.: The distribution of spirochetes in the lesion of acute necrotizing ulcerative gingivitis: an electron microscopic and statistical survey, J. Periodontal. **38:**379, 1967.

Listgarten, M., Mayo, H. E., and Tremblay, R.: Development of dental plaque on epoxy resin crowns in man, J. Periodontal. **46:**10, 1975.

Lynn, B. D.: "The pill" as an etiologic agent in hypertrophic gingivitis, Oral Surg. **24:**333, 1967.

Melnick, M., Shields, E. D., and Bixler, D.: Periodontosis: a phenotypic and genetic analysis, Oral Surg. **42:**32, 1976.

Munford, A. G.: Papillon-Lefevre syndrome: report of two cases in the same family, J. Am. Dent. Assoc. **93:**121, 1976.

Newman, M. G.: The role of bacteroides melaninogenicus and other anaerobes in periodontal infections, Rev. Infect. Dis. **1:**313, 1979.

Newman, M. G.: The role of *bacteroides melaninogenicus* and other anaerobes in periodontal infections, Rev. Infect. Dis. **1:**313, 1979.

Owings, J. R.: An atypical gingivostomatitis: a report of four cases, J. Periodontol. **40:**538, 1969.

Page, L. R., Bosman, C. W., Drummond, J. F., and Ciancio, S. G.: Acute recurrent gingivitis, Oral Surg. **49:**337, 1980.

Ramon, Y., Berman, W., and Bubis, J. J.: Gingival fibromatosis combined with cherubism, Oral Surg. **24:**435, 1967.

Rogers, R. S., III, Sheridan, P. J., and Jordan, R. E.: Desquamative gingivitis, Oral Surg. **42**:316, 1976.

Roth, R. H.: Temporomandibular pain-dysfunction and occlusal relationships, Angle Orthod. **43**:136, 1973.

Selden, H. S.: Pulpoperiapical disease: diagnosis and healing, Oral Surg. **37**:271, 1974.

Silverman, S., Jr., and Lozada, F.: An epilogue to plasma-cell gingivostomatitis (allergic gingivostomatitis), Oral Surg. **43**:211, 1977.

Slots, J.: The predominate cultivable microflora of advanced periodontitis, Scand. J. Dent. Res. **85**:114, 1977.

Slots, J.: Microflora in the healthy gingival sulcus in man, Scand. J. Dent. Res. **85**:247, 1977.

Snyderman, R.: The role of the immune response in the development of periodontal disease, Int. Dent. J. **23**:310, 1973.

Socransky, S. S.: Relationship of bacteria to the etiology of periodontal disease, J. Dent. Res. (Suppl.) **49**:203, 1970.

Socransky, S. S., and Manganiello, A. D.: Bacteriological studies of developing supragingival dental plaque, J. Periodont. Res. **12**:90, 1977.

Stirrups, D. R., and Inglis, J.: Tuberous sclerosis with nonhydantoin gingival hyperplasia, Oral Surg. **49**:211, 1980.

Sutcher, H. D., and Lerman, M. D.: The temporomandibular syndrome, J. Am. Dent, Assoc. **225**:1248, 1973.

Vickers, R. A., and Hudson, C. D.: A clinicopathologic investigation of "plasma cell gingivitis," International Association for Dental Research Abstr. 755, March, 1971.

Vogel, R. E., and Deasy, M. J.: Juvenile periodontitis (periodontosis): current concepts, J. Am. Dent. Assoc. **97**:843, 1978.

Wilson, F. M.: Papillon-Lefevre syndrome, Oral Surg. **28**:488, 1969.

CHAPTER 9
Cysts of jaws

The presence of epithelial tissue within the marrow of the maxilla and the mandible is one of the numerous dissimilarities between the jaws and other bones of the skeleton. The source of this epithelium is both odontogenic and nonodontogenic.

Odontogenic epithelium—which is the remains of the enamel organs of teeth, or the dental lamina—may be present within the jaws as undeveloped or abated enamel organs or as epithelial rests (of Malassez).

Nonodontogenic epithelium is seen only in the upper jaw and is the remains of the epithelium covering the embryonic processes that give rise to the maxilla. As expected, these remnants are found along the line of closure of embryonic processes—that is, along the midline of the palate (line of fusion of palatine processes), in the area between the maxillary canine and lateral incisor (line of fusion of the globular and maxillary processes), and in the area of the base of the nostril (line of closure of the medial and lateral nasal processes with the maxillary process).

Another source of nonodontogenic epithelium in the maxilla is the remains of the vestigial nasopalatine duct, an epithelium-lined canal that in the early fetal life of man and in numerous lower vertebrates connects the nasal and oral cavities. The remains of this duct are seen in the nasopalatine canal and in the area of the incisive papilla.

In the retromolar area of the mandible, and rarely in isolated areas of the maxilla, inclusions of salivary gland epithelium may be seen. Although this epithelium can initiate salivary gland tumors, it does not give rise to cysts and therefore is only of passing interest to the present discussion.

In summary, the jaws contain within their marrow odontogenic and nonodontogenic epithelium. Corresponding to this epithelium, two major types of true cysts (odontogenic and nonodontogenic) arise within the jaws. There is a third group of so-called cysts, which are not cysts in the true sense, because they are not lined by epithelium. With respect to tradition, however, they are included in this chapter.

Odontogenic cysts

1. Primordial
2. Dentigerous
3. Multilocular

   Arise from enamel organ or follicle; therefore, collectively called follicular cysts

4. Radicular
5. Residual

   Arise from epithelial rests of Malassez

6. Odontogenic keratocyst
7. Calcifying odontogenic cyst (keratinizing and calcifying odontogenic cyst; cystic calcifying odontogenic tumor)

   Arise from enamel organ or rests of Malassez

Nonodontogenic cysts

1. Median palatine
2. Median alveolar
3. Globulomaxillary
4. Nasoalveolar
5. Median mandibular

   Arise in area of fusion of facial processes; therefore, collectively called fissural cysts

6. Nasopalatine }   Arise from remnants of nasopalatine duct

Nonepithelial "cysts" (pseudocysts)

1. Traumatic
2. Idiopathic bone cavity
3. Aneurysmal bone

ODONTOGENIC CYSTS

Primordial cyst. The primordial cyst constitutes about 5% of all follicular cysts and 1.75% of all odontogenic cysts (Table 13). It arises from a tooth germ that, instead of forming a tooth, degenerates into a cyst.

Clinically this lesion is always associated with a missing

tooth (unless it arises from a supernumerary tooth germ). The mandible is involved more frequently than the maxilla, and the lesion usually occurs in the second or third decade of life. It may produce an enlargement of the jaw, or it may be asymptomatic. It is painless but, when large, may produce migration of erupted teeth. All teeth in the area are vital. The lesion appears as a well-demarcated area of radiolucency not directly associated with an erupted or unerupted tooth (Fig. 9-1).

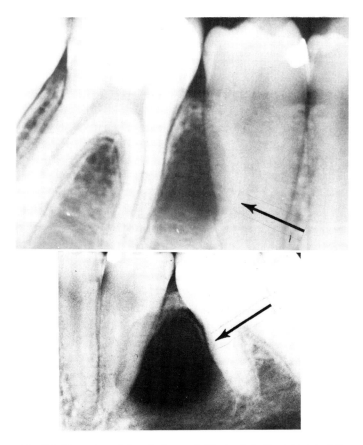

Fig. 9-1. Two primordial cysts (arrows). The teeth in the area are vital.

Microscopic sections show a cystic cavity lined by stratified squamous epithelium and a connective tissue wall that usually, but not always, is free of inflammatory cells and that may contain small islands of odontogenic or ameloblastic epithelium (see discussion of dentigerous cyst).

Primordial cysts are treated by local curettage or excision.

Dentigerous cyst. The dentigerous cyst is the most common of all follicular cysts, constituting about 95% of these lesions and about 34% of all odontogenic cysts (Table 13).

This lesion is slightly more common among males than females and almost 60% occur in the second or third decade of life. About 70% of the lesions occur in the mandible, and 30% in the maxilla. Almost 62% occur in the molar area, 12% in the premolar area, and 12% in the canine area, with the remaining 14% occurring elsewhere in the jaws. The mandibular third molar and maxillary canine are the most frequently involved single teeth.

A dentigerous cyst arises from the enamel organ after partial completion of the crown. The enamel organ around a developing crown undergoes cystic degeneration, and the resultant cyst either completely surrounds or is attached to the crown (Fig. 9-2). The lesion produces enlargement of the jaw that in some instances is quite marked (Fig. 9-3, A).

Table 13. Relative incidence of odontogenic cysts of jaws*

Type	Number	Percent
Primordial	62	1.75
Dentigerous	1,194	33.75
Eruption	19	0.54
Multilocular	4	0.11
Follicular (unclassified)	33	0.93
Radicular	2,046	57.83
Residual	180	5.09
TOTAL	3,538	100.00

*Based on personal analyses of clinical, radiographic, microscopic, and follow-up data on more than 20,000 cases.

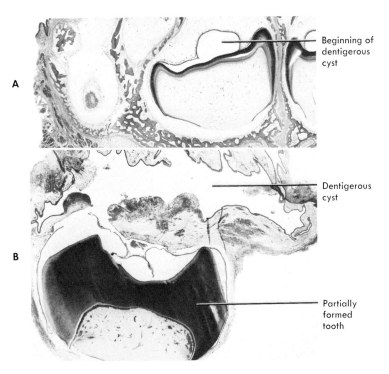

Fig. 9-2. Dentigerous cyst. **A,** Microscopic cystic change in the enamel organ of a developing incisor. **B,** Fully developed cyst. The dark line surrounding the cavity is the epithelial lining.

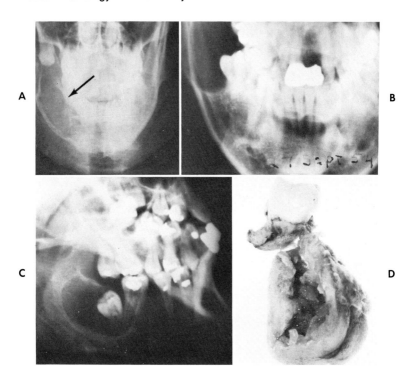

Fig. 9-3. Dentigerous cyst. **A,** Arrow indicates the cyst displacing the tooth toward the ramus. **B** and **C,** Crown of an unerupted tooth surrounded by a clearly demarcated radiolucent area. **D,** Gross specimen. The crown of the tooth is surrounded by a cystic sac.

Radiographs show an unerupted tooth whose crown is surrounded by a clearly demarcated radiolucent area (Fig. 9-3, *B* and *C*). In large cysts of the mandibular third molar region, the radiolucency may extend far into the ramus (Fig. 9-3, *A*). The teeth associated with dentigerous cysts may be pushed out of place—for example, to the lower border of the mandible or the floor of the nose.

Grossly the specimen consists of a tooth whose crown is sur-

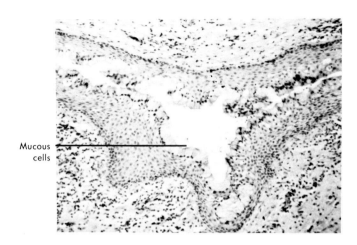

Mucous cells

Fig. 9-4. Lining of a dentigerous cyst. Note the areas of mucous cells.

rounded by a cystic sac (Fig. 9-3, *D*). When the cyst surrounds the crown completely, it is sometimes called a *central dentigerous cyst*. When it is attached to one side of the crown, it is called a *lateral dentigerous cyst*. This distinction, however, is not important or necessary.

Microscopic sections prepared from the lesion reveal that the crown of the tooth is either completely formed or in the process of formation (Fig. 9-2, *B*). The cyst, which may surround the crown completely or be attached to the crown, is lined by stratified squamous epithelium. On rare occasion, the lining may be keratinized, may contain mucous cells (Fig. 9-4), or may be completely or partially lined by granular cells. It has been suggested that cysts that are lined by keratinizing epithelium, (parakeratin or orthokeratin) have a greater chance of recurrence than cysts whose lining is not keratinized (p. 229).

The connective tissue wall consists of collagen bundles and usually shows mild infiltration by plasma cells and lymphocytes. In about 82% of dentigerous and primordial cysts, the connective tissue of the wall contains small islands or rests of odontogenic epithelium. This epithelium is usually inactive but has the potential of giving rise to odontogenic tumors. In rare instances the connective tissue wall of the cyst may contain islands of squamous epithelium. Such islands do not indicate an aggressive potential but represent a squamous metaplasia of the odontogenic islands. In 5% to 6% of cysts, however, the lining of the connective tissue wall shows ameloblastic proliferation (Fig. 9-

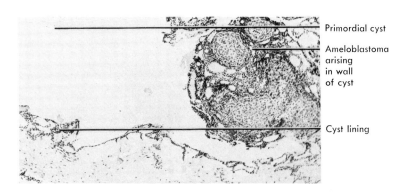

Primordial cyst

Ameloblastoma arising in wall of cyst

Cyst lining

Fig. 9-5. Ameloblastoma arising from the epithelial lining of a primordial cyst.

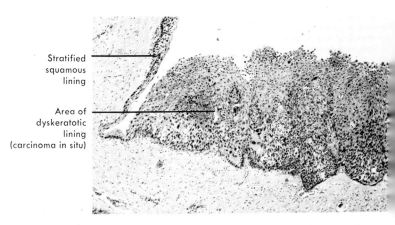

Stratified squamous lining

Area of dyskeratotic lining (carcinoma in situ)

Fig. 9-6. Lining of a dentigerous cyst. Note the area of stratified squamous cells and the carcinoma in situ.

5). These lesions are the precursors of ameloblastomas (p. 252) and require careful removal and follow-up.

Rarely the epithelial lining of a dentigerous cyst may undergo a malignant (dyskeratotic) transformation; carcinoma in situ and squamous cell carcinoma have been shown to arise in these lesions (Fig. 9-6).

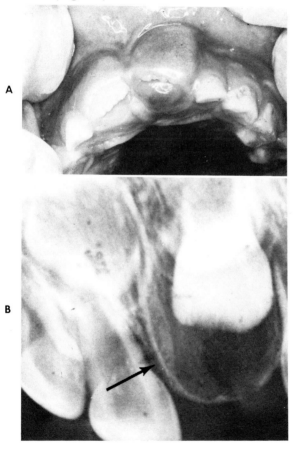

Fig. 9-7. Eruption cyst. **A,** Compressible swelling associated with an erupting tooth. **B,** Note the radiolucency around an erupting central incisor (arrow) in another case.

In children dentigerous cysts often develop with erupting teeth and, just prior to entering the oral cavity, present as bluish, compressible, fluid-containing enlargements on the alveolar ridge. These are called *eruption cysts* (Fig. 9-7). Since eruption cysts are seldom biopsied, their incidence is not accurately reflected in Table 13. Their microscopic features are the same as those of dentigerous cysts. Because the lesions rupture spontaneously as the teeth erupt, no treatment is required. If necessary, they may be incised or marsupialized.

Multilocular cyst. Under rare circumstances a tooth germ may give rise to multiple cysts that, unlike dentigerous cysts, are not associated with a developed tooth. They constitute less than 1% of all follicular cysts.

Clinically this lesion presents as an enlargement of the involved bone. The most common site is the mandibular molar area. Radiographically it has a multicystic or soap bubble appearance. Migration of teeth is common.

Microscopic sections show what appear to be numerous primordial cysts adjoining or communicating with each other. These are lined by stratified squamous epithelium, and their connective tissue walls may have a minimal number of inflammatory cells. In some instances the lining epithelium is keratinized and the cysts contain keratin. Such cysts are identical to the odontogenic keratocyst (see p. 229).

Multilocular cysts require careful local radical excision and curettage.

Multiple jaw cysts are a consistent finding in a developmental anomaly called the *basal cell nevus syndrome* (Figs. 9-8 and 9-9). These cysts individually resemble primordial cysts and are lined by stratified squamous epithelium. The latter may produce keratin, and keratin-producing cysts are called *odontogenic keratocysts* (see p. 229). In addition to the jaw cysts, the patients have multiple basal cell carcinomas and sebaceous cysts of the skin and skeletal deformities (e.g., frontal bossing, splayed ribs, fusion of vertebrae).

Radicular and residual cysts. Radicular and residual cysts are described in Chapter 7.

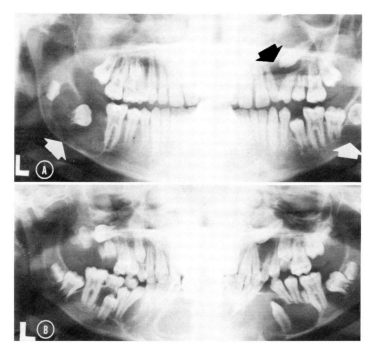

Fig. 9-8. Radiographs of a brother **(A)** and sister **(B)** with multiple cysts of the jaw (arrows). Both children had the basal cell nevus syndrome. (Courtesy A. S. Miller, D. D. S., Philadelphia.)

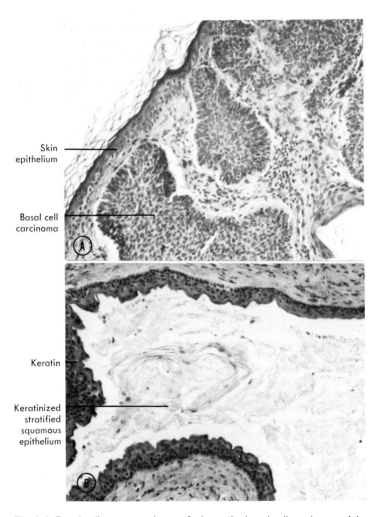

Skin
epithelium

Basal cell
carcinoma

Keratin

Keratinized
stratified
squamous
epithelium

Fig. 9-9. Basal cell nevus syndrome. **A** shows the basal cell carcinoma of the skin and **B,** the wall of one of a number of keratinizing cysts from the jaw. (Courtesy A. S. Miller, D.D.S., Philadelphia.)

Odontogenic keratocyst. About 8% of dentigerous, primordial, and multilocular cysts (and rarely a radicular or residual cyst) show unique histologic features that have led to their classification as *odontogenic keratocysts*. Although cysts are a common feature of the *basal cell nevus syndrome,* about 5% of these are of the odontogenic keratocyst type.

The odontogenic keratocyst is twice as common in the mandible as in the maxilla, and the mandibular third molar area and the ramus are the most frequent site. Lesions are most often seen in the second decade of life, and almost 40% of them are associated with impacted teeth.

The radiographic appearance of an odontogenic keratocyst is not remarkable. When multilocular, lesions resemble the ameloblastoma, for which they may be mistaken.

Microscopic features that have led to a separate name for

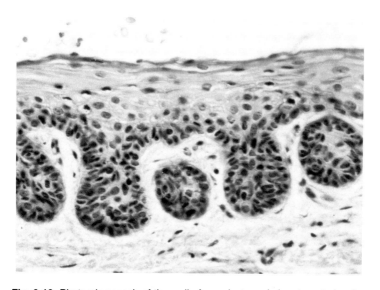

Fig. 9-10. Photomicrograph of the wall of an odontogenic keratocyst showing the budlike proliferation of the basal layer of the epithelial lining. (Courtesy James Adrian, D.D.S., Washington, D.C.)

this cyst include a stratified squamous epithelial lining that produces keratin, a budlike proliferation of the basal layer of the epithelial lining, and the presence of microcysts in the connective tissue wall of the cyst (Figs. 9-9, *B*, and 9-10). It has been suggested that cysts lined by parakeratotic epithelium grow faster than those lined by cells producing orthokeratin.

Since about 45% of odontogenic keratocysts are known to recur, these lesions should be carefully followed after excision.

Calcifying odontogenic cyst (keratinizing and calcifying odontogenic cyst; cystic calcifying odontogenic tumor). This cyst can occur at any age, but more than 50% are seen in patients under 40 years of age (with almost 30% in the second decade). There is no sexual predilection. Almost 80% of lesions occur within the jaws, and 20% in the soft tissue around the jaws. The maxilla and mandible are equally affected. About 25% of the intraosseous lesions are associated with impacted teeth. Clinical features are not different from those of any other odontogenic cyst.

Radiographs show a single or multilocular, well-demarcated radiolucency in which specks of radiopacities can be seen (Fig. 9-11). Lesions range in size from 1 to 8 cm.

Microscopic features of the calcifying odontogenic cyst are unique. The lesion is most often cystic (90%), but it may be solid. It consists of areas of columnar and stellate epithelium (resembling some features of the ameloblastoma), areas of ghost cells (epithelial cells containing keratin-like material), areas of keratin, and focal areas of calcification (Fig. 9-12). Rarely the epithelial cells may contain melanin.

This lesion, whether intraosseous or extraosseous, is benign; and local conservative removal is curative.

•   •   •

Although both the cysts that arise from the enamel organ and those whose lining is derived from the epithelial rests of Malassez are included under the term *odontogenic cysts*, their behavior is dissimilar.

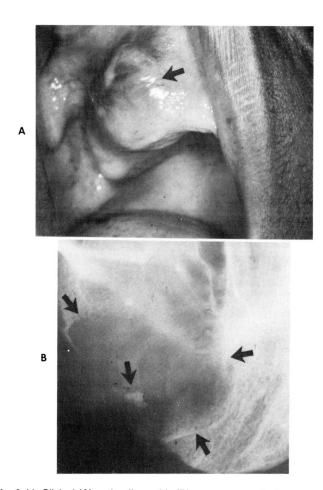

Fig. 9-11. Clinical **(A)** and radiographic **(B)** appearances of a keratinizing and calcifying odontogenic cyst (arrows).

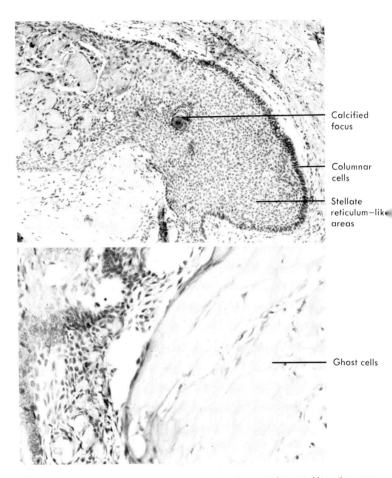

Calcified
focus

Columnar
cells

Stellate
reticulum—like
areas

Ghost cells

Fig. 9-12. Photomicrographs of a calcifying odontogenic cyst. Note the areas of columnar cells, the stellate reticulum—like cells, the ghost cells, and the calcified foci.

Primordial, dentigerous, and multilocular cysts possess the potential of becoming ameloblastomas; and as mentioned previously, 5% to 6% of them show such a change. It has also been estimated that from 25% to 30% of all ameloblastomas arise in these lesions (p. 252). Furthermore, on extremely rare occasion, the lining of a follicular cyst may give rise to a squamous cell carcinoma. For this reason such cysts require very careful removal and postoperative follow-up.

Radicular and residual cysts, on the other hand, do not possess the potential of becoming ameloblastomas.

NONODONTOGENIC CYSTS

Median palatine and median alveolar cysts. The median palatine and median alveolar cysts are midline cysts of the maxilla and constitute only about 7.5% of all nonodontogenic cysts and nonepithelial cysts (pseudocysts) of the jaws (Table 14).

The term *median palatine* is applied to a lesion occurring in the midline of the palate, whereas *median alveolar* refers to a lesion near the alveolar process just posterior to the central incisors. Both lesions arise from the epithelial cells that become

Table 14. Relative incidence of nonodontogenic cysts and nonepithelial cysts (pseudocysts) of jaws*

Type	Number	Percent
Median palatine and median alveolar	20	7.41
Globulomaxillary	46	17.05
Nasoalveolar	7	2.59
Fissural (unclassified)	11	4.07
Nasopalatine (incisive canal and papilla palatina)	147	54.44
Traumatic	35	12.96
Aneurysmal bone	4	1.48
TOTAL	270	100.00

*Based on personal analyses of clinical, radiographic, microscopic, and follow-up data on more than 20,000 cases.

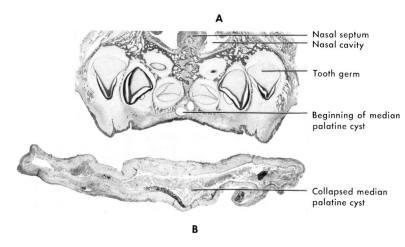

A

Nasal septum
Nasal cavity

Tooth germ

Beginning of median palatine cyst

Collapsed median palatine cyst

B

Fig. 9-13. A, Frontal section through a fetal head. Note the cysts in the midline. **B,** Collapsed median palatine cyst.

trapped in the midline of the maxilla during development (Fig. 9-13).

Clinically both lesions present as a firm swelling in the midline of the palate. The covering mucosa may be pale or blanched, but it is always intact. Ulceration is absent. The lesions are painless but may cause discomfort during mastication and speech.

The lesions are made up characteristically of circumscribed radiolucent areas (Fig. 9-14). Because of its anterior position, a median alveolar cyst may be mistaken for a nasopalatine cyst (p. 238) but can be distinguished from the latter on the basis of its lower and more anterior location.

Microscopic sections prepared from either of these lesions show a cyst lined by stratified squamous or pseudostratified ciliated columnar (respiratory) epithelium. In some cases both types of epithelium can be seen. The cystic cavity contains cellular debris, fluid, or keratin. The periepithelial connective tissue may show mild lymphocytic and plasma cell infiltration.

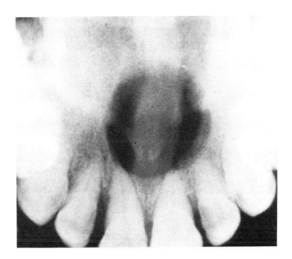

Fig. 9-14. Median alveolar cyst. The teeth in the area are vital. This lesion is often difficult to distinguish from a nasopalatine cyst.

Median palatine and median alveolar cysts are treated by simple enucleation.

Globulomaxillary cyst. The globulomaxillary cyst constitutes about 17% of all nonodontogenic cysts and nonepithelial cysts (pseudocysts) of the jaws (Table 14).

This lesion arises from epithelial remnants left in the line of fusion of the globular and maxillary processes of the embryonic face. It is seen, therefore, between the maxillary canine and lateral incisor, where it may produce an enlargement as well as migration of adjoining teeth. It is otherwise asymptomatic, and all of the regional teeth are vital.

A globulomaxillary cyst characteristically appears as a pear-shaped radiolucency between the canine and lateral incisor. The neck of the "pear" is between the coronal parts of these teeth (Fig. 9-15). The roots of the canine and lateral incisor are usually spread apart by the radiolucency.

Microscopic sections show the same features as are noted in

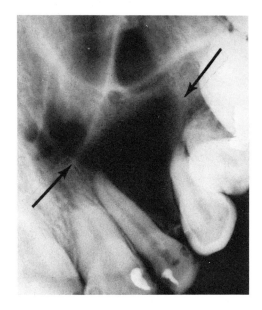

Fig. 9-15. Globulomaxillary cyst. Note the pear-shaped radiolucency (arrows).

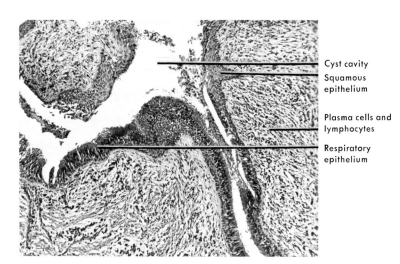

Cyst cavity
Squamous
epithelium

Plasma cells and
lymphocytes

Respiratory
epithelium

Fig. 9-16. Globulomaxillary cyst. Note the lining of both respiratory and squamous epithelium.

median palatine and alveolar cysts—that is, a cystic cavity lined by stratified squamous or respiratory epithelium. The cyst wall shows infiltration by plasma cells and lymphocytes (Fig. 9-16).

Globulomaxillary cysts are treated by enucleation.

Nasoalveolar cyst. The nasoalveolar cyst is really a cyst of soft tissues but is included in this group because it is of fissural origin and because on occasion it does produce resorption of bone. It is one the least common of the nonodontogenic cysts and nonepithelial cysts (pseudocysts) of the jaws and constitutes only about 2.5% of these lesions (Table 14).

The nasoalveolar cyst is seen usually in blacks and is located at the base of the nostril. It produces a swelling that may be seen and felt under the upper lip as well as in the nasal floor. Regional teeth are all vital. Radiographs do not show any bone change. However, if the cyst produces a pressure resorption of bone from the periosteal side, a radiolucency may be evident.

Microscopic features are the same as those described for median and globulomaxillary cysts.

Median mandibular cyst. Rarely a midline cyst of the mandible is observed and is sometimes called a median mandibular cyst (Fig. 9-17). Since no fissural epithelium is seen in this area, the lesion is erroneously termed "fissural." In reality it represents a primordial cyst arising from an accessory tooth germ.

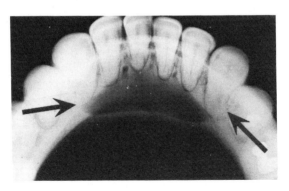

Fig. 9-17. Median mandibular cyst. Arrows outline its periphery.

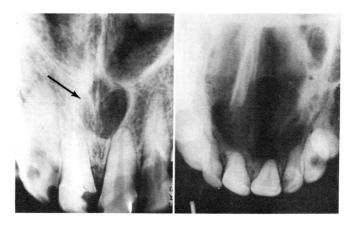

Fig. 9-18. Incisive canal cysts (nasopalatine cysts). In the left figure the shadow of the nasal spine gives the radiolucency a heart-shaped appearance (arrow). The teeth in the area of these cysts are vital.

Nasopalatine cysts. Cysts that arise in the nasopalatine canal constitute about 54% of all nondontogenic cysts and nonepithelial cysts (pseudocysts) of the jaws and are the most common member of this group (Table 14).

Nasopalatine cysts may be divided into two types—*incisive canal cysts* and *cysts of the palatine papilla*—depending on whether they are located in the incisive papilla or within the nasopalatine canal. They may be asymptomatic or may produce an elevation in the anterior part of the palate. The covering mucosa is normal, and the teeth in the area are vital.

An incisive canal cyst appears characteristically as a circumscribed radiolucency in the anterior part of the maxilla (Fig. 9-18). Typically the shadow of the nasal spine is superimposed on the radiolucency so that it assumes a heart-shaped outline. The cyst is located higher than and posterior to the usual location of the median alveolar cyst.

A cyst of the palatine papilla ordinarily does not produce a radiolucency. However, if it erodes the bone from the palatal surface, a corresponding area of radiolucency may be seen.

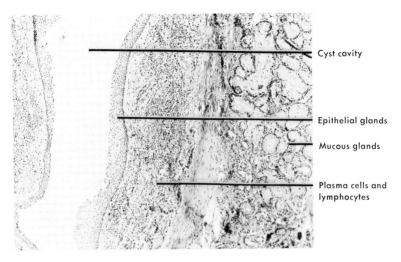

Cyst cavity

Epithelial glands

Mucous glands

Plasma cells and
lymphocytes

Fig. 9-19. Nasopalatine cyst. Note the mucous glands in the wall of the cyst.

Microscopically nasopalatine cysts show a lining of respiration and/or stratified squamous epithelium, the presence of mucous glands and nerves in the connective tissue wall (which distinguishes these lesions from other cysts), and lymphocytic and plasma cell infiltration of the connective tissue (Fig. 9-19).

NONEPITHELIAL CYSTS (PSEUDOCYSTS)

Traumatic cyst. The traumatic cyst, also called solitary bone cyst, hemorrhagic cyst, extravasation cyst, or unicameral cyst, constitutes about 13% of all nonodontogenic cysts and nonepithelial cysts (pseudocysts) of the jaws (Table 14).

This lesion is usually seen in individuals under 20 years of age. Males are affected more often than females. Although sometimes asymptomatic, a traumatic cyst may produce enlargement of the jaw. Pain is rarely associated with the lesion. The area most frequently involved is between the mandibular canines and the ramus. The second favored site is the mandib-

240 Pathology of teeth and jaws

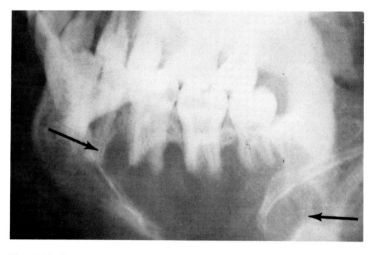

Fig. 9-20. Traumatic cyst. Note the scalloped upper border of the radiolucency (arrows). The teeth are vital.

ular symphysis. Cysts may persist for a long time. The regional teeth are vital. There is usually a history of trauma.

At exploration or surgery, the operator finds that the lesion either is empty or contains a small amount of clear or blood-stained fluid and that the "cyst" is really a large cavity in the bone with very little tissue to line its walls. The inferior alveolar nerve and blood vessels are sometimes seen lying free in the cavity.

A traumatic cyst appears as a large radiolucency that may expand the cortex of the jaw. The radiolucency extends between the teeth and has a scalloped outline. The latter feature is almost unique to the traumatic cyst (Fig. 9-20).

Microscopic sections prepared from the wall of a traumatic cyst show only bone covered by an extremely thin microscopic layer of connective tissue (Fig. 9-21).

The cause of a traumatic cyst is not known, but numerous theories have been proposed—hemorrhage in bone followed by

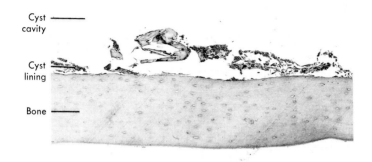

Cyst cavity

Cyst lining

Bone

Fig. 9-21. Traumatic cyst. Section through the wall. There is only a thin layer of connective tissue.

lysis of the blood clot, faulty calcium metabolism, altered resorption and apposition of the bone, and ischemic necrosis of the marrow. Perhaps the most likely mechanism is the development of a benign tumor that undergoes spontaneous lysis and leaves an empty space.

Treatment of traumatic cysts is relatively simple and consists of opening the lesion, curettage, and closure. The resultant blood clot soon undergoes organization, and the bone defect heals rapidly.

Idiopathic bone cavity. This defect in not really a cyst of the jaw. However, because of its clinical and radiographic similarity to cystic lesions, it is included here.

The idiopathic bone cavity is also referred to as *embryonic bone defect* or *lingual mandibular bone cavity*. It occurs in the mandible and is usually located below the inferior dental canal between the mandibular angle and the first molar. However, it may occur in the anterior part of the mandible. It is seen more often in males. Although cases have been reported from the second to the eighth decade of life, most patients are in their fifth or sixth decade.

The lesion is asymptomatic and discovered on routine ex-

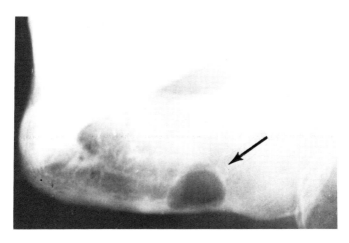

Fig. 9-22. Idiopathic bone cavity. The radiolucency (arrow) is usually located anterior to the angle of the mandible and below the inferior dental canal. (Courtesy Roderick L. Lister, D.D.S., Denver.)

amination. It appears as a well-demarcated radiolucency, usually located below the inferior dental canal, and does not expand the cortical plate (Fig. 9-22). At exploration a defect in the lingual cortical plate and a cavity in the mandible are found. The cavity is usually filled by a portion of the submaxillary gland or sublingual gland or may contain lymphoid or connective tissue. The contents of the cavity are attached via the lingual cortical defect to the soft tissues of the oral floor.

An idiopathic bone cavity is an inclusion defect that occurs during the development and growth of the mandible, but it may not become clinically apparent until adulthood. A portion of the salivary gland is included within the developing mandible; and, except in one area, the bone tissue is formed all around the gland. The lesion requires no treatment.

Aneurysmal bone cyst. This defect constitutes about 1.5% of all nonodontogenic cysts and nonepithelial cysts (pseudocysts) of the jaws (Table 14). It is not a true cyst.

The lesion commonly occurs in individuals under 20 years of

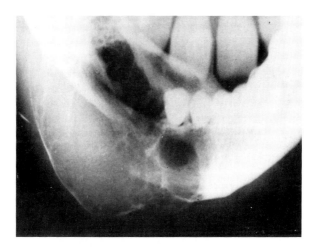

Fig. 9-23. Aneurysmal bone cyst. Note the soap bubble–like radiolucency. The lesion is not always expansile, as seen in this case.

age, and frequently there is a history of trauma. The duration of the lesion is from 1 to 6 months. Usually the mandible is affected. There is a firm, nontender enlargement of the affected site. The mucosal covering is normal. Malocclusion may result from the deformity. At exploration a bone cavity filled by reddish brown liverlike tissue that wells up with blood is found. Curettage produces marked hemorrhage that is not too difficult to control.

The cyst appears characteristically as a radiolucency that may be unilocular but usually has a multilocular or soap bubble appearance (Fig. 9-23). The jaw is expanded, but the cortex is not destroyed.

Microscopic features of the aneurysmal bone cyst are diagnostic (Fig. 9-24). Numerous pools of blood are lined by fusiform connective tissue cells; and the tissue between the blood pools shows fibroblasts, numerous giant cells, foci of hemosiderin, and small blood vessels.

Local curettage of an aneurysmal bone cyst is the treatment of choice and is curative.

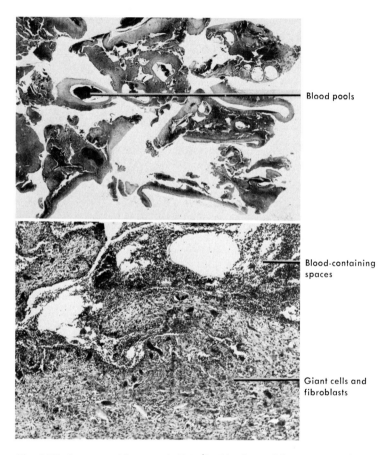

Fig. 9-24. Aneurysmal bone cyst. Note the blood-containing spaces and the intervening stroma of giant cells, capillaries, and fibroblasts.

The aneurysmal bone cyst, as well as the traumatic bone cyst, does not occur exclusively in the jaws. The counterparts of both cysts are seen in other bones of the skeleton.

REFERENCES

Abrams, A. M., Howell, F. V., and Bullock, W. K.: Nasopalatine cysts, Oral Surg. **16:**306, 1963.

Adrian, J. C., Tsaknis, P. J., and German, N. I.: Surgical oral pathology in an Army regional laboratory: a survey, Milit. Med. **141:**82, 1976.

Albers, D. D.: Median mandibular cyst partially lined with pseudostratified columnar epithelium, Oral Surg. **36:**11, 1973.

Altini, M., and Farman, A. G.: The calcifying odontogenic cyst, Oral Surg. **40:**751, 1975.

Anderson, D. E., and Cook, W. A.: Jaw cysts and the basal cell nevus syndrome, J. Oral Surg. **24:**15, 1966.

Angelopoulos, A. P., Tilson, H. B., Steward, F. W., and Jaques, W. E.: Malignant transformation of the epithelial lining of the odontogenic cysts, Oral Surg. **22:**415, 1966.

Anneroth, G., and Nordenram, A.: Calcifying odontogenic cyst, Oral Surg. **39:**794, 1975.

Baker, R. D., D'Onofrio, E. D., Corio, R. L., Crawford, B. E., and Terry, B. C.: Squamous-cell carcinoma arising in a lateral periodontal cyst, Oral Surg. **47:**495, 1979.

Benerjee, S. C.: Squamous-cell carcinoma in a maxillary cyst, Oral Surg. **23:**193, 1967.

Bergenholtz, A., and Persson, G.: Idiopathic bone cavities, Oral Surg. **16:**703, 1963.

Bernier, J. L., and Bhaskar, S. N.: Aneurysmal bone cysts of the mandible, Oral Surg. **9:**1018, 1958.

Bhaskar, S. N.: Oral pathology in the dental office: survey of 20,575 biopsy specimens, J. Am. Dent. Assoc. **76:**761, 1968.

Bhaskar, S. N., Bernier, J. L., and Bodby, F.: Aneurysmal bone cyst and other giant cell lesions of the jaws, J. Oral Surg. **17:**30, 1959.

Biesecker, J. L., and others: Aneursymal bone cysts: a clinicopathologic study of 66 cases, CA **26:**615, 1970.

Bramley, P. A., and Browne, R. M.: Recurring odontogenic cysts, Br. J. Oral Surg. **5:**106, 1967.

Brandao, G. S., Ebling, H., and Souza, I. F.: Bilateral nasolabial cyst, Oral Surg. **37:**480, 1974.

Brannon, R. B.: The odontogenic keratocyst, a clinicopathologic study of 312 cases. I. Clinical features, Oral Surg. **42:**54, 1976.

Brannon, R. B.: The odontogenic keratocyst, Oral Surg. **43:**233, 1977.

Brietenecker, G., and Wepner, F.: A pleomorphic adenoma (so-called mixed tumor) in the wall of a dentigerous cyst, Oral Surg. **36**:63, 1973.

Browne, R. M.: The odontogenic keratocyst, Br. Dent. J. **128**:225, 1970; **131**:249, 1971.

Buchner, A., and Ramon, Y.: Median mandibular cyst—a rare lesion of debatable origin, Oral Surg. **37**:431, 1974.

Buchner, A.: Granular-cell odontogenic cyst, Oral Surg. **36**:707, 1973.

Campbell, R. L., and Burkes, E. J., Jr.: Nasolabial cyst: report of a case, J. Am. Dent. Assoc. **91**:1210, 1975.

Chaves, E., Arnaud, A. C., and Oliveira, A. M.: Calcifying epithelial odontogenic cyst, Oral Surg. **34**:434, 1972.

Chen, S. Y., and Miller, A. S.: Ultrastructure of the keratinizing and calcifying odontogenic cyst, Oral Surg. **39**:769, 1975.

Chretion, P. B., Carpenter, D. F., White, N. S., Harrah, J. D., and Lightbody, P. M.: Squamous carcinoma arising in a dentigerous cyst; presentation of a fatal case and review of four previously reported cases, Oral Surg. **30**:809, 1970.

Christ, T. F.: The globulomaxillary cyst; an embryologic misconception, Oral Surg. **30**:515, 1970.

Courage, G. R., North, A. F., and Hansen, L. S.: Median palatine cysts, Oral Surg. **37**:745, 1974.

David, R., and Buchner, A.: Calcifying odontogenic cysts with intracellular amyloid-like material, Oral Surg. **41**:758, 1976.

Davis, W. M., Jr., Buchs, A. U., and Davis, W. M.: Extravasation cyst diagnostic currettement: a treatment, Oral Surg. **47**:2, 1979.

Ellis, D. J., and Walters, P. J.: Aneurysmal bone cyst of the maxilla, Oral Surg. **34**:26, 1972.

Enriquez, R. E., Ciola, B., and Bahn, S. L.: Verrucous carcinoma arising in an odontogenic cyst, Oral Surg. **49**:151, 1980.

Fantasia, J. E.: Lateral periodontal cyst, Oral Surg. **48**:237, 1979.

Freedman, P. D., Lumerman, H., and Gee, J. K.: Calcifying odontogenic cyst, Oral Surg. **40**:93, 1975.

Generson, R. M., Porter, J. M., and Stratigos, G. T.: Mural odontogenic epithelial proliferations within the wall of a dentigerous cyst: their significance, Oral Surg. **42**:717, 1976.

Goodstein, D. B., and Himmelfarb, R.: Paresthesia and the traumatic bone cyst, Oral Surg. **42**:442, 1976.

Gowgiel, J. M.: Simple bone cyst of the mandible, Oral Surg. **47**:319, 1979.

Hall, A. M.: The solitary bone cyst, Oral Surg. **42**:164, 1976.

Hansen, L. S., Sapone, J., and Sproat, R. C.: Traumatic bone cysts of jaws, Oral Surg. **37**:899, 1974.

Harris, M., and Pannel, G.: Fibrinolytic activity in dental cysts, Oral Surg. **35**:818, 1973.

Hirst, E., McKellar, C. C., Ellis, J. M., and Viner Smith, K.: Malignant aneurysmal bone cyst, J. Bone Joint Surg. **53B:**791, 1970.

Howell, J. B., and Mehregan, A. H.: Pursuit of the pits in the nevoid basal cell carcinoma syndrome, Arch. Dermatol. **102:**586, 1970.

Huebner, G. R., and Turlington, E. G.: So-called traumatic (hemorrhagic) bone cysts of the jaws, Oral Surg. **31:**354, 1971.

Hutton, C. E.: Occurrence of ameloblastoma within a dentigerous cyst, Oral Surg. **24:**147, 1967.

Josell, S. D., Reiskin, A. B., and Gross, B. D.: Dentigerous cysts with mural ameloblastoma, J. Am. Dent. Assoc. **99:**634, 1979.

Keith, D. A.: Macroscopic satellite cyst formation in the odontogenic keratocyst, Oral Surg. **35:**21, 1973.

Kelley, J. E., Hibbard, E. D., and Giansanti, J. S.: Epidermal nevus syndrome, Oral Surg. **34:**774, 1972.

Kopp, W. K., Klatell, J., and Blake, M.: Basal-cell nevus syndrome with other abnormalities, Oral Surg. **27:**9, 1969.

Kramer, H. S., and Scribner, J. H.: Squamous-cell carcinoma arising in a dentigerous cyst, Oral Surg. **19:**555, 1965.

Lalonde, E. R., and Luebke, R. G.: The frequency and distribution of periapical cysts and granulomas, Oral Surg. **25:**861, 1968.

Lipshutz, H., and Abramson, B.: Basal cell nevus syndrome in a Negro, Plast. Reconstr. Surg. **47:**293, 1971.

Mainous, E. G., and Boyne, P. J.: Lingual mandibular bone concavity, J. Am. Dent. Assoc. **90:**666, 1975.

Martinelli, C., Melhado, R. M., and Callestini, E. A.: Squamous-cell carcinoma in a residual mandibular cyst, Oral Surg. **44:**274, 1977.

Meadow, R.: Malignant change in a dental cyst, Oral Surg. **21:**282, 1966.

Miller, A. S., Leifer, C., Pullon, P. A., and Bowser, M. W.: Nevoid basal-cell carcinoma syndrome, Oral Surg. **36:**533, 1973.

Miller, A. S., and Winnick, M.: Salivary gland inclusion in the anterior mandible: report of a case with a review of the literature on aberrant salivary gland tissue and neoplasms, Oral Surg. **31:**790, 1971.

Oliver, L. P.: Aneurysmal bone cyst, Oral Surg. **35:**67, 1973.

Olson, R. E., Thomsen, S., and Lin, L. M.: Odontogenic keratocyst treated by the Partsch operation and delayed enucleation: report of case, J. Am. Dent. Assoc. **94:**321, 1977.

Paul, J. K., Fay, J., and Sample, P.: Recurrent dentigerous cyst evidencing ameloblastic proliferation; report of case, J. Oral Surg. **27:**211, 1969.

Payne, T. F.: An analysis of the clinical and histopathologic parameters of the odontogenic keratocyst, Oral Surg. **33:**538, 1972.

Radden, B. C., and Reade, P. C.: Odontogenic cysts: a review and a clinicopathological study of 368 odontogenic cysts, Aust. Dent. J. **18:**218, 1973.

Redman, R. S.: Nasopalatine duct cyst with pigmented lining suggestive of olfactory epithelium, Oral Surg. **37:**421, 1974.

Reynecke, J. P.: Aneurysmal bone cyst of the maxilla, Oral Surg. **45**:441, 1978.

Riviere, G. R., and Sabet, T. Y.: Experimental follicular cysts in mice, Oral Surg. **36**:205, 1973.

Rud, J., and Pindborg, J. J.: Odontogenic keratocysts: a follow-up study of 21 cases, J. Oral Surg. **27**:323, 1969.

Ruprecht, A., and Reid, J.: Simple bone cyst, Oral Surg. **39**:826, 1975.

Ryan, D. E., and Burkes, E. J.: The multiple basal-cell nevus syndrome in a Negro family, Oral Surg. **36**:831, 1973.

Sapone, J., and Hansen, L. S.: Traumatic bone cysts of jaws: diagnosis, treatment, and prognosis, Oral Surg. **38**:127, 1974.

Sapp, J. P., and Gardner, D. G.: An ultrastructural study of the calcifications in calcifying odontogenic cysts and odontomas, Oral Surg. **44**:754, 1977.

Schofield, I. D. F.: An unusual traumatic bone cyst, Oral Surg. **38**:198, 1974.

Seemayer, T. A., Blundell, J. S., and Wiglesworth, F. W.: Pituitary craniopharyngioma with tooth formation, CA **29**:423, 1972.

Sher, M. R., and Stoopack, J. C.: Odontogenic keratocyst, Oral Surg. **37**:518, 1974.

Smith, J. W., and Nelson, M. A., Jr.: Multiple cysts of the jaws, basal-cell epithelioma of the skin, and bifid ribs, Oral Surg. **22**:306, 1966.

Soskolne, W. A., and Shteyer, A.: Median mandibular cyst, Oral Surg. **44**:84, 1977.

Stanley, H. R., Krogh, H., and Pannkuk, E.: Age changes in the epithelial components of follicles (dental sacs) associated with impacted third molars, Oral Surg. **19**:128, 1965.

Steg, R. F.: Solitary bone cyst of the mandible, Oral Surg. **20**:294, 1965.

Stoelinga, P. J. W., Peters, J. H., van de Staak, W. J. B., and Cohen, M. M., Jr.: Some new findings in the basal-cell nevus syndrome, Oral Surg. **36**:686, 1973.

Symposium: Solitary bone cysts of the mandible, Oral Surg. **8**:903, 1955.

Talman, D. E., and Stafne, E. C.: Developmental bone defects of the mandible, Oral Surg. **24**:488, 1967.

Toller, P.: Epithelial discontinuities in cysts of the jaws, Br. Dent. J. **120**:74, 1966.

Toller, P.: Origin and growth of cysts of the jaws, Ann. R. Coll. Surg. Engl. **40**:306, 1967.

Toller, P.: Newer concepts of odontogenic cysts, Int. J. Oral Surg. **1**:3, 1972.

Uemura, S., and Fuchihata, H.: Radiographic interpretation of the so-called developmental defect of the mandible, Oral Surg. **41**:120, 1976.

Weathers, D. R., and Waldron, C. A.: Unusual multilocular cysts of the jaws (botryoid odontogenic cysts), Oral Surg. **36**:235, 1973.

Whitlock, R. I. H., and Jones, J. H.: Squamous-cell carcinoma of the jaw arising in a simple cyst, Oral Surg. **24**:530, 1967.

Wilson, D. F., and Ross, A. S.: Ultrastructure of odontogenic keratocysts, Oral Surg. **45**:887, 1978.

Winer, R. A., and Doku, H. C.: Traumatic bone cyst in the maxilla, Oral Surg. **46:**367, 1978.

Wright, J. M., Jr.: Squamous odontogenic tumorlike proliferations in odontogenic cysts, Oral Surg. **47:**354, 1979.

Wysocki, G. P., and Sapp, J. P.: Scanning and transmission electron microscopy of odontogenic keratocysts, Oral Surg. **40:**494, 1975.

Zegarelli, D. J., Segarelli-Schmidt, E. C., and Zegarelli, E. V.: Hyaline bodies: some observations on their ultrastructure, Oral Surg. **42:**643, 1976.

CHAPTER 10

Odontogenic tumors of jaws

In the United States, odontogenic tumors constitute about 9% of all tumors of the oral cavity and 2.4% of all lesions biopsied in a dental office (Table 17, p. 474). By contrast, in some parts of Africa, one odontogenic tumor alone (ameloblastoma) constitutes more than 25% of all tumors of the jaws. Thus the incidence of this group of lesions has a geographic variation.

Odontogenic tumors are neoplasms that arise from the dental lamina or any of its derivatives. Besides their origin, they have other features in common. Most of them are benign, but some are locally aggressive (ameloblastoma) and at least one is malignant (ameloblastic fibrosarcoma). With rare exception, these tumors occur within the jaws and are usually slow growing.

Following is a simple, practical classification of the odontogenic tumors:

Epithelial tumors

1. Ameloblastoma
2. Acanthomatous ameloblastoma
3. Odontogenic adenomatoid tumor (adenoameloblastoma)
4. Neuroectodermal tumor of infancy (melanoameloblastoma)

Mesenchymal tumors

1. Cementoma
2. Benign cementoblastoma (true cementoma)
3. Cementifying fibroma
4. Odontogenic myxoma
5. Odontogenic fibroma
6. Dentinoma

250

Mixed tumors (epithelial and mesenchymal)

1. Ameloblastic fibroma
2. Granular cell ameloblastic fibroma
3. Ameloblastic fibro-odontoma
4. Ameloblastic odontoma (odontoameloblastoma)
5. Odontoma (compound, complex, cystic)

Rare odontogenic tumors

1. Granular cell ameloblastoma
2. Calcifying epithelial odontogenic tumor
3. Ameloblastic fibrosarcoma
4. Squamous odontogenic tumor
5. Extraosseous odontogenic tumor

After consideration of the epithelial, mesenchymal, and mixed tumors, with which a student should be familiar, some rare variants of these lesions will be discussed briefly. The latter include the odontogenic tumors that arise in the attached gin-

Table 15. Relative incidence of odontogenic tumors of jaws*

Type	Number	Percent
Ameloblastoma	78	18.18
Odontogenic adenomatoid tumor (adenoameloblastoma)	14	3.26
Neuroectodermal tumor of infancy (melanoameloblastoma)	3	0.70
Cementoma	46	10.73
Odontogenic myxoma	25	5.83
Odontogenic fibroma	98	22.84
Ameloblastic fibroma	11	2.56
Ameloblastic fibro-odontoma	14	3.26
Compound odontoma	43	10.03
Complex odontoma	22	5.13
Cystic odontoma	30	6.99
Odontoma (unclassified)	31	7.23
Odontogenic tumors (rare)	14	3.26
TOTAL	429	100.00

*Based on personal analyses of clinical, radiographic, microscopic, and follow-up data on more than 20,000 cases.

giva. Since the gingiva routinely contains odontogenic epithelium, the origin of these tumors at this site is not unexpected.

Melanin has been described within the epithelial cells of a
number of odontogenic cysts and tumors. These include the calcifying odontogenic cyst, ameloblastic fibroma, ameloblastic
odontoma, calcifying epithelial odontogenic tumor, and ameloblastic fibro-odontoma.

The incidence of various types of odontogenic tumors is included in Table 15.

EPITHELIAL TUMORS

Ameloblastoma. This lesion is the most aggressive of the
odontogenic tumors of the jaws and constitutes about 18% of
these lesions (Table 15).

Like all tumors of its group, the ameloblastoma arises from
the dental lamina or a derivative of the lamina (enamel organ,
epithelial rests, follicular cysts). Consequently it is composed
exclusively of epithelium. It usually occurs between the ages of
20 and 50 years (with the average age being 39). About 80%
occur in the mandible, and the remainder in the maxilla. In
both the mandible and the maxilla the majority (80%) are located in the molar area and a few (10% to 20%) in the premolar
area. Only rarely is the anterior portion of the jaws involved.

The tumor is slow growing, the average duration before
treatment being five to eight years. Clinically the affected site
may appear normal or be enlarged (Fig. 10-1) with displacement
and malocclusion of regional teeth. The mucosa covering the
tumor mass is normal (Fig. 10-2). The lesions are usually painless. About 25% to 30% arise in preexisting follicular cysts, and
5% to 6% of the follicular cysts show ameloblastic proliferation.
Recurrences are common (about 33%), but this is probably due
to incomplete removal.

There may be areas of radiolucency that are unicystic or
multicystic (Fig. 10-3, *A* to *C*). Bony septa may extend into
these areas and impart a soap bubble appearance (Fig. 10-3, *A*
and *B*). Occlusal radiographs show expansion and deformity of

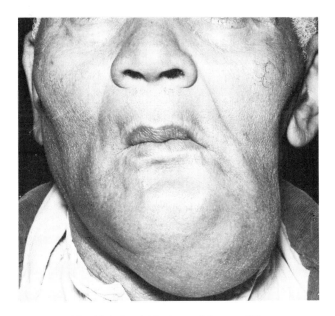

Fig. 10-1. Ameloblastoma of the mandible.

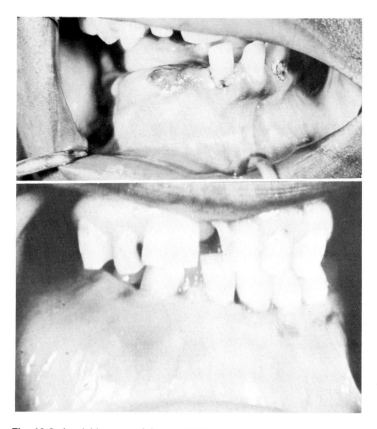

Fig. 10-2. Ameloblastoma of the mandible (two cases). Note the marked enlargement of the mandible.

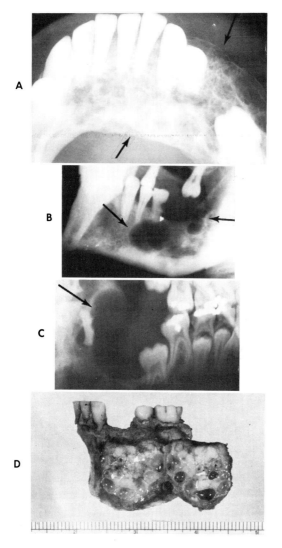

Fig. 10-3. Ameloblastoma of the mandible. **A** and **B,** Soap bubble–like multicystic radiolucencies. **C,** Unicystic lesion. **D,** Gross specimen. Note the multicystic appearance of the lesion.

the cortex, but the latter is seldom destroyed. The tumor may be associated with an impacted tooth and may appear as a radiolucency around the impacted crown (Fig. 10-3, *C*).

Gross specimens usually show a multicystic lesion of the jaw (Fig. 10-3, *D*).

Microscopically an ameloblastoma is exclusively epithelial. The epithelium forms sheets, islands, and cords in which the peripheral layer is formed by columnar or cuboidal cells that resemble ameloblasts, and the central mass is formed usually be stellate cells resembling the stellate reticulum of the enamel organ (Fig. 10-4). Although this is the classic and usual microscopic picture, variations do occur. The stroma of the tumor consists of fibrous connective tissue, and the tumor is not encapsulated. Tumor islands and clusters infiltrate the marrow spaces far beyond the major bulk of the tumor mass. In reality, therefore, the tumor is more extensive than its radiographic shadow and requires a wider excision or curettage than may appear necessary.

Surgical reaction of the tumor is the treatment of choice.

From time to time, case reports of so-called malignant ameloblastomas have appeared in the literature. Many of these lesions are, in reality, intramandibular and intramaxillary adenocarcinomas of minor salivary glands. The latter glands are included within the jaws during embryogenesis. In addition to these cases of mistaken diagnosis, an ameloblastoma may become aspirated during a surgical procedure and may give rise to a secondary focus in the lung. For this reason the metastatic foci of a majority of so-called malignant ameloblastomas have been observed in the lungs; but such lesions are not true metastases. On very rare occasion, however, an ameloblastoma may become malignant and metastasize to regional nodes as well as the lungs.

Acanthomatous ameloblastoma. Except for its microscopic appearance, an acanthomatous ameloblastoma is identical to an ameloblastoma (Fig. 10-5). Part or all of the tumor consists of epithelial islands composed of squamous cells. The latter may

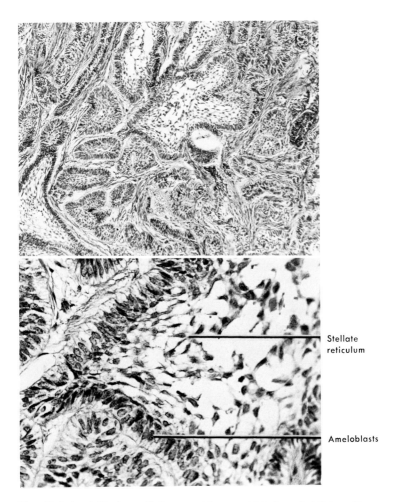

Stellate
reticulum

Ameloblasts

Fig. 10-4. Ameloblastoma. Cells resembling ameloblasts and stellate reticulum can usually be identified.

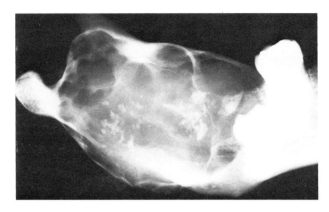

Fig. 10-5. Acanthomatous ameloblastoma. Note the expansile soap bubble–like radiolucency of the mandible.

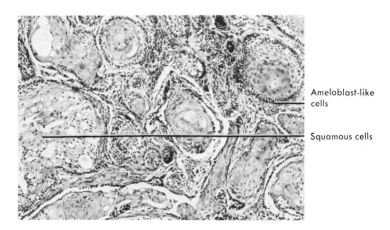

Ameloblast-like cells

Squamous cells

Fig. 10-6. Acanthomatous ameloblastoma. In addition to the other characteristics of an ameloblastoma, the presence of squamous cells is an important feature.

be keratinized and resemble cells of the squamous cell carcinoma (Fig. 10-6). Part of the tumor may show the characteristic ameloblast-like cells, which resemble stellate reticulum.

At one time the acanthomatous ameloblastoma was separated from other ameloblastomas on the assumption that is represented a more aggressive or malignant variety. This assumption is incorrect; as mentioned above, except for its microscopic features just described, the lesion is identical to the ameloblastoma.

Odontogenic adenomatoid tumor (adenoameloblastoma). This lesion is an epithelial odontogenic tumor that constitutes about 3% of all odontogenic tumors of the jaws. It occurs usually in the second decade of life.

Females are afflicted about twice as frequently as males, and the maxilla is involved almost twice as often as the mandible In the maxilla the canine area is the preferred site. The majority (75%) of these tumors are associated with impacted teeth and therefore on radiographs are mistaken for dentigerous cysts (Fig. 10-7). The tumor may be asymptomatic, or it may produce an enlargement in the area (Fig. 10-7, A).

An odontogenic adenomatoid tumor characteristically shows a circumscribed area of radiolucency often associated with an impacted tooth. In some instances the radiolucency has small radiopaque foci. When the tumor is large, the cortex of the involved bone may be slightly expanded (Fig. 10-7); this is the exception, however, rather than the rule.

Unlike other ameloblastomas, an odontogenic adenomatoid tumor may be encapsulated. It is composed of ductlike structures lined by columnar or cuboidal epithelium. The spaces between the ducts are packed with whorls or loosely arranged epithelial cells (Fig. 10-8). Some lesions show microscopic foci of calcification. Because of encapsulation, marrow spaces surrounding the lesion are free of tumor. Most tumors are associated with impacted teeth or irregular masses of calcified material. In many instances, they present as a partially cystic lesion; and the vast majority, if not all, of odontogenic adenomatoid

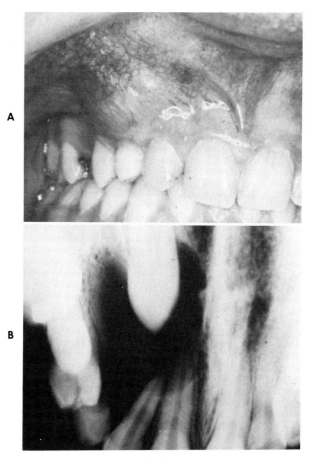

Fig. 10-7. Odontogenic adenomatoid tumor. **A,** Swelling in the area of a retained deciduous canine. **B,** Radiolucency around the impacted permanent canine.

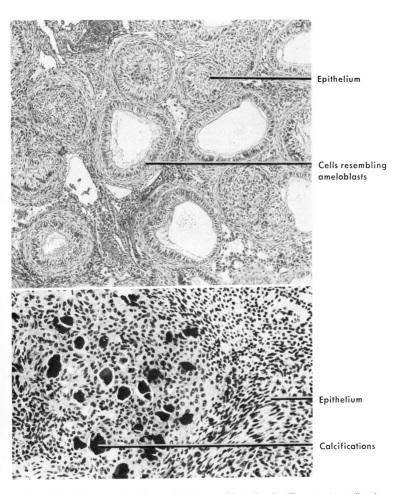

Epithelium

Cells resembling
ameloblasts

Epithelium

Calcifications

Fig. 10-8. Odontogenic adenomatoid tumor. Note the ductlike structures lined
by columnar cells. In between the "ducts," the epithelial cells are densely
packed.

tumors are believed to arise from the epithelial lining of follicular cysts.

Odontogenic adenomatoid tumors are treated by local currettage, following which it does not recur. The lesion therefore is far less aggressive than the ameloblastoma or the acanthomatous ameloblastoma and should be treated most conservatively.

Neuroectodermal tumor of infancy (melanoameloblastoma). This tumor constitutes about 0.7% of all odontogenic tumors of the jaws. It is known by many other names (retinal anlage tumor, anlage tumor, progonoma, pigmented ameloblastoma), each name referring to a different theory of origin. The most favored views are that the tumor arises from neuroectoderm, the precursor of the retina, or that it is odontogenic.

The neuroectodermal tumor of infancy is a rare tumor, with fewer than sixty cases reported in the literature. It is usually benign and occurs during the first year of life, in many instances during the first 6 months. It is seen more commonly in females than in males. Most cases (80%) occur in the maxilla, and the anterior portion is the preferred site (Figs. 10-9 and 10-10). Lesions in areas other than the jaws have been reported (skull, shoulder, uterus, and elsewhere).

Because of the small size of the maxilla in the early months of life, the tumor gives the false impression of being quite extensive. It presents as a relatively rapidly growing swelling of the anterior part of the maxilla (but it may be anywhere in either jaw) (Fig. 10-10, *A*). The swelling elevates the infant's upper lip, making sucking difficult. The overlying mucosa may be intact. In all other respects, the infant appears healthy and normal. Radiolucent areas and displacement of the developing teeth (Fig. 10-10, *B*) may be evident.

Microscopic characteristics of the melanoameloblastoma are diagnostic. The tumor consists of two types of epithelial cells lying in islands and separated by dense connective tissue bundles (Fig. 10-11): one type is a large cuboidal cell with abundant cytoplasm that contains brown melanin granules; the other type consists of a deeply basophilic round nucleus and scanty cyto-

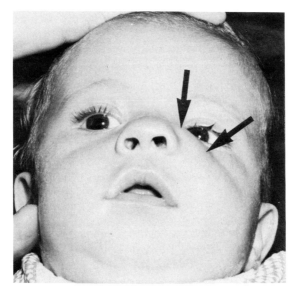

Fig. 10-9. Neuroectodermal tumor of infancy (melanoameloblastoma). Note the enlargement of the anterior left maxilla (arrows).

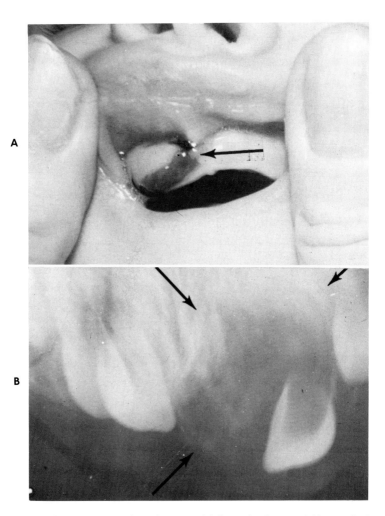

Fig. 10-10. Neuroectodermal tumor of infancy (melanoameloblastoma). **A,** The lesion presents as a swelling in the anterior part of the maxilla. **B,** Note the radiolucency and displacement of the central incisor. (Courtesy Daniel R. Young, D.D.S., Pomona, Calif., and Howard Davis, D.D.S., Bellflower, Calif.)

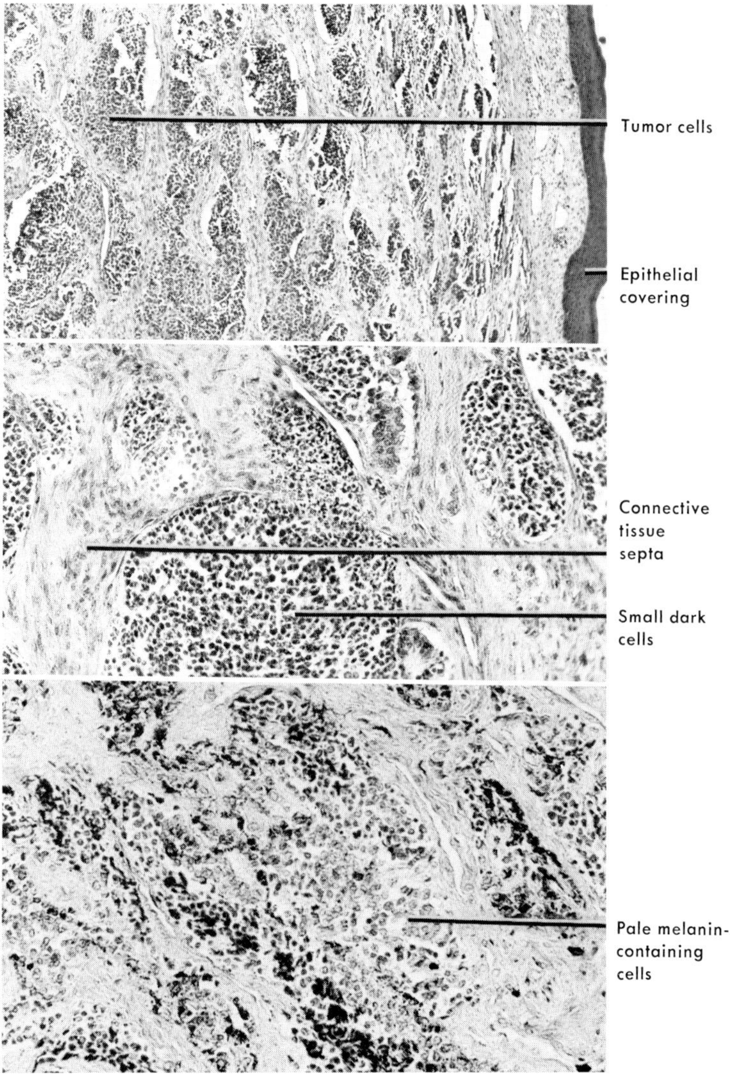
Tumor cells
Epithelial covering
Connective tissue septa
Small dark cells
Pale melanin-containing cells

Fig. 10-11. Neuroectodermal tumor of pregnancy (melanoameloblastoma). This lesion is composed of pigment-containing cells and small cells without pigment. Connective tissue septa intervene between islands of cells.

plasm. The tumor islands may consist of one or both types. Mitoses and pleomorphism are absent.

Neuroectodermal tumors of infancy are usually benign tumors, as mentioned previously, and should be treated by conservative surgical excision. Local recurrences occur in about 15% of cases, and a malignant metastasizing lesion has been reported.

MESENCHYMAL TUMORS

Cementoma. Also known as periapical cemental dysplasia, periapical fibro-osteoma, cementoblastoma, and periapical fibrous dysplasia, the cementoma constitutes a little more than 10% of all odontogenic tumors of the jaws (Table 15).

The cementoma is a periapical lesion (Fig. 10-12) and is

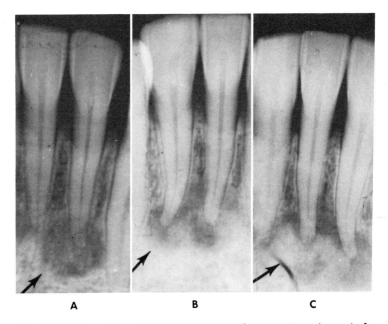

A	**B**	**C**

Fig. 10-12. Three stages in the development of a cementoma (arrows). **A,** Radiolucent stage. **B,** Partly radiolucent and partly radiopaque stage. **C,** Radiopaque stage.

asymptomatic. More than 70% of cases occur in blacks. The lesion is almost ten times as common in females as in males, and the majority of cases occur after the second decade of life. About 92% involve the mandible, usually the incisors. The maxilla rarely is involved. Lesions may be single or multiple (Fig. 10-12). Regional teeth are vital.

The radiographic appearance of a cementoma depends on the stage of development of the tumor. In the first stage a periapical radiolucency is seen that resembles the radiolucency seen with a dental granuloma or radicular cyst (Fig. 10-12, *A*). In the second stage there are radiopaque specks (Fig. 10-12, *B*). In the third stage the lesions appear as circumscribed areas of dense radiopacity (Fig. 10-12, *C*). An average of six years is required for the lesion to progress from the first stage to the third.

Microscopically, in the first stage of development, the lesion consists of young fibroblasts and a moderate amount of collagen fibers (Fig. 10-13, *A*). In the second stage the lesion shows the beginning formation of spicules and islands of a basophilic cellular or moderately cellular calcified tissue that resembles cementum (Fig. 10-13, *B*). In the last stage the entire lesion consists of deeply basophilic calcified masses in which few cells, numerous resting and reversal lines, and almost no small marrow spaces are seen (Fig. 10-13, *C*).

The cementoma is characterized by extremely slow and limited growth. It does not require any treatment.

Benign cementoblastoma (true cementoma). This rare cementum-producing tumor reaches a much larger size than the cementoma and may lead to jaw expansion. It is attached to the root of an erupted permanent tooth and is seen most often in the mandibular molar region. It appears as a dense radiopacity with a peripheral radiolucent border. Patients are under 25 years of age.

Histologic sections show masses of cellular and acellular cementum arranged in a trabecular pattern. Conservative removal is curative.

Cementifying fibroma. The cementifying fibroma is a rare odontogenic tumor that is not related to the apices of the

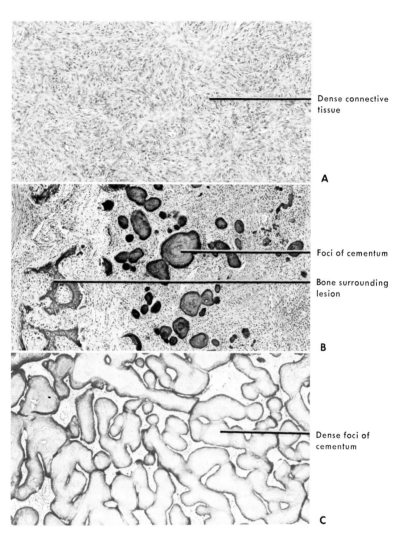

Dense connective tissue

A

Foci of cementum

Bone surrounding lesion

B

Dense foci of cementum

C

Fig. 10-13. Three stages in the development of a cementoma.

teeth—in contradistinction to the cementoma, which is periapical in location. It is usually solitary and may be asymptomatic or produce enlargement of the jaw. It may appear as a radiolucent defect in which radiopaque specks can be seen.

Microscopic sections reveal a tumor comprised of fibroblasts and collagen bundles. Within the fibrous stroma numerous foci of deeply basophilic, relatively acellular calcified material resembling cementum can be seen. Since the cementum and bone are closely related if not identical tissues, distinguishing between them is often impossible. Many of the so-called cementifying fibromas are, in reality, ossifying fibromas in which the bone tissue appears basophilic and superficially resembles cementum.

Odontogenic myxoma. This tumor constitutes about 6% of all odontogenic tumors of the jaws (Table 15) and must be distinguished from the true myxoma. The maxilla is more commonly affected than the mandible. The tumor usually occurs in individuals under 35 years of age and may be associated with an impacted tooth (Fig. 10-14). It is slow growing but eventually may lead to localized expansion of the jaw. It characteristically appears as a well-defined radiolucency (Fig. 10-14).

Microscopic sections show few star-shaped cells with overabundant, lightly basophilic intercellular substance (Fig. 10-15). The ultrastructure of these cells, called the myxoblasts, shows prominent, rough endoplasmic reticulum and prominent Golgi complex, and they produce large amounts of glycosaminoglycans. The latter appear in the light microscope as mucoid basophilic material. Within this tissue isolated foci of epithelium may be seen. The presence of these cells distinguishes this tumor from the true myxoma. Whereas the true myxoma is an infiltrating lesion with great potential for recurrence, the odontogenic myxoma is not as aggressive; and local excision is curative.

Odontogenic fibroma. The odontogenic fibroma constitutes about 23% of all odontogenic tumors of the jaws (Table 15) and is therefore the most common of these lesions. However, its

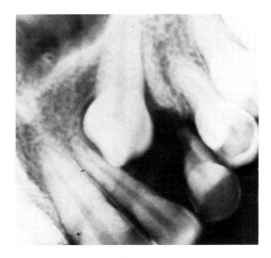

Fig. 10-14. Odontogenic myxoma. These lesions are usually associated with the crowns of unerupted teeth and are often mistaken for dentigerous cysts.

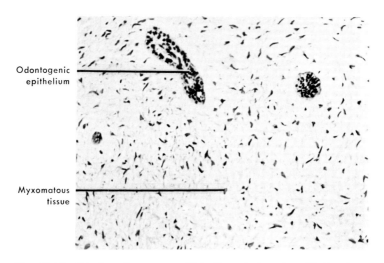

Odontogenic epithelium

Myxomatous tissue

Fig. 10-15. Odontogenic myxoma. Note the odontogenic epithelium in a myxomatous stroma.

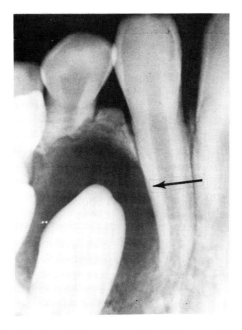

Fig. 10-16. Odontogenic fibroma associated with a mandibular canine.

great frequency has not been well recognized, because radiographically it resembles or is identical to a dentigerous cyst and consequently is misdiagnosed (Fig. 10-16).

The distinction between this lesion and a hyperplastic dental follicle is often arbitrary; therefore, the incidence of this lesion is a matter of dispute. The fibroma occurs with equal frequency in both sexes, usually in the second decade of life. The mandible is affected more commonly than the maxilla, with the third molar and canine areas the most common site of involvement.

Clinically an odontogenic fibroma is asymptomatic or may lead to a slight enlargement of the area and is almost always associated with an impacted tooth. It appears as a radiolucency of varying size associated with the crown of the tooth (Fig. 10-

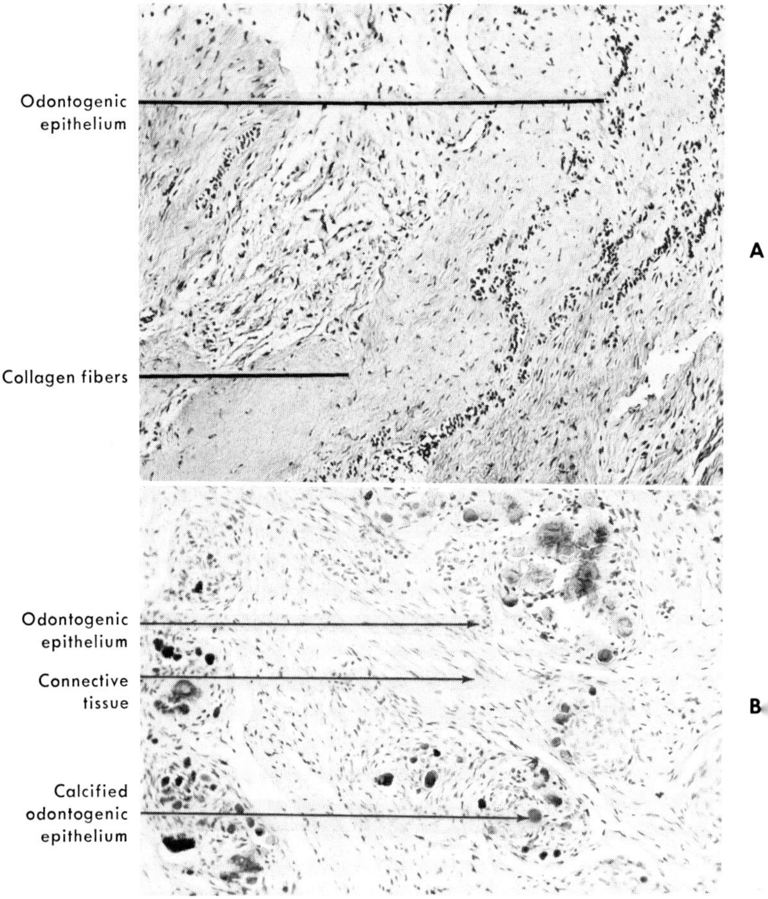

Fig. 10-17. A, Odontogenic fibroma. Note the odontogenic epithelial cells in a mass of dense collagen. B, Calcifying odontogenic fibroma. The lesion is composed of dense fibrous tissue in which calcifying epithelial cells can be seen.

16) and therefore resembles a dentigerous cyst. At exploration or surgery, however, a solid rather than a cystic lesion is found.

Microscopic sections show a circumscribed mass of dense or loosely arranged connective tissue in which strands and islands of epithelium are dispersed (Fig. 10-17, *A*). These epithelial cells do not mimic ameloblasts. In some cases they undergo calcification, and the lesion is called a *calcifying odontogenic fibroma* (Fig. 10-17, *B*). The odontogenic fibroma arises from the tooth follicle (i.e., the connective tissue that surrounds that enamel organ).

Odontogenic fibromas are characterized by limited and slow growth and should be treated only by curettage.

Dentinoma. The dentinoma is believed to be a mesenchymal, odontogenic tumor composed exclusively of dentin. It is extremely rare, if indeed it occurs at all. Lesions called dentinomas are slow growing, occur in the mandible, are radiopaque, and on microscopic examination are seen to consist only of dentinlike material. In reality, they are probably osteomas or odontomas.

MIXED TUMORS (EPITHELIAL AND MESENCHYMAL)

Ameloblastic fibroma. The ameloblastic fibroma is an odontogenic tumor composed of both epithelial and mesenchymal elements. It constitutes about 2.5% of all odontogenic tumors of the jaws (Table 15) and affects a younger age group than does the usual ameloblastoma. The majority of patients are children; 71% are under 20 years of age, and the average age is 15 years. Two out of three patients are male, and the mandible is involved more frequently than the maxilla (9:1).

The premolar and molar area is the preferred site of an ameloblastic fibroma, and the tumor often is associated with an impacted tooth. The lesion is slow growing and may be asymptomatic or produce enlargements of the jaw and migration of teeth. It appears as multiocular areas of radiolucency with expansion of the cortex of the jaw and in some instances displace-

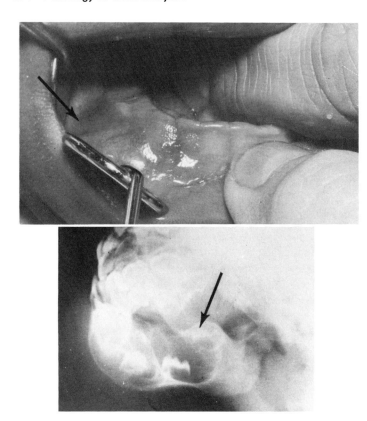

Fig. 10-18. Ameloblastic fibroma. Note the expansion of the jaw and displacement of teeth (arrow).

ment of teeth (Fig. 10-18). Most of the lesions are associated with unerupted teeth.

Microscopic sections show a characteristic picture. There is a background of young, highly cellular mesenchymal tissue that resembles or duplicates the dental papilla of the tooth germ; and within this young mesenchyme are thin strands and islands of odontogenic epithelium (Fig. 10-19). The cells making up

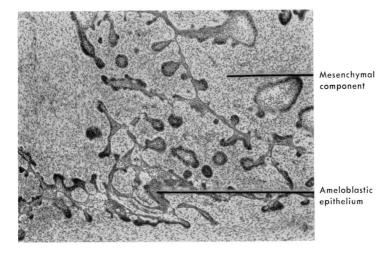

Mesenchymal
component

Ameloblastic
epithelium

Fig. 10-19. Ameloblastic fibroma. Note the proliferation of odontogenic epithelium in an abundant, highly cellular mesenchymal stroma.

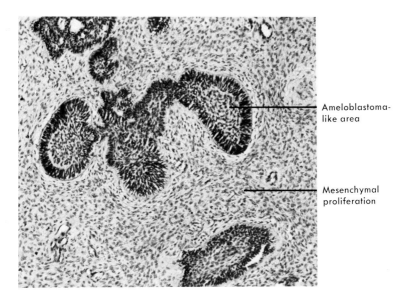

Ameloblastoma-
like area

Mesenchymal
proliferation

Fig. 10-20. Photomicrograph of an ameloblastic fibroma. Note the ameloblastoma-like area and the mesenchymal proliferation.

these strands and islands may be small and closely resemble cells in the dental lamina. In many areas, however, cuboidal and columnar cells resembling ameloblasts and stellate cells resembling stellate reticulum can be seen (Fig. 10-20). The tumor has no calcified tissue component. It is not encapsulated like the odontogenic adenomatoid tumor, and it does not diffusely infiltrate the surrounding marrow spaces like the ordinary ameloblastoma. The tumor tissue extends into the bone as a solid mass.

Ameloblastic fibromas have great potential for recurrence (43%) and can undergo malignant transformation to ameloblastic fibrosarcomas. The treatment of an ameloblastic fibroma should therefore consist of wide excision and careful follow-up.

Granular-cell ameloblastic fibroma. This is a rare odontogenic tumor that is a variant of the ameloblastic fibroma. It occurs usually in the female, is more common in the posterior part of the mandible, is seen in blacks more often than in whites, and patients are usually older than 50 years of age. It usually appears as a radiolucency of long duration, but sometimes radiolucent and radiopaque areas can be seen. Microscopic features consist of islands and strands of odontogenic epithelium (such as that seen in the ameloblastic fibroma) that lie in a stroma of sheets of large granular cells. Ultrastructural examination reveals that these cells are mesenchymal in origin and resemble those seen in granular cell myoblastoma and in congenital epulis of newborn. The lesion is benign, and local removal is curative. There are no recurrences.

Ameloblastic fibro-odontoma. The ameloblastic fibro-odontoma is a benign lesion constituting about 3% of odontogenic tumors of the jaws (Table 15).

This lesion consists of calcified dental tissues as well as actively proliferating odontogenic epithelium and mesenchyme. In essence, it is an ameloblastic fibroma in which hard dental tissues are an additional feature. It occurs in childhood and young adulthood, and almost 75% of patients are less than 20 years of age. The tumors are more common in the mandible than in the maxilla, and more than 90% occur in the posterior part of the jaw. Three males are afflicted for every two females. It is asymptomatic but may enlarge and deform the involved bone.

An ameloblastic fibro-odontoma characteristically appears as an irregular radiopacity surrounded by or associated with a radiolucent zone (Fig. 10-21).

Microscopic sections reveal areas of calcified and uncalcified hard dental tissues (dentin, predentin, enamel, enamel matrix, cementum), islands of mesenchyme that resemble pulp tissue, and numerous islands and cords of odontogenic epithelium that consist of ameloblast-like and stellate reticulum–like cells (Fig. 10-22). In some areas these odontogenic cells cover the enamel matrix the same way the enamel organ covers the enamel. In other areas the odontogenic epithelium resembles the dental lamina.

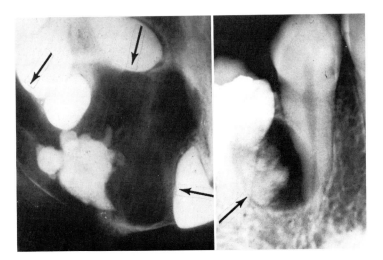

Fig. 10-21. Ameloblastic fibro-odontoma (two cases). This tumor is partly radiolucent and partly radiopaque (arrows) and may be mistaken for a cystic odontoma.

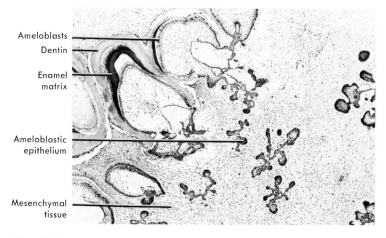

Ameloblasts

Dentin

Enamel
matrix

Ameloblastic
epithelium

Mesenchymal
tissue

Fig. 10-22. Ameloblastic fibro-odontoma. Note the presence of enamel, dentin, epithelium, and pulplike tissue. (Compare with Fig. 10-24.)

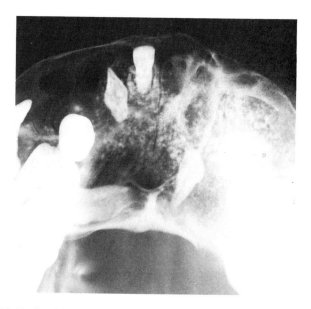

Fig. 10-23. Ameloblastic odontoma. Note the expansion of the jaw, the radiolucency, and the areas of radiopacity.

Microscopic features appear to combine the appearances of an ameloblastic fibroma and an odontoma. In fact, if left undisturbed, this lesion apparently would terminate in a complex odontoma.

The ameloblastic fibro-odontoma, in spite of its name, is not an aggressive lesion. It is often circumscribed, and local conservative removal and curettage are curative.

Ameloblastic odontoma (odontoameloblastoma). This rare mixed odontogenic tumor consists of the simultaneous occurrence of an ameloblastoma and a composite odontoma. It occurs in children, is more common in the mandible, and is usually expansile. It appears as a radiolucency with radiopaque areas (Fig. 10-23).

Histologic features consist of an ameloblastoma (islands of columnar cells around stellate reticulum) with foci and islands of dentin, enamel, enamel matrix, cementum, and pulp tissue (Fig. 10-24). These features are different from those of an ameloblastic fibro-odontoma insofar as the mesenchymal proliferation is not as pronounced, whereas the ameloblastic proliferation is prominent and similar to that seen in the usual ameloblastoma (p. 256).

An ameloblastic odontoma is more aggressive than an ameloblastic fibro-odontoma and requires complete excision.

Odontoma (compound, complex, cystic). Odontomas constitute about 22% of all odontogenic tumors of the jaws (Table 15) and are composed of hard dental tissues.

Odontomas are diagnosed most often in the second decade of life, and 65% of them occur in the maxilla. Compound odontomas (see p. 281) are more common in the anterior maxilla, whereas complex odontomas occur more often in the posterior part of the upper and lower jaws. These tumors occur slightly more often in males, and the most common presenting symptom is an impacted tooth with retention of deciduous teeth. Rarely they assume large sizes and produce deformity of normal jaw contours. They are slow growing and may persist without any symptoms for decades, increasing for a time and then remaining static for the rest of the patient's life.

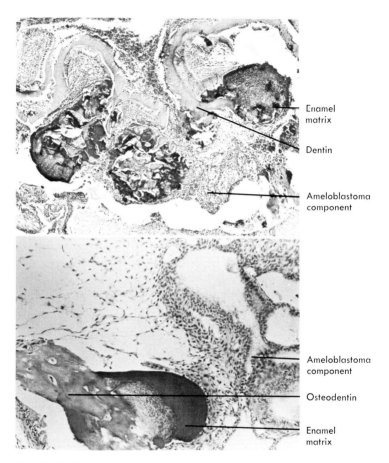

Enamel matrix

Dentin

Ameloblastoma component

Ameloblastoma component

Osteodentin

Enamel matrix

Fig. 10-24. Photomicrograph of an ameloblastic odontoma. Note the amelo-blastoma-like areas and the regions of dentin and enamel. The mesenchymal proliferation is not as marked as in the ameloblastic fibro-odontoma (Compare with Fig. 10-22.)

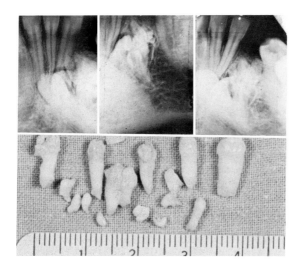

Fig. 10-25. Compound odontoma. This tumor is composed of numerous toothlike structures.

On the basis of gross, radiographic, and microscopic features, two types of odontomas are recognized: *compound* (Fig. 10-25) (or compound composite) and *complex* (Fig. 10-26) (or complex composite). Both types appear as clearly outlined dense radiopacities often surrounded by a thin radiolucent zone. In the compound type crudely formed teeth of varying size and shape may be recognized in the radiopacity (Fig. 10-25). In the complex type the radiopacity does not have a specific shape but appears as a disorganized irregular mass (Fig. 10-26).

Microscopically a compound odontoma shows toothlike structures (Fig. 10-27) consisting of a central core of pulp tissue encased in a shell of dentin and partially covered by enamel. A complex odontoma consists of a haphazard conglomerate of dentin, enamel, enamel matrix, cementum, and pulp tissue (Fig. 10-28).

Compound and complex odontomas are lesions of limited growth whose treatment consists of local removal. Because they

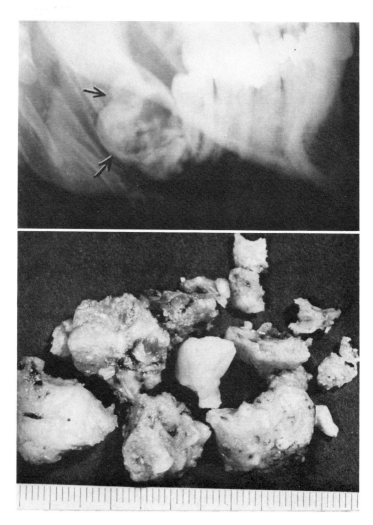

Fig. 10-26. Complex odontoma (arrows). This tumor is composed of a conglomerate mass of dentin, enamel, cementum, and pulp.

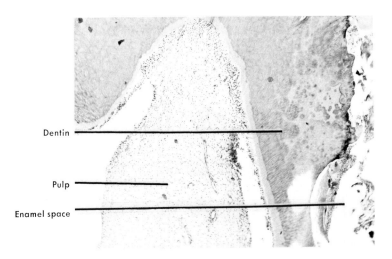

Dentin

Pulp

Enamel space

Fig. 10-27. Compound odontoma. The pulp, dentin, and enamel are arranged to form toothlike structures.

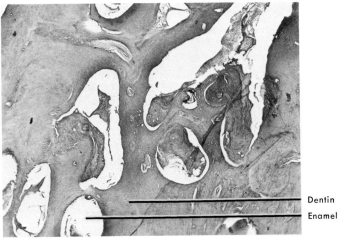

Dentin

Enamel space

Fig. 10-28. Complex odontoma. The dentin and enamel form an ill-organized mass.

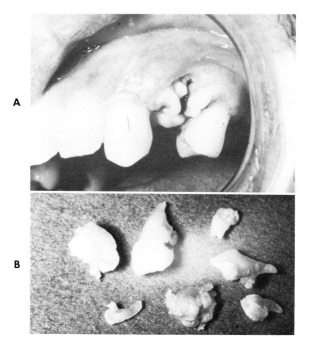

Fig. 10-29. A, Complex odontoma that has erupted into the oral cavity. **B** is the gross specimen after removal.

are separated from the surrounding bone by a zone of connective tissue, they are easily enucleated. They do not recur. In rare instances they may erupt into the oral cavity (Fig. 10-29).

Sometimes an odontoma will be seen in which a cyst is associated with the tumor. This cyst is usually lined by stratified squamous epithelium, and it develops from the enamel organ or organs that gave rise to the odontoma. Such a lesion (i.e., an odontoma with an associated cystic cavity) is called a *cystic odontoma* and constitutes about 7% of all odontogenic tumors of the jaws (Table 15). This lesion behaves as a dentigerous cyst and therefore must be excised.

RARE ODONTOGENIC TUMORS

In addition to the usual odontogenic tumors just described, there are a few rare variants of the lesions that require only brief mention.

Granular cell ameloblastoma. This is a variant of the ameloblastoma that microscopically shows numerous large eosinophilic granular cells (Fig. 10-30, *A* and *B*). These cells form the central mass of epithelial islands and cords. The periphery of the islands is made up of tall, columnar cells. Granular cell ameloblastomas occur predominantly in the posterior part of the mandible, the average age of patients is 41 years, and about 40% of the lesions occur in nonwhites. The lesion recurs with greater frequency than does the ameloblastoma and therefore requires careful follow-up.

Calcifying epithelial odontogenic tumor. This tumor occurs about equally in both sexes. The age range is from 8 to 92 years, with a mean age of about 40 years. There is a marked predilection in the molar-premolar area, and the mandible is involved in about 70% of cases (Fig. 10-31). The majority of lesions are associated with embedded teeth (70%). This tumor can occur in extraosseous locations. The radiograph shows an impacted tooth with a radiolucent area containing small or large radiopaque foci around the crown. Microscopic sections show islands of polyhedral epithelium with foci of calcification and the formation of a hyaline material (which has been shown to be amyloid, Fig. 10-30, *C*). This rare tumor has a low recurrence rate and requires local excision.

Ameloblastic fibrosarcoma. This is a rare malignant odontogenic tumor of the jaws, and less than twenty-five cases have been described. Most reported cases (71%) have occurred during the second, third, and fourth decades of life. There is no sex predilection, but the mandible is involved more often than the maxilla. This tumor is capable of metastasis and is believed to arise in a preexisting benign odontogenic tumor, usually an ameloblastic fibroma. Multiple recurrences following multiple surgical procedures appear to be an important feature in the

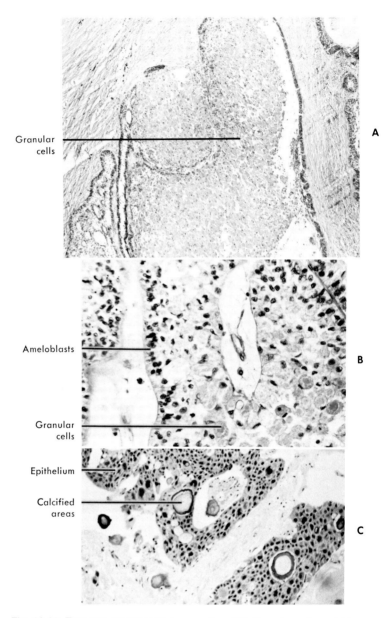

Granular
cells   **A**

Ameloblasts   **B**

Granular
cells

Epithelium

Calcified
areas   **C**

Fig. 10-30. Two rare odontogenic tumors. **A** and **B,** Granular cell ameloblastoma. **C,** Calcifying epithelial odontogenic tumor.

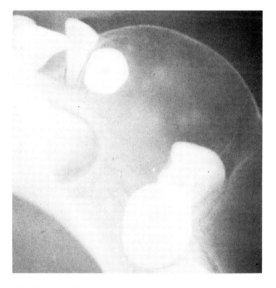

Fig. 10-31. Calcifying epithelial odontogenic tumor. Note the expansion of the buccal cortical plate of the mandible as well as the minute areas of radiopacity in an otherwise radiolucent lesion.

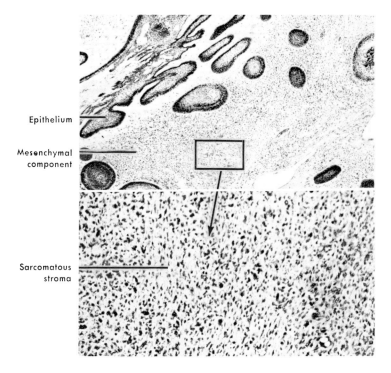

Epithelium

Mesenchymal
component

Sarcomatous
stroma

Fig. 10-32. Ameloblastic fibrosarcoma. Note the proliferation of ameloblasts in a sarcomatous stroma.

transformation of benign odontogenic tumors to malignant ones. The lesion appears as a radiolucency. The microscopic picture is identical to that of an ameloblastic fibroma except the mesenchymal portion of the tumor shows pleomorphism and mitoses (Fig. 10-32). In view of its growth potential, radical resection is recommended. Radiation therapy is of no value.

Squamous odontogenic tumor. This benign odontogenic tumor consists primarily of squamous epithelium. Local excision is curative.

Extraosseous odontogenic tumors. On rare occassion various odontogenic tumors occur outside the jaws; the gingiva is the usual site. They grow slowly and may produce bone resorption from the periosteal surface—in which case they appear as a radiolucent area. Ameloblastomas, odontogenic fibromas, calcifying epithelial odontogenic tumors, and odontogenic adenomatoid tumors have been observed in the soft oral tissues. Local excision is the treatment of choice.

Ameloblastoma-like lesions have been seen in the tibia and are referred to as *adamantinomas of the tibia*. Some of these metastasize widely. Their true nature is not known.

Ameloblastomas and dentigerous cysts can also arise in the area of the pituitary gland. In this location they are known as *craniopharyngiomas* or *suprasellar cysts*. These lesions are of odontogenic origin and may contain teeth or tooth structures. The tumors and cysts originate from oral epithelium, which in the embryo forms a portion of the pituitary gland (Rathke's pouch).

REFERENCES

Abrams, A. M., Kirby, J. W., and Melrose, R. J.: Cementoblastoma, Oral Surg. **38**:394, 1974.

Adekeye, E. O., Edwards, M. B., and Goubran, G. F.: Ameloblastic fibrosarcoma, Oral Surg. **46**:254, 1978.

Anneroth, G., Isacsson, G., and Sigurdsson, A.: Benign cementoblastoma (true cementoma), Oral Surg. **40**:141, 1975.

Balfour, R. S., Loscalo, L. J., and Sulka, M.: Multicentric peripheral ameloblastoma, J. Oral Surg. **31**:335, 1973.

Bedrick, A. E., and Solomon, M. P.: The adenomatoid odontogenic tumor: an unusual clinical presentation, Oral Surg. **48**:143, 1979.

Bhaskar, S. N.: Adenoameloblastoma: its histogenesis and report of 15 new cases, J. Oral Surg. **22**:218, 1964.

Bhaskar, S. N.: Gingival cyst and the keratinizing ameloblastoma, Oral Surg. **19**:796, 1965.

Bhaskar, S. N.: Oral pathology in the dental office: survey of 20,575 biopsy specimens, J. Am. Dent. Assoc. **76**:761, 1968.

Birkholz, H., Sills, A. H., and Reid, R. A.: Peripheral ameloblastoma, J. Am. Dent. Assoc. **97**:658, 1978.

Brekke, J. H., and Gorlin, R. J.: Melanotic neuroectodermal tumor of infancy, J. Oral Surg. **33**:858, 1975.

Buchner, A., and David, R.: Amyloid-like material in odontogenic tumors, J. Oral Surg. **34:**320, 1976.

Budnick, S. D.: Compound and complex odontomas, Oral Surg. **42:**501, 1976.

Castner, D. V., McCully, A. C., and Hiatt, W. R.: Intracystic ameloblastoma in the young patient, Oral Surg. **23:**127, 1967.

Cataldo, E., Nathanson, N., and Shklar, G.: Ameloblastic sarcoma of the mandible, Oral Surg. **16:**953, 1963.

Chandi, S. M., and Simon, G. T.: Calcifying odontogenic cyst: report of two cases, Oral Surg. **30:**99, 1970.

Chaudhry, A. P., Holte, N. D., and Vickers, R. A.: Calcifying epithelial odontogenic tumor, Oral Surg. **15:**843, 1962.

Christ, T. F., Cavalaris, C. J., and Crocker, D. J.: Papilliferous ameloblastic fibroma, Oral Surg. **34:**806, 1972.

Cina, M. T., Dahlin, D. C., and Gores, R. J.: Ameloblastic sarcoma, Oral Surg. **15:**696, 1962.

Corio, R. L., Crawford. B. E., and Schaberg, S. J.: Benign cementoblastoma, Oral Surg. **41:**525, 1976.

Couch, R. D., Morris, E. E., and Vellios, F.: Granular cell ameloblastic fibroma, Am. J. Clin. Pathol. **37:**398, 1962.

Courtney, R. M., and Kerr, D. A.: The odontogenic adenomatoid tumor, Oral Surg. **39:**424, 1975.

Curran, J. B., and Collins, A. P.: Benign (true) cementoblastoma of the mandible, Oral Surg. **35:**168, 1973.

Decker, R. M., and Laffitte, H. B.: Peripheral calcifying epithelial odontogenic tumor, Oral Surg. **23:**398, 1967.

DiBona, M. C., and Cranin, A. N.: Acanthomatous ameloblastoma of the maxilla, Gen. Dentistry. **28:**32, 1980.

Dodge, O. G.: Tumors of the jaw, odontogenic tissues and maxillary antrum (excluding Burkitt lymphoma) in Uganda Africans, CA **18:**205, 1965.

Duckworth, R., and Seward, G. R.: A melanotic ameloblastic odontoma, Oral Surg. **19:**73, 1965.

Dunlap, C. L., and Fritzlen, T. J.: Cystic odontoma with concomitant adenoameloblastoma (adenoameloblastic odontoma), Oral Surg. **34:**450, 1972.

Edwards, M. B., and Gourbran, G. F.: Cystic, melanotic ameloblastic fibroma with granulomatous inflammation, Oral Surg. **49:**333, 1980.

Eversole, L. R., Sabes, W. R., and Dauchess, V. G.: Benign cementoblastoma, Oral Surg. **36:**824, 1973.

Farman, A. G.: The peripheral odontogenic fibroma, Oral Surg. **40:**82, 1975.

Forsberg, A., Lagergren, C., and Martensson, G.: Ameloblastic odontoma, Oral Surg. **14:**726, 1961.

Franklin, C. D., and Pindborg, J. J.: The calcifying epithelial odontogenic tumor, Oral Surg. **42:**753, 1976.

Frissell, C. T., and Shafer, W. G.: Ameloblastic odontoma: report of a case, Oral Surg. **6:**1129, 1953.

Gardner, D. G.: Peripheral ameloblastoma: a study of 21 cases, including 5 reported as basal cell carcinoma of the gingiva, CA **39:**1625, 1977.

Gardner, D. G.: The concept of hamartomas: its relevance to the pathogenesis of odontogenic lesions, Oral Surg. **45:**884, 1978.

Giansanti, J. S., Someren, A., and Waldron, C. A.: Odontogenic adenomatoid tumor (adenoameloblastoma): survey of 111 cases, Oral Surg. **30:**69, 1970.

Goldberg, S. J., and Friedman, J. M.: Ameloblastoma: review of the literature and report of a case, J. Am. Dent. Assoc. **90:**432, 1975.

Goldblatt, L. I.: Ultrastructural study of an odontogenic myxoma, Oral Surg. **42:**206, 1976.

Greer, R. O., Jr., and Richardson, J. F.: Clear-cell calcifying odontogenic tumor viewed relative to the Pindborg tumor, Oral Surg. **42:**775, 1976.

Grenfell, J. W., and Maris, A. M.: Ameloblastic fibroma, Oral Surg. **21:**403, 1966.

Gundlach, K. K. H., and Schulz, A.: Odontogenic myxoma—clinical concept and morphological studies, J. Oral Pathol. **6:**343, 1977.

Hacihanefioğlu, U.: The adenomatoid odontogenic tumor, Oral Surg. **38:**65, 1974.

Hamner, J. E., Gamble, J. W., and Gallegos, G. J.: Odontogenic fibroma, Oral Surg. **21:**113, 1966.

Harrer, W. V., and Patchefsky, A. S.: Mandibular ameloblastoma with intracerebral and pulmonary metastasis, Oral Surg. **29:**893, 1970.

Hartenian, K. M., and Kalfayan, B.: Ameloblastoma containing mucus glands, Oral Surg. **41:**508, 1976.

Hartman, K. S.: Granular-cell ameloblastoma, Oral Surg. **38:**241, 1974.

Hendler, B. H., Abaza, N. A., and Quinn, P.: Odontogenic myxoma, Oral Surg. **47:**203, 1979.

Hoggins, G. S., and Grundy, M. C.: Melanotic neuroectodermal tumor of infancy, Oral Surg. **40:**34, 1975.

Hoke, H. F., Jr., and Harrelson, A. B.: Granular cell ameloblastoma with metastasis to the cervical vertebrae, CA **20:**991, 1967.

Hornova, J.: Adenoameloblastoma in the wall of a dentigerous cyst, Oral Surg. **19:**508, 1965.

Howell, R. M., and Burkes, E. J.: Malignant transformation of ameloblastic fibro-odontoma to ameloblastic fibrosarcoma, Oral Surg. **43:**391, 1977.

Ikemura, K., Tashiro, H., Fujino, H., Ohbu, D., and Nakajima, K.: Ameloblastoma of the mandible with metastasis to the lungs and lymph nodes, CA **29:**930, 1972.

Jones, J. H., McGowan, D. A., and Gorman, J. M.: Calcifying epithelial odontogenic and keratinizing odontogenic tumors, Oral Surg. **25:**465, 1968.

Kalnins, V.: Calcification and amelogenesis in craniopharyngiomas, Oral Surg. **31:**366, 1971.

Khin, U., Sandu, B., Kasper, E., and Adelmen, H.: Adenomatoid odontogenic tumor, J. Oral Surg. **31:**607, 1973.

Klinar, K. L., and McManis, J. C.: Soft-tissue ameloblastoma, Oral Surg. **28**:266, 1969.

Kovi, J., and Laing, W. N.: Tumors of the mandible and maxilla in Acera, Ghana, CA **19**:1301, 1966.

Kramer, I. R. H.: Ameloblastoma: a clinicopathologic appraisal, Br. J. Oral Surg. **1**:13, 1963.

Lash, M., and McCoy, G.: Ameloblastoma of the mandible with pulmonary metastasis, Ann. Otol. **78**:430, 1969.

Lee, K. W., Chin, T. C., and Paul, S.: Peripheral ameloblastoma, Br. J. Oral Surg. **8**:150, 1970.

Leider, A. S., Nelson, J. F., and Trodahl, J. N.: Ameloblastic fibrosarcoma of the jaws, Oral Surg. **33**:559, 1972.

Lopez, J., Jr.: Melanotic neuroectodermal tumor of infancy: review of the literature and report of a case, J. Am. Dent. Assoc. **93**:1159, 1976.

Mader, C. L., and Wendelburg, L.: Benign cementoblastoma, J. Am. Dent. Assoc. **99**:990, 1979.

Martensson, G., Notter, G., and Soderberg, G.: Benign melanotic tumor of the infantile jaw, Oral Surg. **20**:632, 1965.

Matlik, K. C. B.: Atypical adamantinoma: an adamantinoma with cells resembling granular cell myoblastoma, Arch. Pathol. **64**:158, 1957.

Meenaghan, M. A., Appel, B. N., and Green, G. W.: Amyloid-containing odontogenic tumors of man, Oral Surg. **34**:908, 1972.

Mehlisch, D. R., Dahlin, D. C., and Masson, J. K.: Ameloblastoma; a clinicopathologic report, J. Oral Surg. **30**:9, 1972.

Miller, A. S., Lopez, C. F., Pullon, P. A., and Elzay, R. P.: Ameloblastic fibroodontoma, Oral Surg. **41**:354, 1976.

Milobsky, L., Milobsky, S. A., and Miller, G. M.: Adenomatoid odontogenic tumor (adenoameloblastoma), Oral Surg. **40**:681, 1975.

Mincer, H. H., McGinnis, J. P., Jr., and Wyatt, J. R.: Ultrastructure of sclerotic cemental masses, Oral Surg. **43**:70, 1977.

Mohamed, A. H., and Waterhouse, J. P.: A light and electron microscopic study of an atypical calicfying odontogenic tumor containing "amyloid," J. Oral Pathol. **2**:150, 1973.

Mosadomi, A.: Odontogenic tumors in an African population, Oral Surg. **40**:502, 1975.

Nathanson, N. R., and Tedeschi, L. G.: Melanotic progonoma, a tumor of infancy, Oral Surg. **23**:354, 1967.

Olech, E., and Alvares, O.: Ameloblastic odontoma, Oral Surg. **23**:487, 1967.

Papp, P., and Toth, K.: Odontogenic myxoma of the mandible, Oral Sur. **20**:82, 1965.

Patterson, J. T., Martin, T. H., DeJean, E. K., and Burzynski, N. J.: Extraosseous calcifying epithelial odontogenic tumor; report of a case, Oral Surg. **27**:363, 1969.

Peterson, L. J.: Granular-cell tumor, Oral Surg. **37**:728, 1974.

Pindborg, J. J.: The calcifying epithelial odontogenic tumor, Acta Odontol. Scad. **24**:419, 1966.

Pontiers, E. E., Aziobis, M. D., and Foster, J. A.: Multicentric melanoamelo-blastoma of the maxilla, CA **18**:387, 1965.

Porter, J., Miller, R., and Stratigos, G. T.: Ameloblastoma of the maxilla, Oral Surg. **44**:34, 1977.

Potdar, G. G.: Ameloblastoma of the jaw as seen in Bombay, India, Oral Surg. **28**:297, 1969.

Pullon, P. A., Shafer, W. G., Elzay, R. P., Kerr, D. A., and Corio, R. L.: Squamous odontogenic tumor, Oral Surg. **40**:616, 1975.

Regezi, J. A., Courtney, R. M., and Kerr, D. A.: Keratinization in odontogenic tumors, Oral Surg. **39**:447, 1975.

Rockoff, H. M.: A statistical analysis of ameloblastoma, Oral Surg. **16**:1100, 1963.

Schmidseder, R., and Hausaman, J.: Multiple odontogenic tumors and other anomalies, Oral Surg. **39**:249, 1975.

Sciubba, J. J., and Zola, M. B.: Odontogenic epithelial hamartoma, Oral Surg. **45**:261, 1978.

Sedano, H. O.: Ameloblastic fibroma, Oral Surg. **17**:475, 1964.

Sehdev, M. K., Huvos, A. G., Strong, E. W., Gerold, F. P., and Willis, G. W.: Ameloblastoma of maxilla and mandible, CA **33**:324, 1974.

Seymour, R. L., Funke, F. W. and Irby, W. B.: Adenoameloblastoma, Oral Surg. **38**:860, 1974.

Simes, R. J., Barros, R. E., Klein-Szanto, A. J. P., and Cabrini, R. L.: Ultra-structure of an odontogenic myxoma, Oral Surg. **39**:640, 1975.

Simpson, H. E.: Basal-cell carcinoma and peripheral ameloblastoma, Oral Surg. **38**:233, 1974.

Slavin, G., and Cameron, H. M.: Ameloblastomas in Africans from Tanzania and Uganda, Br. J. Cancer **23**:31, 1969.

Small, I. A., and Waldron, C. A.: Ameloblastomas of the jaws, Oral Surg. **8**:281, 1955.

Smith, J. F., and Blankenship, J.: The calcifying odontogenic cyst, Oral Surg. **20**:624, 1965.

Solomon, M. P., Vuletin, J. C., Pertschuk, L. P., Gormley, M. B., and Rosen, Y.: Calcifying epithelial odontogenic tumor, Oral Surg. **40**:522, 1975.

Sugimura, M., Yamauchi, T., Yashikawa, K., Takeda, N., Sakita, M., and Miyazaki, T.: Malignant ameloblastoma with metastasis to the lumbar ver-tebra: report of a case, J. Oral Surg. **27**:350, 1969.

Tanaka, S., Mitsui, Y., Mizuno, Y., and Emori, S.: Recurrent ameloblastic fi-broma, Oral Surg. **33**:944, 1972.

Trodahl, J. N.: Ameloblastic fibroma, Oral Surg. **33**:547, 1972.

Tsukada, Y., De La Pava, S., and Pickren, J. W.: Granular-cell ameloblastoma and metastasis to the lungs: report of a case and review of the literature, CA **18**:916, 1965.

Vegh, T.: Multiple cementomas (periapical cemental dysplasia), Oral Surg. **42**:402, 1976.

Vuletin, J. C., Solomon, M. P., and Pertschuk, L. P.: Peripheral odontogenic tumor with ghost-cell keratinization, Oral Surg. **45**:406, 1978.

Wallen, N. G.: Extraosseous ameloblastoma, Oral Surg. **34**:95, 1972.

Wertheimer, F. W., and Sabin, M.: Calcifying odontogenic fibroma: report of a case, J. Oral Surg. **30**:367, 1972.

Wertheimer, F. W., and Stroud, D. E.: Peripheral ameloblastoma in a papilloma with recurrence; report of a case, J. Oral Surg. **30**:47, 1972.

Wesley, R. K., Wysocki, G. P., and Mintz, S. M.: The central odontogenic fibroma, clinical and morphologic studies, Oral Surg. **40**:235, 1975.

Westwood, R. M., Alexander, R. W., and Bennett, D. E.: Giant odontogenic myxofibroma, Oral Surg. **37**:83, 1974.

White, D. K., Chen, S. Y., Hartman, K. S., Miller, A. S., and Gomez, L. F.: Central granular-cell tumor of the jaws (the so-called granular-cell ameloblastic fibroma), Oral Surg. **45**:396, 1978.

White, D. K., Chen, S. Y., Mohnac, A. M., and Miller, A. S.: Odontogenic myxoma, Oral Surg. **39**:901, 1975.

Yazdi, I., and Nowparast, B.: Extraosseous adenomatoid odontogenic tumor with special reference to the probability of the basal-cell layer of oral epithelium as a potential source of origin, Oral Surg. **37**:249, 1974.

Young, D. R., and Robinson, M.: Ameloblastomas in children, Oral Surg. **15**:1155, 1962.

Zegarelli, E. V., Kutschner, A. H., Napoli, N., Iurono, F., and Hoffman, P.: The cementoma, Oral Surg. **17**:219, 1964.

CHAPTER 11

Nonodontogenic tumors and pseudotumors of jaws

Tumors of the jaws that do not arise from the dental lamina or its derivatives are classified as nonodontogenic and may be benign or malignant.

Benign tumors

1. Giant cell granuloma (central)
2. Giant cell tumor
3. Myxoma
4. Chondroma
5. Central fibro-osseous lesions (fibroma; ossifying fibroma; monostotic fibrous dysplasia; fibroma with ossification; fibroma with calcification)
6. Osteoblastoma
7. Cherubism (familial intraosseous fibrous swellings of jaws)
8. Osteoma
9. Tori
10. Hemangioma of bone
11. Fibroma

Malignant tumors

1. Osteogenic sarcoma
2. Chondrosarcoma
3. Multiple myeloma and solitary myeloma
4. Ewing's tumor
5. Reticulum cell sarcoma
6. Burkitt's sarcoma (tumor)
7. Metastatic tumors
8. Rare tumors

BENIGN TUMORS

Giant cell granuloma (central). This tumor or tumorlike growth may be located within the jaw (central) or involve the gingiva (peripheral). The latter is discussed with the lesions of the soft tissues (p. 497).

The central giant cell granuloma is seen predominantly in patients under 20 years of age and occurs more commonly in females than in males. The mandible is involved more often than the maxilla, and in the mandible the premolar and molar areas are the preferred sites. Although at times the lesion is asymptomatic, it usually is expansile—that is, it produces a clinically or radiographically discernable enlargement (Fig. 11-1, *A*). The regional teeth may migrate. The covering mucosa is intact and normal. A history of trauma in the area, including tooth extraction, is not rare. Radiographs show a single cystic area or a soap bubble-like deformity (Fig. 11-1, *B*). At operation

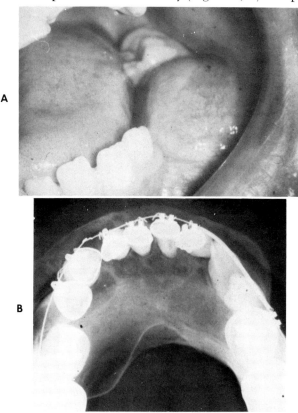

A

B

Fig. 11-1. Two central giant cell granulomas. **A,** Swelling in the canine and premolar area. **B,** A tumor in the anterior of the mandible has produced a large deformity.

the jaw defect is seen to be filled by a solid reddish or reddish gray tissue that resembles liver and bleeds easily.

Microscopically a giant cell granuloma has an unmistakable morphology (Fig. 11-2) consisting of numerous multinucleated giant cells dispersed throughout the specimen, numerous small blood vessels, an abundance of young fibroblasts that have ovoid vesicular nuclei, foci of hemosiderin unevenly dispersed throughout the lesion, and areas of bone trabeculae. Careful observation frequently reveals phagocytosis in the giant cells.

The soap bubble–like radiographic appearance of this lesion is not diagnostic, because the ameloblastoma, the aneurysmal bone cyst, and the myxoma may also appear as soap bubble-like lesions. However, the ameloblastoma occurs in an older age group, and the myxoma is extremely rare. When a giant cell granuloma appears as a single area of radiolucency, diagnosis from the radiograph is impossible.

Microscopically a central giant cell granuloma closely resembles a peripheral giant cell granuloma, from which it is distinguished by its location. It also resembles a giant cell tumor, but

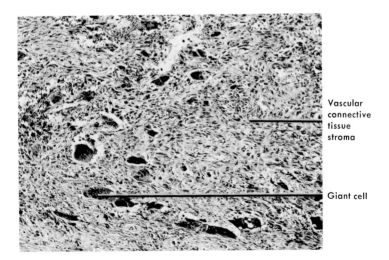

Vascular connective tissue stroma

Giant cell

Fig. 11-2. Giant cell granuloma.

fortunately the latter lesion occurs rarely, if ever, in the jaws. It is differentiated from an aneurysmal bone cyst by the absence of blood pools seen in the bone cyst (p. 242). Finally, sometimes a giant cell granuloma is indistinguishable histologically from the brown nodes of hyperparathyroidism (p. 669). However, the brown nodes are associated with the excessive secretion of parathormone, generalized bone destruction, increased blood calcium and alkaline phosphatase, lowered blood phosphorus, and other generalized symptoms.

If a central giant cell granuloma should recur more than once, as a precautionary measure it is advisable to check the blood calcium and phosphorus levels.

Local curettage is the treatment of choice. Even lesions of the size shown in Fig. 11-1 can be treated by local curettage. Prognosis is excellent. Recurrences following local curettage are rare. Radiation or radical surgery is contraindicated.

Giant cell tumor. A giant cell tumor rarely, if ever, occurs in the jaws. It is found in the long bones, particularly the lower end of the radius and femur and the upper end of the tibia. In the *long* bones it may behave in a benign manner (about 50%), be locally aggressive (about 33%), or metastasize (about 17%). In these locations, therefore, it is a dangerous lesion.

Microscopically a giant cell tumor may be indistinguishable from a giant cell granuloma; and it is not possible to distinguish between the benign, the locally aggressive, and the malignant forms. Since it rarely, if ever, occurs in the oral regions, it is of little importance in the differential diagnosis of radiolucent lesions of the jaws.

Myxoma. A true (nonodontogenic) myxoma of the jaws must be distinguised from an odontogenic myxoma. The former may occur in any part of the skeleton or soft tissues.

Since the jaws are the most common site for lesions involving the bones, a true myxoma is of importance to the dentist. In the jaws it has neither sexual nor age preference and may involve either the mandible or the maxilla. It is slow growing but produces enlargement of the involved area. Migration and loosening of teeth also occur (Figs. 11-3, *A*, and 11-4).

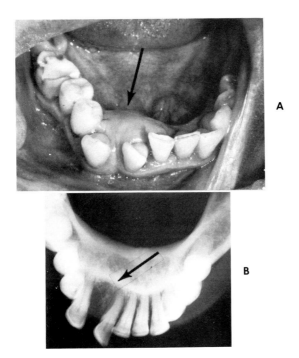

Fig. 11-3. Myxoma (arrows) of the mandible. The lateral incisor and canine were loose.

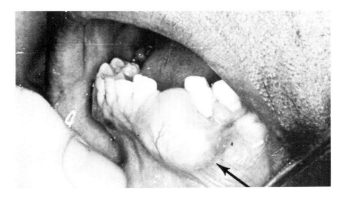

Fig. 11-4. Myxoma (arrow) of the mandible. The tumor arose within the jaw and produced migration of teeth.

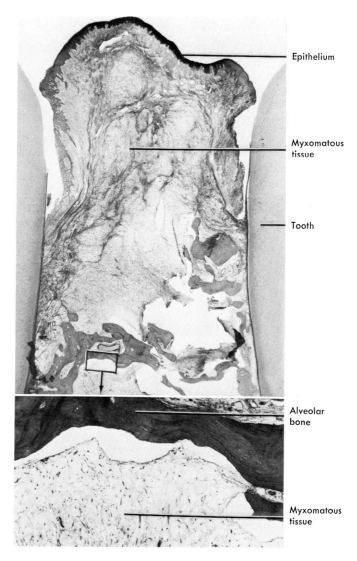

Epithelium

Myxomatous
tissue

Tooth

Alveolar
bone

Myxomatous
tissue

Fig. 11-5. Myxoma of the mandible (same lesion as shown in Fig. 11-4). Myxomatous tissue has replaced the interdental septum as well as the gingiva.

The lesion appears as either a single or a soap bubble-like area of radiolucency. The cortex is thinned and may be expanded (Fig. 11-3, *B*).

Grossly the tumor is seen to have the consistency of jelly. Microscopic sections are diagnostic, showing numerous stellate cells in an overabundant stroma of mucoid material. The tumor cell is the myxoblast, which produces large amounts of glycosaminoglycans. The latter is the mucoid material that gives the tumor its gelatinous consistency. The tumor is not encapsulated and infiltrates the marrow spaces (Fig. 11-5). It is benign and does not metastasize. Because of its consistency and infiltrative nature, it may be difficult to eradicate. It is more aggressive than the odontogenic myxoma; and unless excision is complete, recurrence is most likely.

Chondroma. The chondroma is a benign tumor of bone that usually arises in tubular bones of the skeleton. Its occurrence in the jaws is rare. It may arise in the mandible or the maxilla and, though slow in growth, may produce enlargement, tooth migration, and tooth resorption (Fig. 11-6).

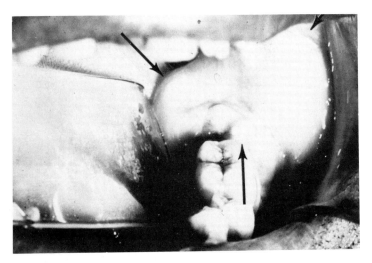

Fig. 11-6. Chondroma (arrows) arising in the retromolar area of the mandible.

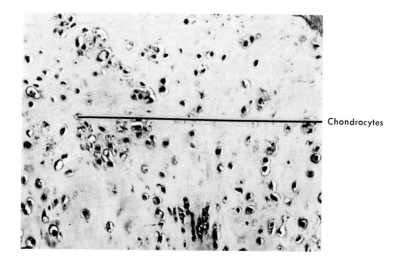

Chondrocytes

Fig. 11-7. Chondroma. Normal chondrocytes form the major part of the tumor.

The lesion characteristically appears as a radiolucency alone or as a radiolucency with radiopaque foci. Microscopic sections reveal hyaline cartilage with normal chondrocytes (Fig. 11-7). Areas of calcified cartilage may also be present.

The chondroma is dangerous for several reasons: (1) it may become malignant; (2) it infiltrates the marrow spaces and is difficult to eradicate; (3) in spite of the seemingly innocent microscopic appearance, it often behaves as a low-grade chondrosarcoma (p. 320). For all these reasons, chondromas of the jaws should be treated by radical local excision.

Central fibro-osseous lesions (fibroma; ossifying fibroma; monostotic fibrous dysplasia; fibroma with ossification; fibroma with calcification). Central fibro-osseous lesions of the jaws are characterized microscopically by young fibrous connective tissue and varying amounts of bone. They have been given a wide variety of names, and considerable confusion exists regarding their terminology. From the clinical, histologic, and therapeutic viewpoint, however, these discussions are superfluous.

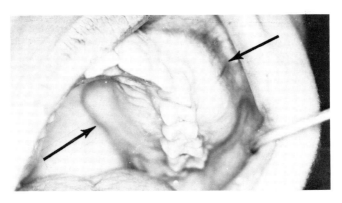

Fig. 11-8. Ossifying fibroma (arrows). Note the enlargement of the jaw. Migration of teeth is not conspicuous in this case but is often present.

Clinically the lesions may occur at any age but are most common in children and young adults. They are slow growing and painless but usually produce buccal or labial enlargement of the jaw and facial deformity (Fig. 11-8). The maxilla is affected more often than the mandible. Tooth migration may be present.

Central fibro-osseous lesions may appear as an area of radiolucency with radiopaque foci or as an entirely radiopaque mass (Fig. 11-9). Rarely the very early stages of the lesion may be completely radiolucent. The jaws are usually expanded. The cortex is thinned but intact. Tooth migration may be apparent. Lesions of the maxilla may extend and replace part or all of the maxillary sinus.

Microscopically the most important feature is the presence of fibrous connective tissue of varying degrees of maturity (Fig. 11-10). This means that the lesions may consist exclusively of young proliferating fibroblasts, may show fibroblasts and collagen fibers, or may be predominantly collagenous. The second most important feature is the presence of a calcified material (usually bone) that varies in quantity from just a few isolated foci to a dense network of trabeculae (Fig. 11-10). The bone

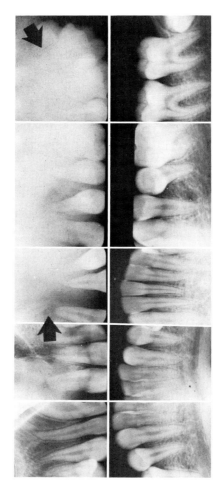

Fig. 11-9. Ossifying fibroma (arrows) of the maxilla.

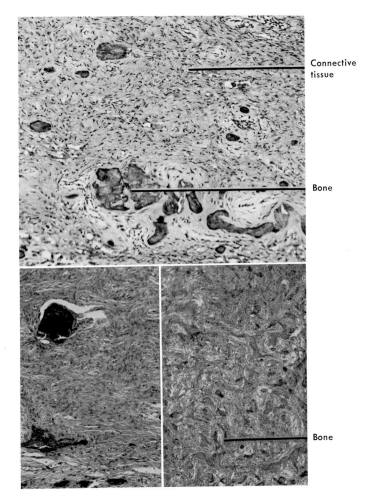

Fig. 11-10. Ossifying fibroma. Note the fibrous tissue and bone. These two components occur in varying proportions.

tissue forms foci of varying pattern. The surfaces of bone trabeculae show bone apposition and resorption. The periphery of
the tumors shows resorption of cortex.

These fibro-osseous lesions vary greatly in their behavior,
but all are benign and do not metastasize or undergo malignant
change. They may be slow growing, and curettage may prevent
recurrence; or they may recur numerous times (those of the
maxilla extending into the sinuses and the orbit). Highly cellular
lesions are usually more aggressive. Lesions in children appear
to grow more rapidly.

Since these lesions do not metastasize and many respond
well to curettage, local conservative treatment should be given
first preference. This is especially true in children, in whom a
relatively small lesion may occupy a relatively large area of the
jaw and therefore give an impression of poor prognosis. Radiation of these lesions is contraindicated and dangerous.

Osteoblastoma. This rare, solitary, painful lesion of the long
bones and vertebrae may also involve the jaws. Patients are between 10 and 35 years of age. The lesion is characterized by
solitary radiopacities of varying density. Microscopic features include bone trabeculae with osteoid borders in a rich fibrous tissue stroma. Many osteoblasts line the trabeculae.

The osteoblastoma is a benign lesion, and local conservative
removal is the treatment of choice. The lesion must be distinguished from the osteogenic sarcoma, for which it is sometimes
mistaken.

Cherubism (familial intraosseous fibrous swellings of jaws).
Cherubism is a familial disease involving only the jaws. It begins in childhood (3 to 5 years of age). It is usually bilateral and
involves the premolar and molar regions and coronoid process
of the mandible. However, a single lesion may start in the anterior part of the mandible and later appear in the molar area;
or the maxilla may be involved.

Swelling of the jaws is progressive, produces an enlargement
of the face (giving the patient a cherubic appearance), and is
painless and firm to touch (Fig. 11-11). Migration of teeth and

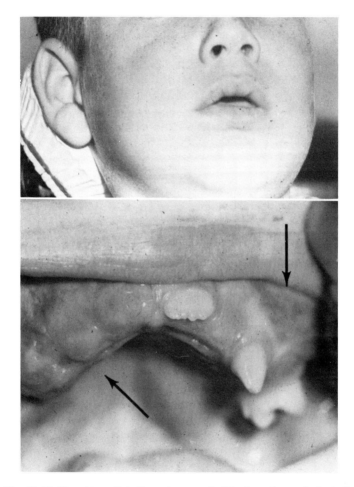

Fig. 11-11. Cherubism. Note the enlargement of the face. Arrows indicate the enlarged alveolar ridges and abnormal eruptive pattern.

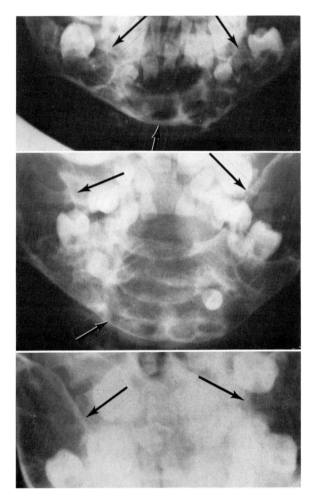

Fig. 11-12. Cherubism. Arrows denote the progressive enlargement of radio-lucent areas and the migration of teeth in a patient at $2^{1}/_{2}$, $4^{1}/_{2}$, and $7^{1}/_{2}$ years of age.

tooth germs may be apparent. The patient may have cervical lymphadenopathy. The lesion grows rapidly for two to three years, then subsides, and finally ceases. Usually there is no trace of the deformity by the time the patient reaches adulthood.

Radiographs of the involved area show a multilocular lesion (Fig. 11-12). Both erupted and unerupted teeth are displaced (Fig. 11-13); the teeth may be malformed or absent and (if erupted) may be loose. Root resorption is often present. The cortex is thinned and expanded but intact.

Microscopically lesions of cherubism show giant cells (simi-

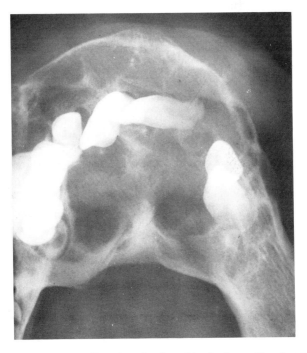

Fig. 11-13. Cherubism. Note the migration of teeth, the multilocular radiolucency, and the expansion of the mandible.

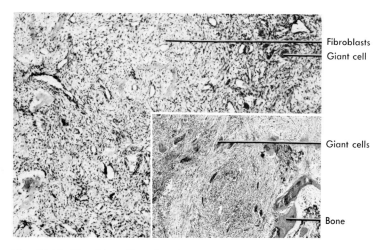

Fibroblasts
Giant cell

Giant cells

Bone

Fig. 11-14. Cherubism. Note the giant cells, fibrous connective tissue, and bone trabeculae.

lar to those seen in giant cell granuloma), fibrous connective tissue that may be highly cellular or show abundant collagen with few cells, and spicules of bone (Fig. 11-14).

Since the lesion is self-limiting and usually improves spontaneously, it should be left untreated until after the child reaches puberty. Any residual deformity may be corrected by conservative surgical contouring. However, when swelling interferes with function, surgical intervention may be necessary much earlier.

Osteoma. This lesion is a benign tumor that may be endosteal or periosteal in location. It grows extremely slowly and may cease growth spontaneously.

Radiographs show an osteosclerotic mass, and microscopic sections show dense mature lamellated bone. If the tumor is removed, it does not recur. Differentiation between tori, exostoses, enostoses, and osteoma is often arbitrary.

In a hereditary disturbance called *Gardner's syndrome,* os-

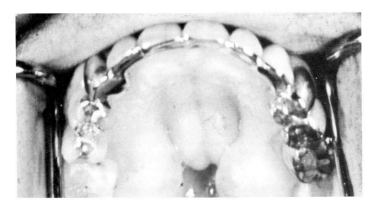

Fig. 11-15. Torus palatinus. Note the expansile lesions in the midline of the palate. Exostoses of the tuberosities are also present.

teomas of the maxilla, mandible, and other facial bones are associated with polyps of the large intestines, odontomas, and epidermal cysts of the skin. Approximately fifteen years after onset, 40% of polyps in the large bowel develop adenocarcinomas.

Tori. Bone excrescences on the periosteal surface of the maxilla and mandible are called tori (exostoses) (Fig. 11-15). Although they may occur in either jaw, in any location, and at any age—they usually present characteristic features.

The midline of the palate is the most frequent site (about 20% of the American population) and in this location the lesion is referred to as *torus palatinus* (Fig. 11-15). The torus palatinus occurs in females twice as frequently as in males and starts before 30 years of age.

The second most common site is the mandible (about 8% of the population), where the lesion is usually on the lingual aspect of the premolar and molar area. In this location the lesion is designated *torus mandibularis* (Fig. 11-16). Like the torus palatinus, it occurs before 30 years of age and affects both sexes equally.

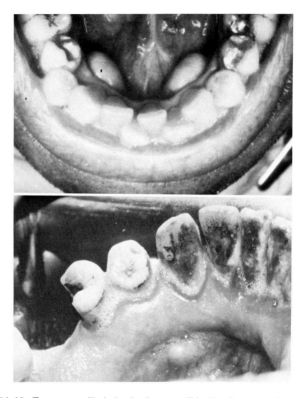

Fig. 11-16. Torus mandibularis. In the mandible the lingual surface of the premolars is the usual location.

Both the torus palatinus and the torus mandibularis are asymptomatic. Microscopic sections show a mass of dense normal bone or a peripheral layer of cortical bone with a central area of marrow and bone trabeculae. If tori interfere with function or the proper adaptation of a denture, they should be removed. They do not recur.

Hemangioma of bone. A central hemangioma of the jaws is extremely rare and extremely dangerous. In less than forty reported cases, the mandible was affected twice as frequently as the maxilla. These lesions may be slow growing and asymptomatic; or they may grow rapidly, expand the cortical plate, and lead to loosening of the teeth. Teeth that become loose can be pumped in and out of their sockets. The cervical area of the teeth may show oozing of blood. In some instances pulsation can be felt over the jaw lesions, but this is not a constant finding. Lesions may involve both the soft tissues and the bone (Fig. 11-17).

A hemangioma of bone may appear as a radiolucency that is honeycombed or unremarkable (Fig. 11-18). In some cases radiolucencies with linear trabeculations have been described. Clinical diagnosis is difficult; but when the lesion is suspected, aspiration is of great value. On tooth extraction bleeding is profuse and often uncontrollable. Ligation of the external carotid arteries, packing, and finally jaw resection may be necessary. Microscopic sections show numerous blood-containing spaces or vessels in the bone marrow (Figs. 11-17, *B* and *C*, and 11-19).

Fibroma. Central fibroma of the jaws is a very rare tumor. It resembles ossifying fibroma in all respects, except that microscopically the lesion has no osseous component. An aggressive, fibrous tumor–like growth of the jaw called *juvenile fibromatosis* has been described. It usually involves the mandible, is rapidly growing, occurs in children, and microscopically shows cellular interlacing bundles of elongated fibroblasts; but there is no pleomorphism. The lesion does not metastasize, and local excision is curative.

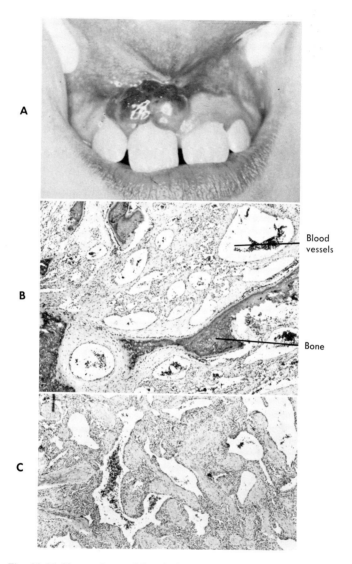

Fig. 11-17. Hemangioma of the gingiva and underlying bone. Note the blood vessel proliferation in the bone marrow spaces (**B** and **C**).

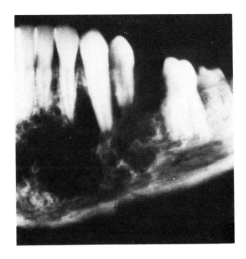

Fig. 11-18. Hemangioma of the mandible. Usually the radiograph has a honeycombed appearance.

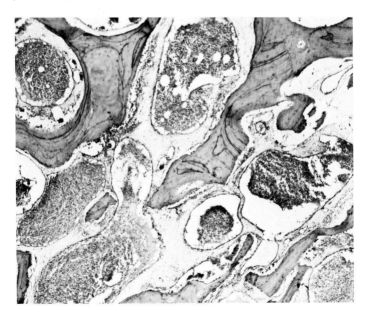

Fig. 11-19. Hemangioma of bone. Note the presence of numerous blood vessels in between the bone trabeculae.

MALIGNANT TUMORS

Osteogenic sarcoma. The osteogenic sarcoma is a malignant tumor of bone, and about 6.5% of reported cases have occurred in the jaws. The jaw tumors occur about a decade later than tumors in other parts of the skeleton, and the mean age is 30 years.

This lesion more commonly afflicts males (twice as frequently as females), and the mandible is involved more often than the maxilla. The tumor presents as a rapidly growing swelling that may be associated with vague pain and paresthesia. Often there is a history of tooth extraction or trauma. Teeth in the area may be loose and show migration and root resorption. The mucosa and skin covering the lesion may appear erythematous. Spontaneous pathologic fractures may occur.

The osteogenic sarcoma appears as a radiopacity in which bone trabeculae radiate from the periphery of the lesion, producing a "sun ray" effect (Fig. 11-20). The appearance may be of irregular radiopaque and radiolucent areas or of an entirely radiolucent area. In some instances widening of the periodontal space is the earliest radiographic sign and when present is considered highly suggestive of this malignancy (Fig. 11-21).

The microscopic appearance of an osteogenic sarcoma is varied but usually consists of highly atypical bone trabeculae and a stroma of pleomorphic cells resembling osteoblasts and fibroblasts (Fig. 11-22). These mesenchymal cells show numerous mitoses, hyperchromatic nuclei, and giant cells. Some osteogenic sarcomas are composed predominantly of the stroma, whereas others contain a great deal of abnormal bone. It is apparent, therefore, why different tumors have different radiographic appearances.

An osteogenic sarcoma is highly malignant, metastasizes widely, and has a poor prognosis. Only 25% of patients with such a tumor of the jaws survive beyond five years. However, this is better than the 16% survival rate for patients with an osteogenic sarcoma of other bones. For the jaw lesions a radical resection with or without chemotherapy and radiation therapy are the recommended modes of treatment. The worst prognosis is associated with maxillary tumors that involve the antrum (pa-

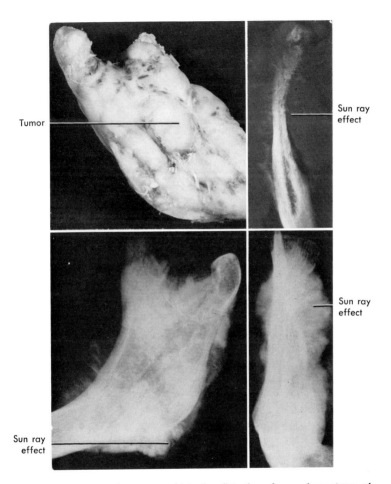

Fig. 11-20. Osteogenic sarcoma. Note the distortion of normal countours of the mandible in the gross specimen. Radiographs show radiating lines from the cortex of the mandible—called the sun ray effect.

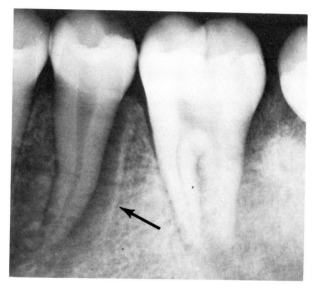

Fig. 11-21. Osteogenic sarcoma (radiopacity). Widening of the periodontal ligament (arrow) is an early diagnostic feature.

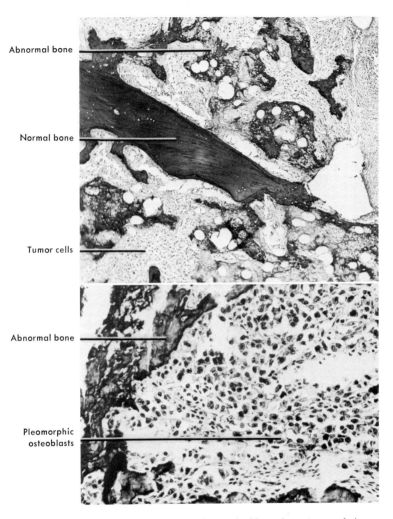

Abnormal bone

Normal bone

Tumor cells

Abnormal bone

Pleomorphic
osteoblasts

Fig. 11-22. Osteogenic sarcoma. Note the atypical bone in a stroma of pleomorphic mesenchymal cells (osteoblasts and fibroblasts).

tients survive less than one year), and the best with those of the mandibular symphysis (patients survive more than six years). Survival of patients with maxillary tumors that do not involve the sinus is about three years.

Chondrosarcoma. Like the osteogenic sarcoma, the chondrosarcoma is a rare tumor of the jaws. It has a slight preference for the maxilla and usually occurs between 25 and 50 years of age. It grows rapidly and may present the same clinical and radiographic symptoms described for the osteogenic sarcoma. (The sun ray effect is usually absent, Fig. 11-23.) Microscopically, however, sheets and islands of atypical chondrocytes in various stages of differentiation can be seen (Fig. 11-24), rang-

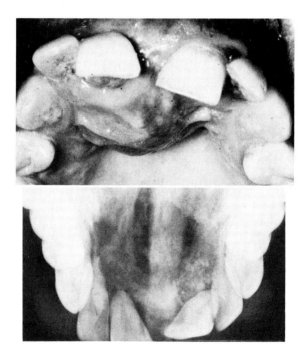

Fig. 11-23. Chondrosarcoma of the maxilla. The clinical photograph shows an enlargement and migration of the incisors. The radiograph shows root resorption and a partly radiopaque lesion.

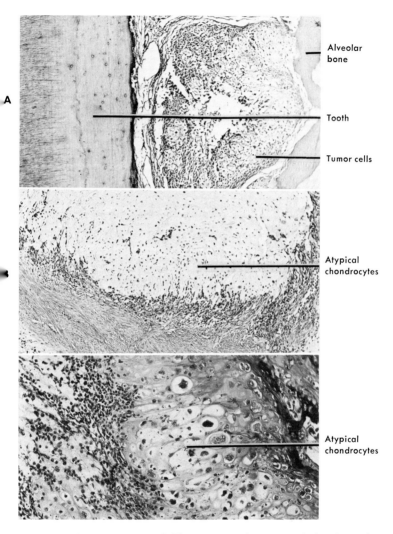

A

Alveolar bone

Tooth

Tumor cells

Atypical chondrocytes

Atypical chondrocytes

Fig. 11-24. Chondrosarcoma. **A,** The tumor can be seen replacing the periodontal ligament. **B** and **C,** Tumor cells in different stages of development.

ing from young mesenchymal cells to cells that resemble mature chondrocytes. Small foci or large areas of bone may be seen.

The tumor does not metastasize as readily as the osteogenic sarcoma. However, tumors of the mandible may extend along the structures of the neck into the mediastinum, and tumors of the maxilla may extend into the base of the brain.

Radical surgery is the only possible treatment. The prognosis in chondrosarcoma of the jaws is poorer than that in chondrosarcoma of the long bones; and only about a third of the patients survive more than five years.

Multiple myeloma and solitary myeloma. Multiple myeloma and solitary myeloma are malignant tumors of bone marrow. Although there are some finer differences between the two, in essence the solitary type is only an early manifestation of the multiple form and may precede it by many years. In this discussion, therefore, only multiple myeloma will be considered.

Multiple myeloma is a malignant tumor of bone marrow. More than 80% of cases occur in patients past 45 years of age, and males are afflicted twice as frequently as females. The bones usually involved are the skull (Fig. 11-25), jaws, vertebrae, pelvis, and femur. General symptoms are pain in the back and pathologic fractures.

Laboratory findings may include leukopenia; anemia; elevated gamma globulin; the presence of Bence Jones proteins in the urine (a protein in urine that coagulates between 40° and 60° C and disappears on boiling); deposition of amyloid-like (paramyloid) material in the body tissues, including the gingiva and tongue (Fig. 11-26 and p. 660); and hypercalcemia.

Multiple myeloma may have a number of oral manifestations. Jaw lesions occur in about 30% of cases, and in 12% to 15% of all cases the jaw lesion is the primary manifestation. The mandible is involved far more frequently than the maxilla, and the lesions are multiple (Fig. 11-25). The sites usually affected are the premolar-molar region and the coronoid process. Some clinical features of the oral lesions are pain, swelling, numbness, loosening of the teeth, and formation of soft tissue plasmacytomas (p. 525).

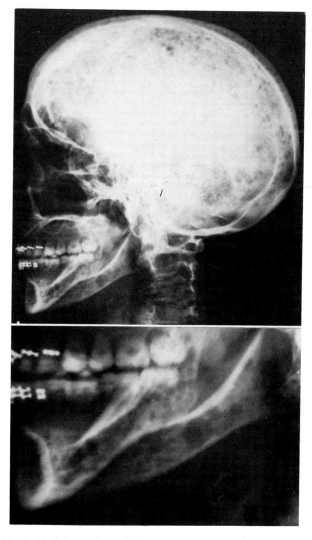

Fig. 11-25. Multiple myeloma. Note the numerous punched-out radiolucent areas in the skull and mandible.

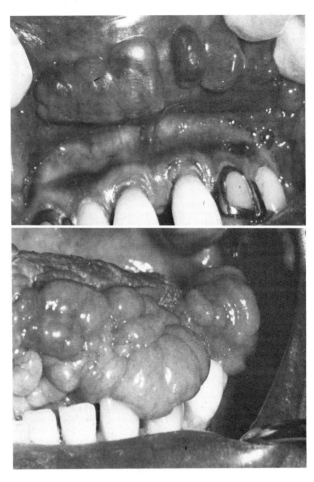

Fig. 11-26. Multiple amyloid deposits (tumors) in the lip and tongue of a patient with multiple myeloma. (Courtesy R. A. Kraut, D.D.S., J. Buhler, D.D.S., J. LaRue, D.D.S., and A. Acevado, D.D.S.—all of the U.S. Army dental corps.)

Multiple myelomas usually present multiple clear-cut, punched-out areas of radiolucency (Fig. 11-25). These areas do not show any peripheral osteosclerotic bone reaction. Root resorption and loss of lamina dura may also be seen. Microscopic sections reveal a solid tumor mass composed exclusively of atypical cells closely resembling plasma cells (Fig. 11-27). Abnormal

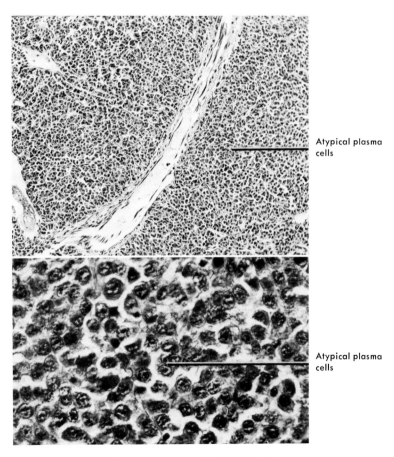

Atypical plasma cells

Atypical plasma cells

Fig. 11-27. Multiple myeloma. Note the atypical plasma cells.

immunoglobulins (myeloma proteins), which can be detected in the serum by electrophoresis, and polypeptides (Bence Jones proteins), which are detected in the urine, are secreted by these tumor cells. Electron microscopic studies can show the presence of these abnormal globulins in the cytoplasm of tumor cells (as crystalline structures). These cells have all the features of a secreting cell, such as prominent rough endoplasmic reticulum, Golgi complex, and dilated cisternae. In those cases of plasma cell tumors in which these secretory features of the tumor cells are absent, Bence Jones protein and abnormal serum immunoglobulins cannot be detected. Such myelomas are sometimes referred to as *"nonsecretory" myeloma*.

Radiation and chemotherapeutic agents are used in the management of this disease, but the prognosis is poor.

In addition to multiple myeloma and solitary myeloma, two other lesions, the soft tissue myeloma (plasmacytoma) and plasma cell granuloma are composed of cells that resemble plasma cells. These lesions may or may not be related to multiple myeloma and are described on pp. 525 and 528.

Ewing's tumor. This is a rare lesion of the jaws, with fewer than fifty cases having been reported in the literature.

The tumor is believed to be more common in the Far East than in the United States. It occurs with greater frequency in males than in females, involves the mandible much more often than the maxilla, and usually afflicts individuals under 20 years of age. It grows rapidly and is accompanied by pain, fever, and swelling. The teeth in the area become loose and migrate, and the cortical plate of bone is destroyed.

Microscopic sections show broad sheets or bands of ill-defined polyhedral dark-staining cells with sparse cytoplasm. The sheets are separated by connective tissue septa (Fig. 11-28). The tumor is radiosensitive, and radiation followed by surgical excision is the treatment of choice.

For some reason, lesions of the maxilla have a better prognosis than do those of the mandible.

Reticulum cell sarcoma. Also called histiocytic lymphoma, a

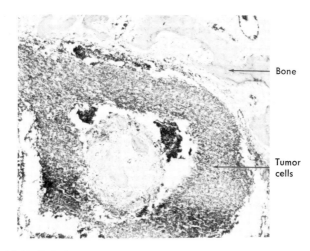

Fig. 11-28. Ewing's sarcoma. Note the infiltration of bone by sheets of small dark-staining cells.

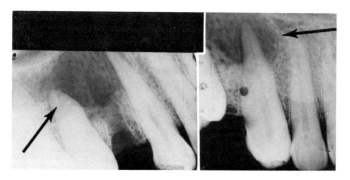

Fig. 11-29. Reticulum cell sarcoma of the maxilla (arrows). The radiolucency is often associated with pain.

reticulum cell sarcoma of the oral regions may involve either the soft tissues or the jaws or both.

Lesions of the jaws are associated with toothache, loosening of teeth, and an ill-defined radiolucency of the area (Fig. 11-29). If due to erroneous diagnosis the teeth are extracted, the sockets fail to heal. Tumors of the maxilla involve the maxillary sinus, extend into the nasal floor, and produce symptoms of nasal obstruction. Patients are usually under 40 years of age. Males are afflicted more frequently than females, and the mandible is the preferred site.

Microscopic features of both the soft tissue lesion and the jaw lesion are identical. The tumor is composed of almost solid sheets of pale-staining cells with oval or round pale nuclei. These cells form a syncytium and show mitoses (Fig. 11-30). Silver stains reveal a fine network of reticular (argyrophilic) fibers between and around the tumor cells.

The prognosis of reticulum cell sarcoma of bone is believed to be better than in such lesions of the soft tissue. Lesions of both types are radiosensitive, and surgery with radiation is the treatment of choice. The jaw lesions respond favorably to radiation and chemotherapy.

Burkitt's sarcoma (tumor). Burkitt's sarcoma, Burkitt's lymphoma or tumor, occurs most frequently between the ages of 3 and 8 years, with patients seldom older than 15 years; males are afflicted more often than females. The condition is characterized by the occurrence of multiple simultaneous tumors and involves various parts of the body. The most common site is the jaws (50% of cases), but lesions also occur in the kidneys, liver, testes, ovaries, thyroid gland, salivary glands, and abdominal lymph nodes. Although the majority of cases occur in tropical Africa, where it is the most common form of malignant tumor of childhood, it has also been observed in temperate zones throughout the world.

Burkitt's sarcoma occurs most frequently in areas with an altitude below 5,000 feet and a temperature above 60° F. Although it is not certain, there is considerable evidence that it is caused by a virus (reovirus 3 and viruses of the herpes group).

The maxilla is affected twice as often as the mandible, and the molar areas are the primary site of involvement. Clinical features consist of loosening and exfoliation of the teeth, swelling, rapid growth, and destruction of the cortical plate.

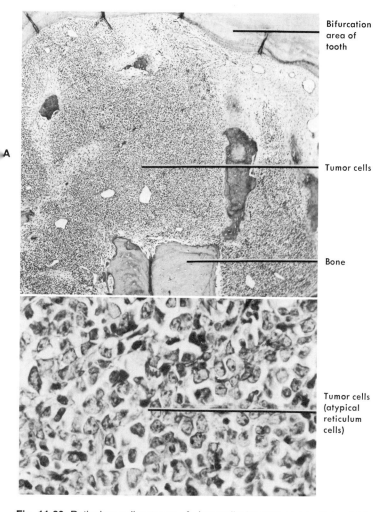

Fig. 11-30. Reticulum cell sarcoma. **A,** Interradicular area of a tooth in which the supporting bone has been almost completely replaced by tumor. **B,** High-power view of the tumor cells. Note the syncytial arrangement.

The lesion is characterized by single or multiple ill-defined radiolucencies.

Microscopically the tumor is composed of sheets of large round or oval cells of the lymphoid series with scanty cytoplasm (Fig. 11-31). In between the lymphoid cells many large clear histiocytes can be seen, and these give the lesion the so-called "starry sky" appearance (Fig. 11-31). The tumor infiltrates all areas of the jaw; and when the cortical plate is destroyed, tumor cells can be seen in oral soft tissues.

Treatment of Burkitt's sarcoma consists of chemotherapy.

Metastatic tumors. Metastatic tumors to the oral region are far less frequent than primary tumors. It is estimated that 1% of all malignant tumors of the body metastasize to the jaws, about 1% of all oral malignancies represent metastases, and about 33% of oral metastases represent the first clinical indication of the primary malignancy elsewhere.

Roughly 72% of oral metastases occur in the mandible and

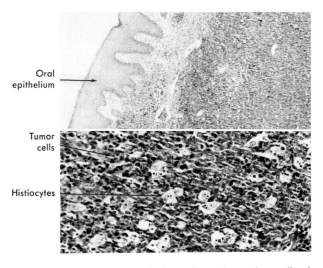

Oral epithelium

Tumor cells

Histiocytes

Fig. 11-31. Burkitt's sarcoma. In the lower figure large clear cells give the lesion a "starry sky" appearance.

18% in the maxilla (the remaining 10% occur in soft tissues; p. 567). In the jaws the preferred sites are the areas of hematopoietic marrow, and therefore the metastatic foci are generally seen in the premolar and molar areas of the mandible and maxilla.

Patients are usually between 40 and 60 years of age, and almost 60% are females. About 20% of jaw metastases are from

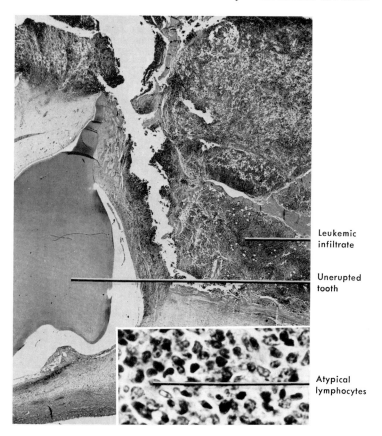

Leukemic infiltrate

Unerupted tooth

Atypical lymphocytes

Fig. 11-32. Massive leukemic infiltrate in the jaw of an infant with acute leukemia. Inset, High-power view of tumor cells. (Courtesy Harold Fullmer, D.D.S., Washington, D.C.)

a primary cancer in the breast, 15% are from the thyroid gland, 13% are from the kidney, 12% are from the lungs, 10% are from the urogenital system, 9% are from the gastrointestinal tract, and 21% are from a variety of other organs. Besides the metastatic tumors, patients with acute leukemia almost invariably have leukemic infiltrates in the jaws (Fig. 11-32).

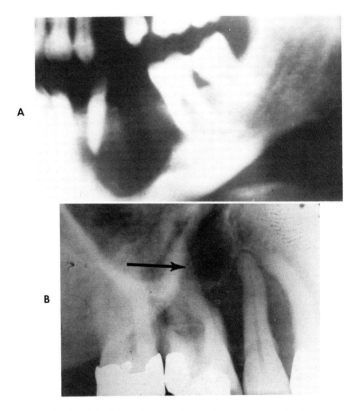

Fig. 11-33. A, Metastatic adenocarcinoma to the jaw from the large intestine. **B,** Metastatic lesion (arrow) to the premolar area of the maxilla from carcinoma of the breast.

Clinically the metastatic lesion may produce swelling, pain, pressure, loosening of teeth, and paresthesia; or it may be asymptomatic. It is usually characterized by one or more areas of radiolucency that may have ill-defined borders and a "moth-eaten" appearance (Fig. 11-33). In some patients with prostate or breast tumors, a radiopacity can be seen. Final diagnosis, of course, is made only at biopsy (Fig. 11-34). Any of the symptoms described that cannot be readily explained obviously should be thoroughly investigated.

Rare tumors. A squamous cell carcinoma or a malignant salivary gland tumor may arise within the jaws, but this is extremely uncommon. The mandible is the usual site. A squamous cell carcinoma within the jaw probably arises from the epithelial rests of Malassez or the lining of an odontogenic cyst. A malignant salivary gland tumor may arise from ectopic salivary gland tissue, which is often seen in the jaws (p. 575).

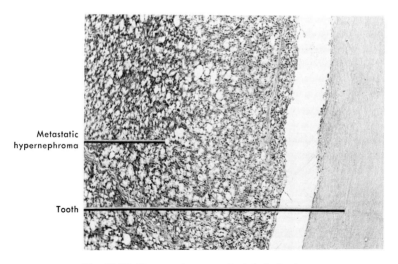

Fig. 11-34. Hypernephroma metastatic to the jaw.

REFERENCES

Adatia, A. K.: Dental tissues and Burkitt's tumor, Oral Surg. **25**:221, 1968.

Adkins, K. F., Martinez, M. G., and Robinson, L. H.: Cellular morphology and relationships in giant-cell lesions of the jaws, Oral Surg. **28**:216, 1969.

Adkins, K. F., Martinez M. G., and Romaniuk, K.: Ultrastructure of giant cell lesions, Oral Surg. **33**:775, 1972.

Afshin, H., and Sharmin, R.: Hemangioma involving the maxillary sinus, Oral Surg. **38**:204, 1974.

Ajagbe, H. A., Samuel, I., and Daramola, J. O.: Giant-cell tumor of the maxilla, Oral Surg. **46**:759, 1978.

Allan, J. H., and Scott, J.: Osteochondroma of the mandible, Oral Surg. **37**:556, 1974.

Anderson, D. E., and McClendon, J. L.: Cherubism—hereditary fibrous dysplasia of the jaws: I. Genetic considerations, Oral Surg. **15**(Suppl. 2):5, 1962.

Astacio, J. N., and Mendez, J. E.: Benign cementoblastoma (true cementoma), Oral Surg. **38**:95, 1974.

Badger, G. A., Syed, A. A., and Malby, F. C.: Desmoplastic fibroma of the mandible, Can. J. Otolaryngol. **3**:605, 1974.

Banerjee, S. C.: Metastasis to the mandible, Oral Surg. **23**:71, 1967.

Barker, B. F., Jensen, J. L., and Howell, F. V.: Focal osteoporotic bone marrow defects of the jaws, Oral Surg. **38**:404, 1974.

Barr, G. S., Zweig, B., and Itkin, A. B.: Intraoral corroboration of systemic plasma-cell myeloma, Oral Surg. **42**:22, 1976.

Barros, R. E., Domingeuz, F. V., and Cabrini, R. L.: Myxoma of the jaws, Oral Surg. **27**:225, 1969.

Bell, W., and Hinds, E. C.: Fibrosarcoma complicating polyostotic fibrous dysplasia, Oral Surg. **23**:299, 1967.

Bertelli, A. P., Costa, F. Q., and Miziara, J. E. A.: Metastatic tumors of the mandible, Oral Surg. **30**:21, 1970.

Bhansali, S. K., and Desai, P. B.: Ewing's sarcoma: observations on 107 cases, J. Bone Joint Surg. **45-A**:541, 1963.

Bhaskar, S. N.: Oral manifestation of metastatic tumors, Postgrad. Med. **49**:155, 1971.

Bhaskar, S. N., Bernier, J. L., and Godby, F.: Aneurysmal bone cyst and other giant cell lesions of the jaws; report of 104 cases, J. Oral Surg. **17**:30-41, 1959.

Bhaskar, S. N., and Dubit, J.: Central and peripheral hemangioma, Oral Surg. **23**:385, 1976.

Bhoweer, A. L., and Shirwatkar, L. G.: Central hemangioma of the mandible, J. Oral Med. **30**:111, 1975.

Brady, C. L., and Browne, R. M.: Benign osteoblastoma of the mandible, CA **30**:329, 1972.

Brady, F. A., Sapp, J. P., and Christensen, R. E.: Extracondylar osteochondromas of the jaws, Oral Surg. **46:**658, 1978.

Browand, B. C., and Waldron, C. A.: Central mucoepidermoid tumors of the jaws, Oral Surg. **40:**631, 1975.

Burkitt, D.: Etiology of Burkitt's lymphoma: an alternative hypothesis to a vectored virus, J. Natl. Cancer Inst. **42:**19, 1969.

Burkitt, D.: Host defence mechanisms in Burkitt's lymphoma and Kaposi's sarcoma: the clinical evidence, Br. Med. J. **4:**424, 1970.

Burkitt, D., Hunt, S. R., and Wright, D. H.: The African lymphoma (preliminary observations on response to therapy), CA **18:**399, 1965.

Burland, J. G.: Cherubism: familial bilateral osseous dysplasia of the jaws, Oral Surg. **15**(suppl.):43, 1962.

Campbell, R. L., Kelly, D. E., and Burkes, E. J., Jr.: Primary reticulum-cell sarcoma of the mandible, Oral Surg. **39:**918, 1975.

Carson, C. P., Ackerman, L. P., and Maltby, J. D.: Plasma cell myeloma: a clinical, pathologic and roentgenologic review of 90 cases, Am. J. Clin. Pathol. **25:**849, 1955.

Cataldo, E., and Meyer, I.: Solitary and multiple plasma cell tumors of the jaws and oral cavity, Oral Surg. **22:**628, 1966.

Chaudhry, A. P., Robinovitch, M. R., Mitchell, D. F., and Vickers, R. A.: Chondrogenic tumors of the jaws, Am. J. Surg. **102:**403, 1961.

Chen, S. Y.: Ultrastructure of a plasma-cell myeloma in the mandible, Oral Surg. **48:**57, 1979.

Christopherson, W. M., and Miller, A. J.: A re-evaluation of solitary plasma-cell myeloma of bone, CA **3:**240, 1950.

Cohen, M. H., and others: Burkitt's tumor in the United States, CA **23:**1259, 1969.

Colombo, C. S., and Boivin, Y.: Myxoma of the jaws, Oral Surg. **21:**431, 1966.

Cranin, A. N., Berman, S., and Tucker, N.: Renal-cell carcinoma of the mandibular periodontium, Oral Surg. **21:**626, 1966.

Cranin, A. N., and Gross, E. R.: Severe oral and perioral amyloidosis as a primary complication of multiple myeloma, Oral Surg. **23:**158, 1967.

Deeb, M. E., Waite, D. E., and Jaspers, M. T.: Fibrous dysplasia of the jaws, Oral Surg. **47:**312, 1979.

De Lathouwer, C., and Verhest, A.: Malignant primary intraosseous carcinoma of the mandible, Oral Surg. **37:**77, 1974.

De-The, G., Geser, A., Day, N. E., Tukei, P. M., Williams, E. H., Beri, D. P., Smith, P. G., Dean, A. G., Bronkamm, G. W., Feorino, P., and Henle, W.: Epidemiological evidence for causal relationship between Epstein-Barr virus and Burkitt's lymphoma from Ugandan prospective study, Nature **274:**756, 1978.

Dorfman, R. F.: Diagnosis of Burkitt's tumor in the United States, CA **21:**563, 1968.

Ebling, H., and Goldenberg, N.: Central angioma, Oral Surg. **21**:9, 1966.

Ebling, H., and Wagner, J. E.: Recurrent myxoma, Oral Surg. **21**:94, 1966.

Ellis, D. J., and Winslow, J. R.: Reticulum-cell sarcoma of the mandible, Oral Surg. **42**:570, 1976.

Epker, B., Merrill, R. G., and Henny, F. A.: Breast adenocarcinoma metastatic to the mandible, Oral Surg. **28**:471, 1969.

Eversole, L. R., Saves, W. R., Beandebura, J., and Massey, G. B.: Medulloblastoma; extradural metastasis to the jaw, Oral Surg. **34**:634, 1972.

Farman, A. G., Nortje, C. J., Grotepass, F. W., Farman, F. J., and Van Zyl, J. A.: Myxofibroma of the jaws, Br. J. Oral Surg. **15**:3, 1977.

Flick, W. G., and Lawrence, F. R.: Oral amyloidosis as initial symptom of multiple myeloma, Oral Surg. **49**:18, 1980.

Freedman, P. D., Cardo, V. A., Kerpel, S. M., and Lumerman, H.: Desmoplastic fibroma (fibromatosis) of the jawbones, Oral Surg. **46**:386, 1978.

Gamez-Araujo, J. J., Toth, B. B., and Luna, M. A.: Central hemangioma of the mandible and maxilla: review of a vascular lesion, Oral Surg. **37**:230, 1974.

Gandhi, R. K., Kinare, S. G., Parulkar, G. B., and Sen, P. K.: Hemangiosarcoma (malignant hemangioendothelioma) of the mandible in a child, Oral Surg. **22**:359, 1966.

Gardner, D. G., and Mills, D. M.: The widened periodontal ligament of osteosarcoma of the jaws, Oral Surg. **41**:652, 1976.

Garrington, G. E., Scofield, H. H., Cornyn, J., and Hooker, S. P.: Osteo-sarcoma of the jaws, CA **20**:377, 1967.

Ghosh, B. C., Huvos, A. G., Gerold, F. P., and Miller, T. R.: Myxoma of the jaw bones, CA **31**:237, 1973.

Gomez, A. C., Youmans, R. D., and Chambers, R. G.: Osteogenic sarcoma of the mandible; a method of treatment, Am. J. Surg. **100**:613, 1960.

Goveia, G., and Bahn, S.: Asymptomatic hepatocellular carcinoma metastatic to the mandible, Oral Surg. **45**:424, 1978.

Griffin, E. R., Bell, T. M., and Adatia, A. K.: Virus infection of teeth in Burkitt's tumour. East Afr. Med. J. **44**:67, 1967.

Hardt, N. P.: Metastatic neuroblastoma in the mandible, Oral Surg. **41**:314, 1976.

Hasleton, P. S., Simpson, W., and Craig, R. D. P.: Myxoma of the mandible— a fibroblastic tumor, Oral Surg. **46**:396, 1978.

Henefer, E. P., Bishop, H. C., and Brown, A.: Juvenile fibromatosis with invasion of the mandible: report of two cases, J. Oral Surg. **36**:965, 1978.

Jacobs, H., Ruben, M. P., and Lyon, J.: Renal-cell carcinoma metastatic to the mandible and gingiva, Oral Surg. **22**:649, 1966.

James, R. B., Alexander, R. W., and Traver, J. G.: Osteochondroma of the mandibular coronoid process, Oral Surg. **37**:189, 1974.

Jones, W. A.: Cherubism, Oral Surg. **20**:648, 1965.

Kafuko, G. W., and Burkitt, D. P.: Burkitt's lymphoma and malaria, Int. J. Cancer **6**:1, 1970.

Kangur, T. T., Dahlin, D. C., and Turlington, E. G.: Myxomatous tumors of the jaws, J. Oral Surg. **33:**523, 1975.

Kolas, S., Halperin, V., Jefferis, K., Huddleston, S. D., and Robinson, H. B. G.: The occurrence of torus palatinus and torus mandibularis in 2,478 dental patients, Oral Surg. **6:**1134, 1953.

Kraut, R. A., Buhler, J. E., LaRue, J. R., and Acevedo, A.: Amyloidosis associated with multiple myeloma, Oral Surg. **43:**63, 1977.

Lainson, P. A., Khowassah, M. A., and Tewfik, H. H.: Seminoma metastatic to the jaws, Oral Surg. **40:**404, 1975.

Large, N. D., Niebel, H. H., and Fredricks, W. H.: Myxoma of the jaws, Oral Surg. **13:**1462, 1960.

Levy, B., and Smith, W. K.: A jaw metastasis from the colon, Oral Surg. **38:**769, 1974.

Lewin, R., and Cataldo, E.: Multiple myeloma discovered from oral manifestations: report of a case, J. Oral Surg. **25:**68, 1967.

Linkous, C. M., and Welch, J. T.: Metastatic malignant tumors of the jaws, Oral Surg. **38:**703, 1974.

MacMahon, B.: Epidemiologic aspects of acute leukemia and Burkitt's tumor, CA **21:**558, 1968.

Melrose, R. J., and Abrams, A. M.: Juvenile fibromatosis affecting the jaws, Oral Surg. **49:**317, 1980.

Milobsky, S. A., Milobsky, L., and Epstein, L. I.: Metastatic renal adenocarcinoma presenting as periapical pathosis in the maxilla, Oral Surg. **39:**30, 1975.

Mori, M., Murakami, M., Hirose, I., and Shimozato, T.: Histochemical studies of myxoma of the jaws., J. Oral Surg. **33:**529, 1975.

Neal, C. J., Jr.: Multiple osteomas of the mandible associated with polyposis of the colon (Gardner's syndrome), Oral Surg. **28:**628, 1969.

Newland, J. R., and Ayala, A. G.: Parosteal osteosarcoma of the maxilla, Oral Surg. **43:**727, 1977.

Orlean, S. L., and Blewitt, G.: Multiple myeloma with manifestation of a bony lesion in the maxilla, Oral Surg. **19:**817, 1965.

Perriman, A., Uthman, A., and Kuzair, K. Y.: Central hemangiomas of the jaws, Oral Surg. **37:**502, 1974.

Peters, W. J. N.: Cherubism: a study of twenty cases from one family, Oral Surg. **47:**307, 1979.

Pickle, D. E., Gordon, R., Scopp, I. W., and Mittelman, G. J.: Multiple myeloma: its oral manifestations, Oral Surg. **21:**347, 1966.

Polte, H. W., Kolodny, S. C., and Hooker, S. P.: Intraosseous angiolipoma of the mandible, Oral Surg. **41:**637, 1976.

Potdar, G. G.: Ewing's tumors of the jaws, Oral Surg. **29:**505, 1970.

Potdar, G. G.: Osteogenic sarcoma of the jaws, Oral Surg. **30:**381, 1970.

Potdar, G. G., and Srikhande, S. S.: Chondrogenic tumors of the jaws, Oral Surg. **30:**649, 1970.

Pullon, P. A., and Cohen, D. M.: Oral metastasis of retinoblastoma, Oral Surg. **37**:583, 1974.

Ramsey, H. E., Strong, E. W., and Frazell, E. L.: Progressive fibrous dysplasia of the maxilla, J. Am. Dent. Assoc. **81**:1388, 1970.

Rapoport, A., Sobrinho, J. A., Carvalho, M. B., Magrin, J., Costa, F. Q., and Quadros, J. V.: Ewing's sarcoma of the mandible, Oral Surg. **44**:89, 1977.

Reed, R. J., and Hagy, D. M.: Benign nonodontogenic fibro-osseous lesions of the skull, Oral Surg. **19**:214, 1965.

Remagen, W., and Prein, J.: Benign osteoblastoma, Oral Surg. **39**:279, 1975.

Roca, A. N., Smith, J. L., MacComb, W. S., and Jing, B. S.: Ewing's sarcoma of the maxilla and mandible, Oral Surg. **25**:194, 1968.

Saw, D.: Fibrosarcoma of maxilla, Oral Surg. **47**:164, 1979.

Schmaman, A., Smith, I., and Ackerman, L. V.: Benign fibro-osseous lesions of the mandible and maxilla, CA **26**:303, 1970.

Schofield, I. D. F.: An aggressive fibrous dysplasia, Oral Surg. **38**:29, 1974.

Shawkat, A. H., and Phillips, J. D.: Multiple myeloma, Oral Surg. **37**:969, 1974.

Shear, M.: Primary intra-alveolar epidermoid carcinoma of the jaw, J. Pathol. **97**:645, 1969.

Sidhu, S. S., Sukhija, D. S., and Parkash, H.: Burkitt's lymphoma, Oral Surg. **39**:463, 1975.

Siguira, I.: Desmoplastic fibroma: case report and review of the literature, J. Bone Joint Surg. **58A**:126, 1976.

Simon, G. T., Kendrick, R. W., and Whitlock, R. I. H.: Osteochondroma of the mandibular condyle, Oral Surg. **43**:18, 1977.

Singh, K. R. B., Vanniasingham, P. C., Sreenevasan, G. A., Kutty, M. K., and Omar-Ahmad, U. D.: Burkitt's lymphoma: report of five cases in West Malaysia, Far East Med. J. **5**:261, 1969.

Sirsat, M. V., Sampat, M. B., and Shrikhande, S. S.: Primary intraalveolar squamous-cell carcinoma of the mandible, Oral Surg. **35**:366, 1973.

Slootweg, P. J., and Muller, H., Malignant fibrous histiocytoma of the maxilla, Oral Surg. **44**:560, 1977.

Small, E. W.: Malignant chordoma, Oral Surg. **37**:863, 1974.

Sobel, R. S., and Goldberg, N. L.: Lymphoma metastatic to the mandible, J. Dent. Child. **39**:262, 1972.

Soloman, M. P., Biernacki, J., Slippen, M., and Rosen, Y.: Parosteal osteogenic sarcoma of the mandible, Arch. Otolaryngol. **101**:754, 1975.

Stewart, S. S., Baum, S. M., Arlen, M., and Elguezabal, A.: Myxoma of the lower jaw, Oral Surg. **36**:800, 1973.

Straith, F. E.: Metastatic adenocarcinoma of mandible, Oral Surg. **24**:1, 1967.

Tanner, H. C., Dahlin, D. C., and Childs, D. S.: Sarcoma complicating fibrous dysplasia, Oral Surg. **14**:837, 1961.

Tasanen, A., Konow, L. V., and Nordling, S.: Central giant-cell lesion in the mandibular condyle, Oral Surg. **45**:532, 1978.

Todd, I. D. H.: Treatment of solitary plasmocytoma, Clin. Radiol. **16:**395, 1965.

Topazian, R. G.: Central hemangioma of the mandible, Oral Surg. **18:**1, 1964.

Torres, J. S., and Vinas, F.: Central mandibular hemangioma, Oral Surg. **37:**509, 1974.

Toth, B. B., Byrne, P., and Hinds, E. C.: Central adenocarcinoma of the mandible, Oral Surg. **39:**436, 1975.

Unni, K. K., Dahlin, D. C., Beabout, I. W., and Ivins, J. C.: Parosteal osteogenic sarcoma, CA **37:**2466, 1976.

van der Kwast, W. A. M., and van der Waal, I.: Jaw metastases, Oral Surg. **37:**850, 1974.

Waldron, C. A., and Giansanti, J. S.: Benign fibro-osseous lesions of the jaws: a clinical-radiologic-histologic review of sixty-five cases, Oral Surg. **35:**340, 1973.

Webb, H. E., Devine, K. D., and Harrison, E. G.: Solitary myeloma of the mandible, Oral Surg. **22:**1, 1966.

Yip, W. K., and Lee, H. T. L.: Benign osteoblastoma of the maxilla, Oral Surg. **38:**259, 1974.

Zimmerman, D. C., and Dahlin, D. C.: Myxomatous tumors of the jaws, Oral Surg. **11:**1069, 1958.

CHAPTER 12

Diseases of jaws

A heterogeneous group of diseases of the jaws, most of unknown cause and not discussed elsewhere, are described in this chapter.

1. Paget's disease (osteitis deformans)
2. Osteopetrosis (Albers-Schönberg disease; marble bone disease)
3. Leontiasis ossea
4. Engelmann's disease (Camurati-Engelmann disease; multiple diaphyseal sclerosis)
5. Osteogenesis imperfecta (Lobstein's disease; brittle bone; fragilitas ossium; osteopsathyrosis)
6. Caffey's disease (infantile cortical hyperostosis)
7. Garré's disease (osteomyelitis)
8. Condensing osteitis
9. Chronic sclerosing osteomyelitis
10. Fibrous dysplasia (osteitis fibrosa disseminata; fibrous osteodystrophy; polyostotic fibrous dysplasia)
11. Histiocytosis X
    a. Eosinophilic granuloma
    b. Hand-Schüller-Christian disease
    c. Letterer-Siwe disease
12. Gaucher's disease
13. Niemann-Pick disease
14. Osteomyelitis
15. Hematopoietic marrow
16. Gorham's disease
17. Osteoradionecrosis

Paget's disease (osteitis deformans). Paget's disease, a generalized bone disease of unknown cause, is named after the man who first described it (in 1876).

Generally the disease occurs after 40 years of age, and males are affected slightly more frequently than females. It is believed to affect about 3% of the population over 40 years of age. Major involvement occurs in the skull (Fig. 12-1) and the weight-bearing parts of the skeleton. The tibia is bent anteriorly and the femur outward, causing the patient to assume a waddling gait. Enlargement of the head, pain, headaches, mental disturbances, and loss of hearing and eyesight (because of involve-

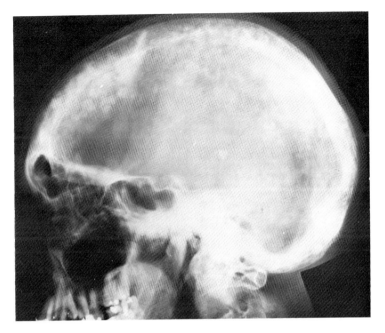

Fig. 12-1. Skull in Paget's disease. Note the cotton wool appearance of the radiopacities.

ment of the cranial base and pressure on the cranial nerves) are the chief complaints. The alkaline phosphatase level of blood is markedly increased.

Oral involvement is common, and the jaws frequently are affected. Enlargement of the alveolar ridge in an edentulous patient, which causes dentures to gradually lose their fit, may be the first symptom of the disease. The maxilla is affected more often than the mandible. Teeth may migrate and occasionally loosen, and diastemas may develop (Fig. 12-2).

Radiographic findings depend on the stage of the disease. In the early stages an irregular radiolucency is evident. This progressively turns to radiopacity and finally to dense, irregular, highly radiopaque areas resembling cotton wool (Fig. 12-3). The

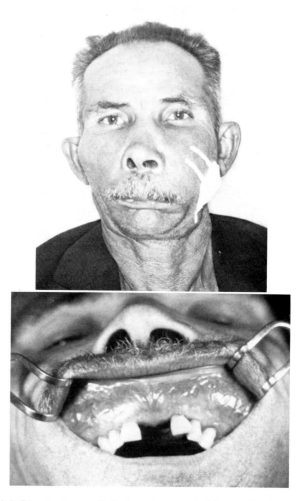

Fig. 12-2. Paget's disease. Note the enlargement of the maxilla, the migration of teeth, and the diastema.

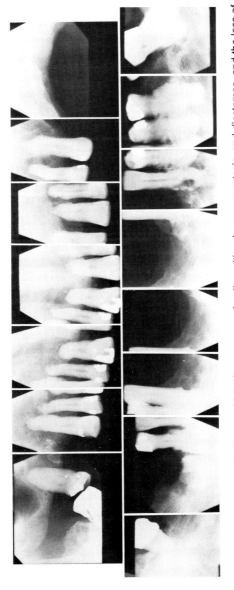

Fig. 12-3. Jaws in Paget's disease. Note the presence of radiopacities, hypercementosis, and diastemas, and the loss of lamina dura.

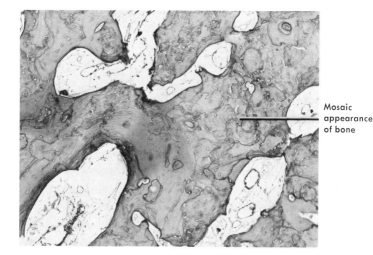

Mosaic
appearance
of bone

Fig. 12-4. Paget's disease. Note the mosaic appearance of the bone.

teeth show hypercementosis, pulp calcifications, and loss of lamina dura (Fig. 12-3). Other conditions with loss of lamina dura are hyperparathyroidism and fibrous dysplasia.

The microscopic appearance of Paget's disease is almost pathognomonic and consists of a mosaic or jigsaw pattern that is a result of successive waves of bone destruction and bone apposition (Fig. 12-4). There are numerous osteoclasts and areas of bone resorption as well as osteoblasts and areas of bone formation. Bone resorption and apposition occur in a chaotic manner, thus weakening the affected bone. The marrow shows fibrosis and marked vascularity.

There is no treatment for Paget's disease. Some cases undergo spontaneous remission. About 25% of patients with this condition, develop osteogenic sarcomas. In such cases the prognosis is poor.

Osteopetrosis (Albers-Schönberg disease; marble bone disease). Osteopetrosis is a hereditary disease that is transmitted

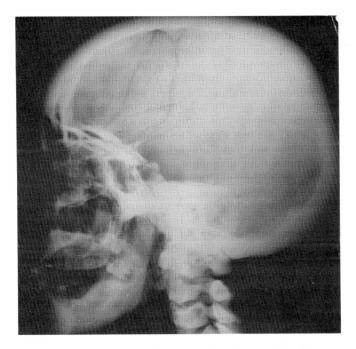

Fig. 12-5. Osteopetrosis. The bones show dense radiopacities.

as a recessive mutation and is characterized by normal bone formation in the absence of bone resorption.

The disease affects the entire skeleton but especially the bones of the extremities. The bones are dense and heavy. There is obliteration of red marrow, which leads to anemia.

Pressure on the nerve foramina causes neurologic disturbances (e.g., paralysis, optic and acoustic impairment). Spontaneous fractures occur. Dense radiopacities are observed (Fig. 12-5). Teeth may fail to erupt or may erupt late or in abnormal sites. Roots and crown may be malformed. Healing of extraction wounds is retarded, and there is formation of sequestra. Osteomyelitis is a common occurrence after surgery.

Microscopic sections prepared from the affected bones show a remarkable increase in the number of bone trabeculae. Osteoclasts are present but are not effective. The hematopoietic marrow is replaced by fibrous marrow. Because of the lack of bone resorption, the bony crypts impinge on the enlarging tooth germs (which become markedly distorted).

There is no treatment for osteopetrosis.

Leontiasis ossea. Leontiasis ossea is a developmental disturbance that is a form of fibrous dysplasia. It affects primarily the upper face. It is essentially a hyperostosis (i.e., a disorder characterized by the presence of dense bone tissue). Lesions therefore are characterized by dense areas of radiopacity in the maxilla, nasal bones, frontal bones, temporal bones, and zygomatic bones. The accessory sinuses are also replaced by bone tissue.

The disease starts in childhood and is progressive, leading to blindness or deafness, and usually fatal. The loss of sight and hearing is due to compression of the optic and acoustic nerves by the excessive bone at the optic foramina and the internal acoustic meatus.

Engelmann's disease (Camurati-Engelmann disease; multiple diaphyseal sclerosis). Engelmann's disease is hereditary and affects primarily the diaphyses of long bones. The bones are heavy. There is marked osteosclerosis, and a few instances of osteosclerotic mandibles have been described.

Osteogenesis imperfecta (Lobstein's disease; brittle bone; fragilitas ossium; osteopsathyrosis). Osteogenesis imperfecta is a hereditary disease representing a mutation. It may develop in utero and therefore be apparent at birth (osteogenesis imperfecta congenitalis), or it may develop during childhood and adolescence (osteogenesis imperfecta tarda).

The essential defect is in the mesenchyme, resulting in bone tissue that is of abnormal quality and quantity. This leads to multiple fractures, which heal only to fracture again. Almost all cases are associated with dentinogenesis imperfecta. Some are associated with "blue sclerae" because the pigmented choroid membrane of the eyes appears blue when seen through a thin sclera.

The mandible is more severely affected than the maxilla. Microscopic sections show thin trabeculae of immature bone tissue. The prognosis is poor, and there is no known treatment for the disease. Death may occur in utero, at birth, or in infancy; or the patient may survive with multiple deformities.

Caffey's disease (infantile cortical hyperostosis). Caffey's disease is characterized by enlargement of the affected bone and some systemic symptoms. Its cause is not known. Patients are usually under 6 months of age.

In certain instances the disease is associated with fever, leukocytosis, an increased sedimentation rate, and elevated alkaline phosphatase. Although any bone may be involved, the most common sites are the mandible (Fig. 12-6), the ulna, and the clavicle. The mandible is involved in more than 75% of cases. Children with this disease are irritable. Swelling over the affected bone appears suddenly and disappears in 3 to 12 months without suppuration.

Radiographs taken sometime after the clinical appearance of swelling show thickening of the cortex and bulging of the lower border of the mandible (Fig. 12-6). Some cases of cortical thickening as seen in this disease have been associated with child abuse.

Microscopic sections show edema and thickening of the periosteum and apposition of a large number of thin bone trabeculae that are laid down parallel to each other (Fig. 12-7).

The prognosis in Caffey's disease is good, and the lesion requires nothing more than symptomatic therapy. Surgery is not necessary, but corticosteroids have been used to alleviate symptoms.

Garré's disease (osteomyelitis). In some patients with osteomyelitis, there is a marked growth of new bone tissue underneath the periosteum. This type of proliferative or sclerosing reaction on the periosteal side of inflammatory lesions in bone has been called Garré's osteomyelitis.

The mandible is involved more frequently than the maxilla, and the lesion commonly occurs in children or young adults. There is usually an inflammatory lesion within the jaw (e.g.,

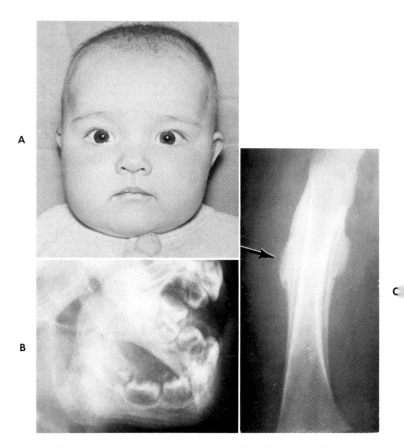

Fig. 12-6. Caffey's disease. **A** and **B,** Mandible. Note the thickness of the lower border. **C,** Femur. The cortical bone is thickened. (**A** and **B** from Bethart, H., and Fitch, H. B.: Oral Surg. **16:**622, 1963; **C** courtesy Hector Bethart, D.D.S.)

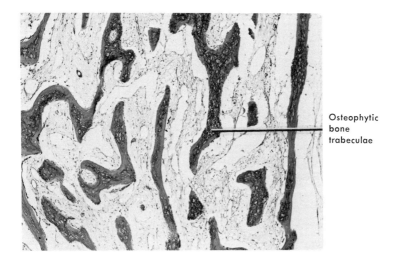

Fig. 12-7. Caffey's disease with osteophytic bone trabeculae.

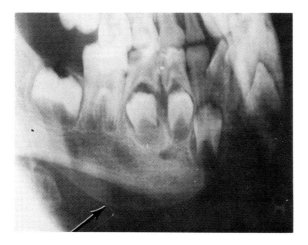

Fig. 12-8. Reactive exostosis of the mandible. (Garré's disease, or osteomyelitis). Note the thickening of the lower border of the mandible (arrow).

periapical abscess, radicular cyst), and the periosteal surface of the bone opposing this area is markedly thickened (Fig. 12-8).

Microscopic sections show elevation of the periosteum, new bone formation as parallel trabeculae of bone, fibrous marrow, and the presence of plasma cells and lymphocytes in the marrow spaces.

Treatment of Garré's disease consists of removal of the cause.

Condensing osteitis. Also called the focal type of sclerosing osteomyelitis, this condition is a localized low-grade chronic inflammation of the bone marrow. It is associated with bone formation rather than bone destruction. It occurs in the middle age, and the mandibular molar area is the most commonly affected site. Usually there are no symptoms. Condensing osteitis is associated with a tooth having pulp or periapical pathology or is seen in an old extraction site.

The lesions appear as localized radiopacities (Fig. 12-9). Microscopic sections show dense bone trabeculae, narrow marrow spaces, and mild infiltration by plasma cells and lymphocytes. The lesion requires no treatment.

Chronic sclerosing osteomyelitis. This condition is also called diffuse sclerosing osteomyelitis (DSO), multiple enostosis, sclerosing osteitis, gigantiform cementomas, or sclerotic cemental masses of the jaws. It occurs predominantly in females, in the third decade of life or later, and is more common in blacks than in whites.

The mandible is involved far more frequently than the maxilla, and the premolar and molar areas are the usual sites. Teeth may or may not be present in the area. The lesions range in duration from a few months to many years and often last for the life of the patient. The affected area may be enlarged. Some patients have repeated episodes of pain around the jaws, swelling, and trismus; or the lesions may be asymptomatic.

Multiple, well-defined or diffuse, dense radiopacities may be surrounded by radiolucencies (Fig. 12-10). Jaw lesions have a cotton wool or pagetoid appearance (Fig. 12-11) with the rest of the skeleton not involved.

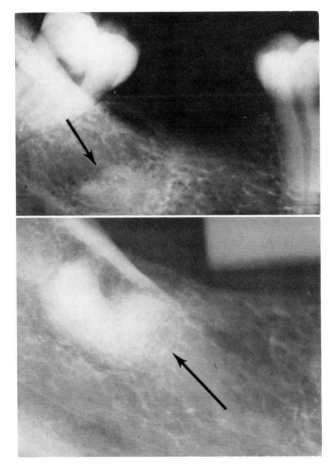

Fig. 12-9. Condensing osteitis is characterized by localized, usually asymptomatic areas of radiopacity (arrows).

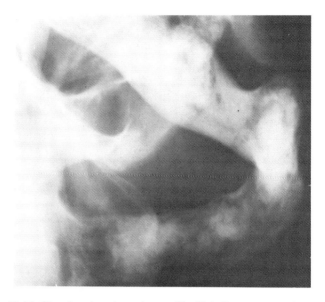

Fig. 12-10. Chronic sclerosing osteomyelitis. Note the presence of many radiopacities in this edentulous mandible.

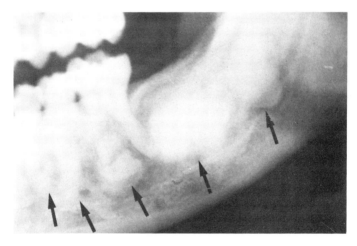

Fig. 12-11. Chronic sclerosing osteomyelitis (arrows) in the mandible. The lesion has a cotton wool appearance.

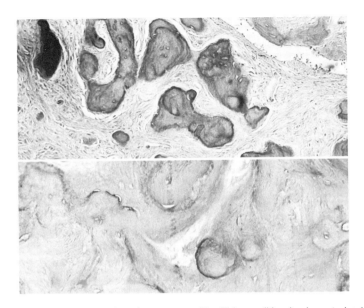

Fig. 12-12. Chronic sclerosing osteomyelitis. This condition is characterized by dense lamellated bone tissue with many basophilic lines.

Microscopically multiple enostoses are characterized by areas of dense lamellated bone with numerous basophilic resting and reversal lines (Fig. 12-12). Bone tissue configuration may resemble the jigsaw pattern of Paget's disease; but lesions are restricted to the jaws, and the alkaline phosphatase level is within normal limits. The marrow spaces are sparse and filled by a fibrous marrow that, in ulcerated lesions, contains plasma cells, neutrophils, and lymphocytes.

Since the disease is extensive but self-limiting, it is neither possible nor necessary to remove all lesions. Foci of the disease that are near the crest of an edentulous ridge are subject to ulceration and sequestration. If a patient wears a denture over one of these areas, secondary inflammation is a common sequela. For this reason, lesions that are secondarily inflamed or are near the crest of a ridge should be surgically removed.

Since the cause of this disease is not known, other treatments such as antibiotic therapy, cortisone therapy, and decortication have been tried with questionable results.

Fibrous dysplasia (osteitis fibrosa disseminata; fibrous osteodystrophy; polyostotic fibrous dysplasia). Fibrous dysplasia is a disease of childhood or adolescence that involves many bones.

Although the lesions are commonly unilateral, they may occur bilaterally. Fibrous dysplasia sometimes is associated with hypergonadism in females and with brown spots on the skin (café au lait spots). When fibrous dysplasia occurs with pigmentation and sexual disturbances, it is called *Albright's syndrome.* The affected bone is enlarged and deformed, the jaws are enlarged and deformed, teeth and tooth germs are displaced, and malocclusion follows (Fig. 12-13).

Radiographs may show enlargement of the jaw, expansion of the cortex, a radiolucency, reduced radiopacity, or a mottled

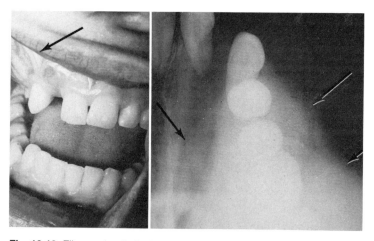

Fig. 12-13. Fibrous dysplasia. Note the characteristic enlargement of the jaw, the radiopacity, and the migration of teeth (arrows). Furthermore, other bones in the skeleton are involved.

appearance (Fig. 12-13). Microscopic sections show replacement of normal bone by an essentially fibroblastic lesion in which numerous regularly arranged trabeculae of bone can be seen (Fig. 12-14). Without the clinical features the lesion is often difficult to distinguish from an ossifying fibroma and other fibro-osseous lesions.

Treatment of fibrous dysplasia consists of conservative surgical excision.

Histiocytosis X. The term histiocytosis X is applied to a group of three manifestations of one disease process: eosinophilic granuloma, Hand-Schüller-Christian disease, and Letterer-Siwe disease. This grouping is based on the assumption that the three entities are all associated with involvement of the reticuloendothelial system (reticulum cells of the bone marrow, spleen, lymph nodes, and liver, and histiocytes and macrophages of connective tissue).

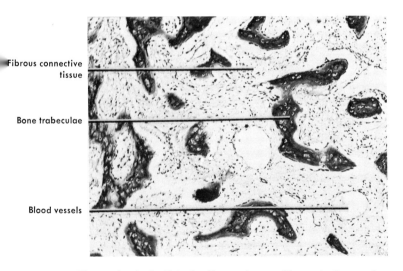

Fibrous connective
tissue

Bone trabeculae

Blood vessels

Fig. 12-14. Fibrous dysplasia. Note the fibrous stroma with evenly dispersed bone trabeculae.

Eosinophilic granuloma is known as histiocytosis localized in bone, Hand-Schüller-Christian disease as chronic disseminated histiocytosis X, and Letterer-Siwe disease as acute or subacute disseminated histiocytosis X. Almost 65% of patients are under 6 years of age. Although gingival or jaw lesions are found in about 35% of patients, in 15% of patients the oral lesions are the primary clinical manifestation and the dentist is the first to see the case.

The most important clinical, radiographic, and microscopic features of these diseases are given in the ensuing discussions.

Eosinophilic granuloma. This manifestation, localized in bone, occurs in the second and third decades of life (median age about 20 years), affects males far more commonly than females, and is the chronic localized form of histiocytosis X.

Usually the lesions are in bones and are solitary (monostotic). However, multiple lesions may occur in bone (polyostotic) as well as in soft tissues. With the exception of the hands and feet, any bone may be affected. The mandible is involved three times as often as the maxilla, and the posterior portion of the jaws is the preferred site. General symptoms are fever, malaise, anorexia, and headache. Lesions of the jaws are not uncommon and may be the *first* and *only signs of the disease*.

Oral lesions consist of a sore mouth, fetid breath, pus, pain, swelling, loosening of the teeth, retarded healing after extraction, an unpleasant taste, and swollen gingiva (Fig. 12-15).

Radiographs show single or multiple areas of complete radiolucency in the jaws. When the lesions involve the alveolar bone, regional teeth appear to "hang in air" (Fig. 12-16).

Microscopic sections are pathognomonic. Lesions consist of two types of cells: histiocytes and eosinophils (Fig. 12-17). The histiocytes, or reticulum cells, are large cells with light-staining cytoplasm and a vesicular nucleus, and they form almost solid sheets. The eosinophils are dispersed singly and in clusters throughout the lesion. Histiocytes and eosinophils replace bone tissue and marrow of the jaw, thus causing loosening of the teeth.

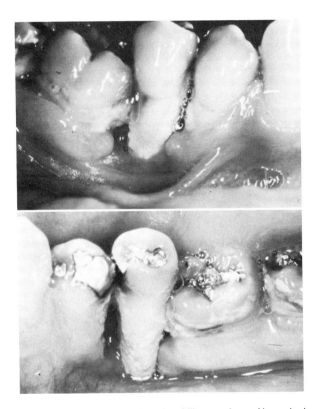

Fig. 12-15. Clinical appearance of eosinophilic granuloma. Necrosis, loosening of teeth, and ulceration are common features. (Courtesy Milton J. Knapp, D.D.S., Portland, Ore.)

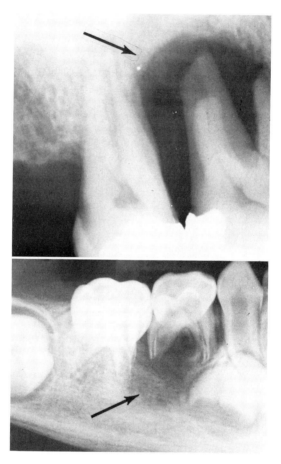

Fig. 12-16. Eosinophilic granuloma (two cases). The classic radiographic appearance is that of teeth "hanging in air" (arrows).

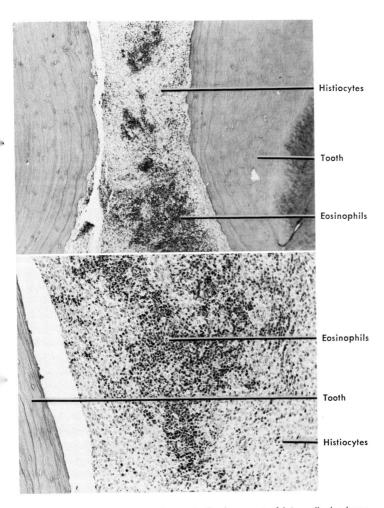

Fig. 12-17. Eosinophilic granuloma. **A,** Replacement of interradicular bone. **B,** High-power view of the cellular components, consisting of histiocytes and eosinophils.

360 Pathology of teeth and jaws

Eosinophilic granuloma responds favorably to surgical curettage, following which less than 16% of lesions recur.

Hand-Schüller-Christian disease. This disease, or chronic disseminated histiocytosis X, occurs in the first decade of life. It primarily involves the bones, in which areas of normal marrow are replaced by proliferating macrophages. The skull is most frequently affected (Fig. 12-18).

Besides the lesions in bone, there may be papular rashes or petechial eruptions on the skin, ulceration and necrosis of oral

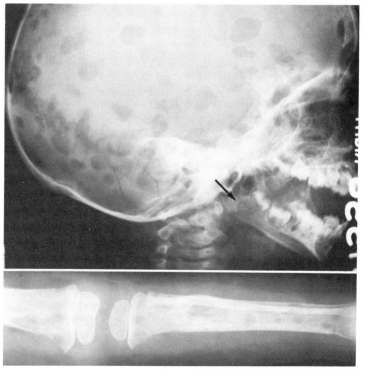

Fig. 12-18. Hand-Schüller-Christian disease. Lesions occur in the skull, jaws (arrow), and long bones.

mucosa, and enlargement of the liver, lymph nodes, and spleen. A few patients have a triad of symptoms: (1) bone lesions; (2) exophthalmos, which results from a lesion in the orbit displacing the eyeball outward; and (3) diabetes insipidus, which results from a lesion in the body of the sphenoid extending to the pituitary gland and replacing its posterior lobe (Fig. 12-18). These three symptoms together constitute the *Hand-Schüller-Christian syndrome*.

Clinically and radiographically the oral lesions are identical to those of eosinophilic granuloma. Microscopic sections show many large vacuolated foam cells as well as smaller nonvacuolated cells. These are lipid-containing (cholesterol) and non lipidized histiocytes (Fig. 12-19). The lesions may respond favorably to radiation therapy, regress, or be progressive and prove ultimately fatal.

Letterer-Siwe disease. This manifestation, acute or subacute disseminated histiocytosis X, is the most severe form of the

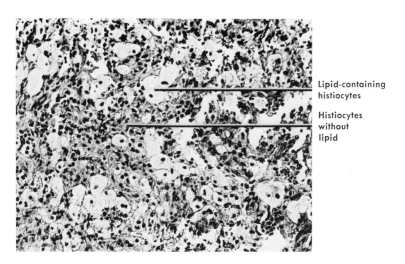

Lipid-containing histiocytes

Histiocytes without lipid

Fig. 12-19. Hand-Schüller-Christian disease. Note the lipid-containing and lipid-free histiocytes.

three manifestations of histiocytosis and is invariably fatal. It usually occurs before the age of 2 years and primarily involved the viscera—resulting in enlargement of the spleen, liver, and lymph nodes, and involvement of the lungs, bone marrow, and skin. Replacement of bone marrow leads to anemia and petechiae.

Jaw lesions are less common in Letterer-Siwe disease than in eosinophilic granuloma or Hand-Schüller-Christian disease. However, the skull, skeleton, and jaws may be involved the same as in Hand-Schüller-Christian disease (Fig. 12-20). Microscopic sections show marked proliferation of nonlipidized histiocytes.

Gaucher's disease. In this disease of the reticuloendothelial system—a lipid (kerasin) is deposited in the reticular cells of the liver, spleen, lymph nodes, and bone marrow. It can occur at any age, and females have a greater predilection than males. The skin shows brown pigmentation.

Lesions in the oral regions are rare. Because of replacement of marrow and thrombocytopenia, there is gingival bleeding. Microscopically the presence of large foam cells with striations, called Gaucher's cells, is pathognomonic.

Niemann-Pick disease. This disorder, characterized by accumulation of a lipid (sphingomyelin) in cells of the reticuloendothelial system, is limited to infants. The patients are usually of Hebrew descent, and the disease is fatal within two years.

Oral lesions, which are rare, consist of radiolucent areas in the jaws. Involvement of the brain and optic nerve leads to idiocy and blindness.

Osteomyelitis. In a strict sense, any inflammatory lesion that involves the bone marrow can be referred to as osteomyelitis. By usage, however, the term osteomyelitis is limited to pus-producing inflammatory lesions of the bones.

The disease can occur at any age and is most common in males. Although in infancy the maxilla is usually involved, during childhood and later life the mandible is the preferred site. Acute exacerbation of periapical lesions and fractures are the

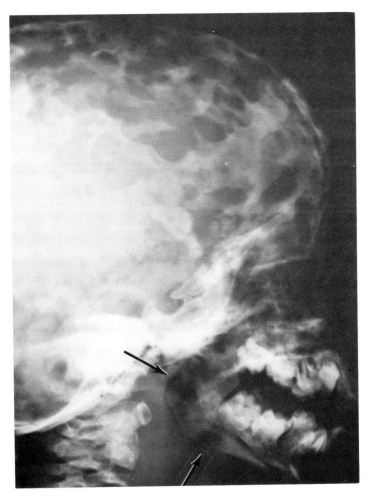

Fig. 12-20. Letterer-Siwe disease. Note the presence of numerous radiolucencies in the skull and jaws (arrows).

precipitating factors. Staphylococci and streptococci are the usual causative organisms, but osteomyelitis may be caused by other organisms such as *Actinomyces israelii* and the tubercle bacillus.

Clinically there is swelling and pain and sometime redness of the skin overlying the area of involvement. Fever, malaise, leukocytosis, and lymphadenopathy are present. The breath may be fetid and the teeth loose.

In the early stages, radiographic findings are negative; but in a week or two, diffuse irregular areas of radiolucency may be apparent (Fig. 12-21).

Microscopic sections show dense, diffuse infiltration of the marrow by neutrophils (Fig. 12-22). Further away from the area of involvement, the infiltrate consists predominantly of lymphocytes and plasma cells. Bone trabeculae in the involved area show empty lacunae. Bone devoid of osteocytes (i.e., dead bone) is called a *sequestrum*. By a process of bone resorption, the living connective tissue surrounding the dead bone segregates it from the remainder of the jaw. (Normal bone surrounding a sequestrum is called an *involucrum*.) Small sequestra are exfoliated slowly and spontaneously, but larger ones require surgical intervention.

Treatment of osteomyelitis consists of drainage, antibiotics, and, if necessary, surgical removal of the sequestra.

Hematopoietic marrow. Although hematopoietic marrow is not a pathologic process, it is included here because of its radiographic appearance.

In some patients foci of red bone marrow large enough to present as radiolucencies develop in certain areas of the jaws. Since these are asymptomatic, they are found on routine examination. The mandible is involved far more frequently than the maxilla, and the premolar and molar areas are the preferred sites (Fig. 12-23). Hematopoietic marrow is seen in females more often than in males. The lesions can occur at any age, but about 25% appear in the fourth decade of life.

Microscopically the specimen reveals typical hematopoietic

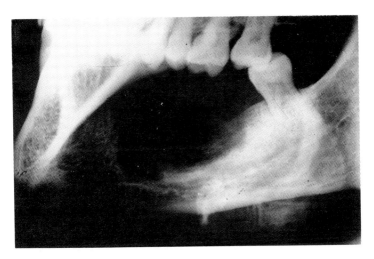

Fig. 12-21. Osteomyelitis. Note the irregular destruction of the mandible. The clinical presence of pus is a constant finding.

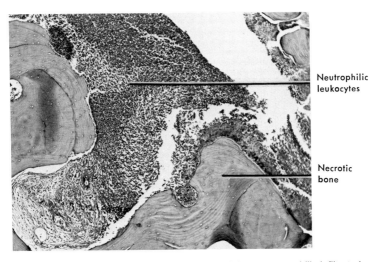

Neutrophilic leukocytes

Necrotic bone

Fig. 12-22. Osteomyelitis. Note the presence of dense neutrophilic infiltrate in the marrow spaces.

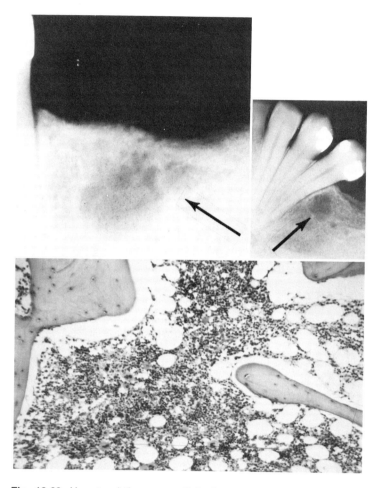

Fig. 12-23. Hematopoietic marrow. Note the asymptomatic radiolucencies (arrows). In the lower figure the microscopic features consist of the usual components of red bone marrow—fat, megakaryocytes, and various types of immature blood cells of the white and red series.

marrow, including fat, megakaryocytes, and immature cells of the polymorphonuclear and erythrocytic series (Fig. 12-23). Since clinically these foci cannot be distinguished from other radiolucent lesions, their surgical exploration is necessary.

Physiologic osteoporosis of the jaws occurs in most elderly individuals and is usually generalized, but in some cases it appears as localized diffuse radiolucencies.

Gorham's disease. In this rare condition a large portion of a bone disappears without any apparent cause. Although it usually affects the scapula, any bone of the skeleton may be involved.

Cases with disappearance of the ramus and parts of the mandibular body have been reported. Patients are usually children or young adults, and a history of trauma (e.g., beating or tooth extraction) is often elicited. No treatment is effective, and bone resorption can cease spontaneously.

Osteoradionecrosis. Radiation of the jaws during treatment of head and neck cancer can lead to long-lasting damage to vascular, connective, and bone tissues. This damage lowers the re-

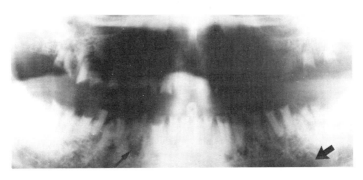

Fig. 12-24. Osteoradionecrosis in a patient who received radiation therapy for a squamous cell carcinoma of the tongue. There are multiple periapical lesions that followed radiation caries (left arrow). Arrow on the right shows radiolucencies that represent bone destruction due to radiation and subsequent inflammation.

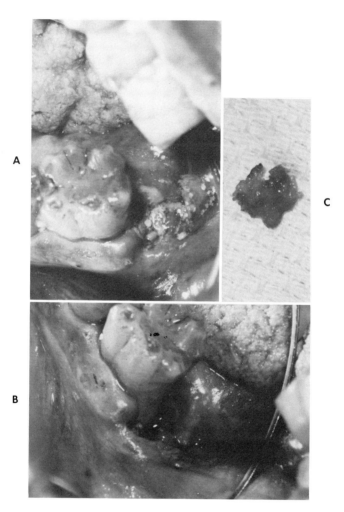

Fig. 12-25. Osteoradionecrosis. Sequestrum distal to a lower second molar before **(A)** and after **(B)** removal. The removed bone is shown in **C.**

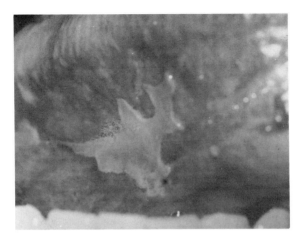

Fig. 12-26. Necrosis on the ventral surface of the tongue of a patient who received large doses of radiation for squamous cell carcinoma of the area.

sistance of bone to infection and injury. Thus extraction of teeth or soft tissue infection following damaging radiation can produce prolonged and catastrophic bone destruction called osteoradionecrosis. There is a positive correlation between dental disease present before radiation therapy and the subsequent incidence of osteoradionecrosis. Therefore, as much dental disease as practical should be eradicated before radiation therapy.

Roentgenograms of radiated jaws show an early stage of radiopacity that is soon accompanied by radiolucent areas (Fig. 12-24). Sequestion of bone, fistulae, and ulceration of mucosa may be present, and the lesions are often associated with pain (Figs. 12-25 and 12-26). Teeth in the area may show cervical or root caries called radiation caries. Caries may lead to pulp necrosis and periapical lesions (Fig. 12-24). Patients with teeth have a much higher incidence of osteoradionecrosis than those who are edentulous (2:1).

Microscopic sections reveal sequestra (areas of bone without osteocytes), neutrophils, and lymphocytic infiltrate of bone marrow; endarteritis; foci of sclerosis of bone; and connective tissue necrosis.

The incidence of osteoradionecrosis can be reduced by maximal eradication of dental disease before radiation and meticulous oral hygiene and dental care after radiation.

REFERENCES

Bethart, H., and Fitch, H. B.: Caffey's disease, Oral Surg. **16:**622, 1963.

Bhaskar, S. N.: Hemopoietic marrow (unpublished data).

Bhaskar, S. N., and Cutright, D. E.: Multiple enostosis, J. Oral Surg. **26:**321, 1968.

Boyne, P. J.: Incidence of osteosclerotic areas in the mandible and maxilla, J. Oral Surg. **18:**486, 1960.

Braham, R. L.: Multiple congenital abnormalities with diaphyseal dysplasia (Camurati-Engelmann's syndrome), Oral Surg. **27:**20, 1969.

Brunner, H.: Eosinophilic granuloma of mouth, pharynx, and nasal passages, Oral Surg. **4:**623, 1951.

Brustein, H. C., and Mautner, R. L.: Osteogenesis imperfecta, Oral Surg. **42:**42, 1976.

Caffey, J.: Infantile cortical hyperostoses, J. Pediatr. **29:**541, 1946.

Collins, E. M., Schmale, J., and Kiersch, T. A.: Chronic disseminated histiocytosis X treated with vinblastine sulfate and prednisone, Oral Surg. **38:**388, 1974.

Cunningham, J.: Hand-Schüller-Kay-Christian disease and Kay's triad, N. Engl. J. Med. **282:**1325, 1970.

Cutler, L. S., and Krutchkoff, D.: An ultrastructural study of eosinophilic granuloma: the Langerhans cell—its role in histogenesis and diagnosis, Oral Surg. **44:**246, 1977.

Cutright, D. E.: Osseous and chondromatous metaplasia caused by dentures, Oral Surg. **34:**625, 1972.

Dick, H. M., and Simpson, W. J.: Dental changes in osteopetrosis, Oral Surg. **34:**408, 1972.

Ellis, D. J., Winslow, J. R., and Indovina, A. A.: Garré's osteomyelitis of the mandible, Oral Surg. **44:**183, 1977.

El-Mofty, S.: Atrophy of the mandible (massive osteolysis), Oral Surg. **31:**690, 1971.

El-Mofty, S.: Chronic diffuse sclerosing osteomyelitis, Oral Surg. **36:**898, 1973.

Enriquez, P., Dahlin, D. C., Hayles, A. B., and Henderson, E. D.: Histiocytosis X; a clinical study, Mayo Clin. Proc. **42:**88, 1967.

Goldstein, B. H., Sciubba, J. J., and Laskin, D. M.: Actinomycosis of the maxilla: review of literature and review of case, J. Oral Surg. **30:**362, 1972.

Gorham, L. W., Wright, A. W., Shultz, H. H., and Maxon, F. C.: Disappearing bones: a rare form of massive osteolysis, Am. J. Med. **17:**674, 1954.

Hartman, K. S.: Histiocytosis X: a review of 114 cases with oral involvement, Oral Surg. **49:**38, 1980.

Jacobsson, S., and Heyden, G.: Chronic sclerosing osteomyelitis of the mandible, Oral Surg. **43:**357, 1977.

Jacobsson, S., and Hollender, L.: Treatment and prognosis of diffuse sclerosing osteomyelitis (DSO) of the mandible, Oral Surg. **49:**7, 1980.

Jacobsson, S., Hollender, L., Lindberg, S., and Larsson, A.: Chronic sclerosing osteomyelitis of the mandible, Oral Surg. **45:**167, 1978.

Jones, G. B., Midgley, R. L., and Smith, G. S.: Massive osteolysis—disappearing bones, J. Bone Joint Surg. **40B:**494, 1958.

Kanter, H. M., Lin, L. M., Goepp, R. A., and Olson, R. E.: Mandibular histiocytosis X and acute lymphoblastic leukemia, Oral Surg. **42:**221, 1976.

Keen, E. G., Sammartino, C. A., and Johnson, E. S.: Chronic sclerosing osteomyelitis of the mandible, J. Am. Dent. Assoc. **76:**597, 1968.

Lichenstein, L.: Histiocytosis X; integration of eosinophilic granuloma of bone, "Letterer-Siwe disease," and "Schüller-Christian disease" as related manifestations of a single nosologic entity, Arch. Pathol. **56:**84, 1953.

Michanowicz, A. E., Michanowicz, J. P., and Stein, G. M.: Gaucher's disease, Oral Surg. **23:**36, 1967.

Moch, W. S.: Gaucher's disease with mandibular bone lesions, Oral Surg. **6:**1250, 1953.

Murphy, J. B., Segelman, A., and Doku, C.: Osteitis deformans, Oral Surg. **46:**765, 1978.

Murray, C. G., Daly, T. E., and Zimmerman, S. O.: The relationship between dental disease and radiation necrosis of the mandible, Oral Surg. **49:**99, 1980.

Musser, L. B., Tulumello, T. N., and Hiatt, W. R.: Actinomycosis of the anterior maxilla, Oral Surg. **44:**21, 1977.

Pappas, G. C.: Bone changes in osteoradionecrosis; a review, Oral Surg. **27:**622, 1969.

Pell, G. J., Shafer, W. G., Gregory, G. T., Ping, R. S., and Spear, L. B.: Garré's osteomyelitis of the mandible, J. Oral Surg. **13:**248, 1955.

Phillips, R. M., Bush, O. B., and Hall, H. D.: Massive osteolysis (phantom bone, disappearing bone), Oral Surg. **34:**886, 1972.

Rabe, W. C., Angelillo, J. C., and Leipert, D. W.: Chronic sclerosing osteomyelitis: treatment considerations in an atypical case, Oral Surg. **49:**117, 1980.

Ramon, Y., and Buchner, A.: Camurati-Englemann's disease affecting the jaws, Oral Surg. **22:**592, 1966.

Reitzik, M., and Lownie, J. F.: Familial polyostotic fibrous dysplasia, Oral Surg. **40:**769, 1975.

Sedano, H. O., Cernea, P., Hosxe, G., and Gorlin, R. J.: Histiocytosis X, Oral Surg. **27:**760, 1969.

Sleeper, E. L.: Eosinophilic granuloma of bone; its relationship to Hand-

Schüller-Christian and Letterer-Siwe's diseases, with emphasis upon oral symptoms and findings, Oral Surg. 4:896, 1951.

Smith, N. H. H.: Albers-Schönberg disease (osteopetrosis), Oral Surg. **22:**699, 1966.

Smith, R. M.: Osteopetrosis (Albers-Schönberg disease, marble bones, osteosclerosis fragilis generalisata), Oral Surg. **20:**298, 1965.

Smith, S. N., and Farman, A. G.: Osteomyelitis with proliferative periostitis (Garre's osteomyelitis), Oral Surg. **43:**315, 1977.

Stenhouse, D.: Intraoral actinomycosis, Oral Surg. **39:**547, 1975.

Trapnell, D. H.: Periodontal manifestations of osteopetrosis, Br. J. Radiol. **41:**669, 1968.

Waldron, C. A., Giansanti, J. S., and Browand, B. C.: Sclerotic cemental masses of the jaws (so-called chronic sclerosing osteomyelitis, sclerosing osteitis, multiple enostosis, and gigantiform cementoma), Oral Surg. **39:**590, 1975.

Weinger, J. M., and Holtrop, M. E.: An ultrastructural study of bone cells: the occurrence of microtubules, microfilaments, and tight junctions, Calcif. Tissue Res. **14:**15, 1974.

White, S. C., and Prey, N. W.: An estimation of somatic hazards to the United States population from dental radiography, Oral Surg. **43:**152, 1977.

PART IV

PATHOLOGY OF ORAL MUCOSA, TONGUE, AND SALIVARY GLANDS

CHAPTER 13

Surface lesions of oral mucosa

The surface lesions of the oral mucosa and tongue are classified according to their clinical appearance.

White lesions

1. Desquamative gingivitis
2. Benign hyperkeratosis (pachyderma oris; pachyderma oralis; focal keratosis)
3. Leukoplakia with dyskeratosis (dysplastic leukoplakia)
4. Verrucous leukoplakia
5. Carcinoma in situ
6. Erythroplakia
7. Squamous cell carcinoma
8. White sponge nevus (naevus spongiosis albus mucosae, white folded gingivostomatitis; congenital leukokeratosis mucosae oris; leukoedema exfoliativum mucosae oris)
9. Hereditary benign intraepithelial dyskeratosis (red eye)
10. Lichen planus
11. Stomatitis nicotina (leukokeratosis nicotini palati, nicotinic stomatitis)
12. White hairy tongue (lingua villosa alba)
13. Candidiasis (moniliasis; thrush)
14. Fordyce's disease
15. Chemical burn
16. Geographic tongue
17. Epstein's pearl (Bohn's nodule)

Vesicular lesions

1. Primary herpetic gingivostomatitis
2. Secondary herpetic lesions (herpes labialis)
3. Aphthous ulcers
4. Periadenitis mucosa necrotica recurrens (Sutton's disease; Mikulicz's ulcer; periadenitis aphthae; aphthous major)
5. Herpes zoster (shingles)

373

Vesicular lesions—cont'd

6. Erythema multiforme
   a. Behçet's syndrome
   b. Stevens-Johnson syndrome
   c. Ectodermosis erosiva pluriorificialis
7. Reiter's syndrome
8. Pemphigus
9. Benign mucous membrane pemphigus (pemphigoid)
10. Smallpox
11. Chickenpox
12. Measles (rubeola)
13. Herpangina
14. Hand-foot-and-mouth disease
15. Epidermolysis bullosa
16. Allergic reactions (stomatitis venenata, stomatitis medicamentosa)
17. Mucocele

Pigmented lesions

1. Amalgam tattoo
2. Addison's disease
3. Normal pigmented patches
4. Jeghers' syndrome
5. Melanotic macule
6. Focal melanosis
7. Nevi
8. Melanoma
9. Miscellaneous pigmentations

Miscellaneous surface lesions

1. Submucosal fibrosis
2. Geographic tongue (wandering rash; glossitis migrans; migratory glossitis; glossitis areata exfoliativa)
3. Perléche
4. Denture stomatitis
5. Leukoedema
6. Palatal erythema, ecchymoses, and petechiae
7. Mucocutaneous lymph node syndrome
8. Hereditary mucoepithelial dysplasia

WHITE LESIONS

Desquamative gingivitis. Desquamative gingivitis appears as a white lesion of the gingiva that can be wiped off with ease. It is described earlier in the book (p. 186).

Benign hyperkeratosis (pachyderma oris; pachyderma oralis; focal keratosis). Benign hyperkeratosis is the most common white lesion of the oral cavity and constitutes about 71% of all white lesions.

Roughly 7.5% of all lesions biopsied in a dental office represent benign hyperkeratosis. It is about twice as common in males as in females and has an average duration of approximately 28 months. The vast majority occur in the fifth and sixth decades of life, with the average age at occurrence being 48 years.

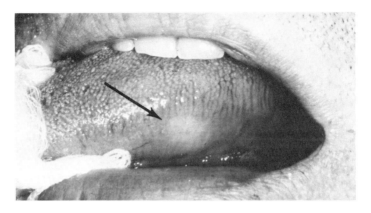

Fig. 13-1. Benign hyperkeratosis. Arrow points to a flat white area on the lateral border of the tongue.

Benign hyperkeratosis is seen in the following areas, which are listed in the order of frequency of involvement: mandibular mucosa, cheek, lip, palate, floor of mouth, maxillary, mucosa, tongue. The lesion may be elevated or flat (Fig. 13-1). It may be associated with an apparent cause, such as habitual cheek biting (pathomimia, morsicatio buccarum) or lip biting, or the cause may be obscure.

Microscopically benign hyperkeratosis is characterized by a thickened layer of keratin (hyperkeratosis) or parakeratosis (Fig. 13-2). The latter term is used when the keratin layer shows remnants of epithelial nuclei. There may be thickening of epithelial ridges and the stratum malpighii (acanthosis) with elongation of ridges, but the individual epithelial cells are normal. The connective tissue beneath the epithelium may appear normal or show infiltration by plasma cells and lymphocytes. The prognosis is excellent. If the cause is eliminated, the lesion may disappear spontaneously in 2 or 3 weeks. Lesions do not recur after excision unless the cause persists.

Leukoplakia with dyskeratosis (dysplastic leukoplakia). In a clinical sense the term leukoplakia has been used for a variety

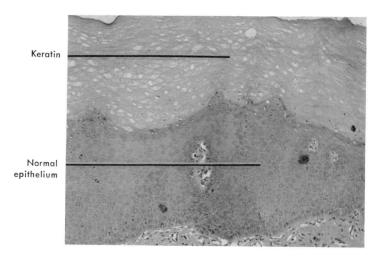

Fig. 13-2. Benign hyperkeratosis. The epithelium is normal but is covered by a thick layer of keratin.

of white lesions on the mucosal surfaces. Leukoplakia with dyskeratosis (dysplastic leukoplakia), however, represents a premalignant lesion.

As with benign hyperkeratosis, leukoplakia with dyskeratosis—or dysplastic leukoplakia—usually consists of elevated or flat white lesions of the oral mucosa that may be fissured (Figs. 13-3 and 13-4); but some lesions are represented by an ulcer or an area of erythema. The disease constitutes about 13% of all white lesions of the oral mucous membrane, and 1% of lesions biopsied in a dental office are leukoplakia with dyskeratosis. Males are afflicted more frequently than females (3:2), with the average duration of the lesion being 30 months. The vast majority of lesions occur in the fifth and sixth decades of life, and the average age at occurrence is 53 years. Leukoplakia with dyskeratosis can be seen in the following areas, which are listed in the order of frequency of involvement: cheek, lip, mandibular mucosa, floor of the mouth, tongue, palate, and maxillary mucosa.

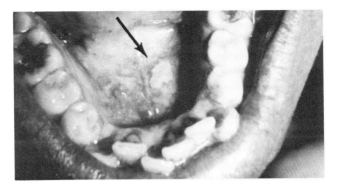

Fig. 13-3. Leukoplakia with dyskeratosis (arrow). Clinically this condition cannot be distinguished from benign hyperkeratosis.

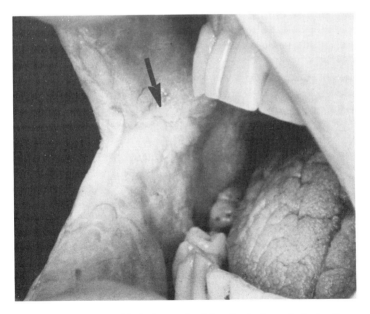

Fig. 13-4. Leukoplakia with dyskeratosis of the cheek. Arrow indicates fissuring, but this is of no diagnostic significance.

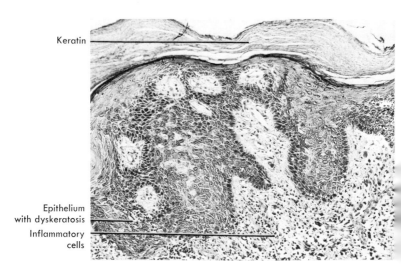

Keratin

Epithelium
with dyskeratosis
Inflammatory
cells

Fig. 13-5. Leukoplakia with dyskeratosis. A thick keratin layer lies over the area of dyskeratotic epithelium.

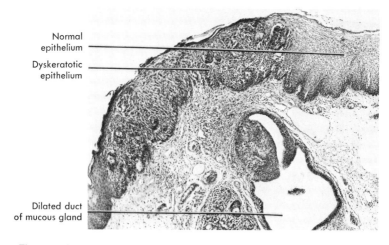

Normal
epithelium
Dyskeratotic
epithelium

Dilated duct
of mucous gland

Fig. 13-6. Leukoplakia with dyskeratosis. Note the transition between the normal and the dyskeratotic epithelium (on the surface as well as in the duct of the mucous gland).

The microscopic features of leukoplakia with dyskeratosis are the same as those described for benign hyperkeratosis except that the epithelial cells show dyskeratosis (Figs. 13-5 and 13-6). The term *dyskeratosis* is used to imply a number of cellular aberrations usually associated with malignant tumors. Epithelium showing hyperchromatic nuclei, abnormal mitoses, abnormal arrangement of cell layers (i.e., loss of polarity), disruption of nuclear-cytoplasmic ratio, keratinization of individual cells, and other similar abnormalities in the cell or its environment is referred to as *dyskeratotic* (i.e., epithelial dysplasia).

Leukoplakia with dyskeratosis is a premalignant lesion; in other words, if left untreated, some of the lesions progress to carcinoma. Untreated dysplastic leukoplakia of the floor of the mouth and base of the tongue becomes invasive carcinoma more than 90% of the time, whereas untreated lesions of the lip do so less than 25% of the time. Since both clinically and microscopically it is impossible to distinguish between those leukoplakias that will become invasive and those that will not, the

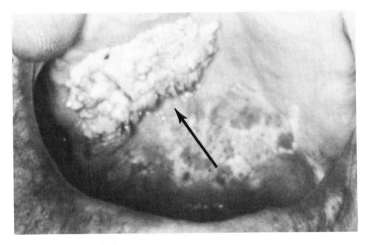

Fig. 13-7. Verrucous leukoplakia of the palate. The lesion is white, and its surface is thrown into folds (verrucous) (arrow). Microscopic features are those of leukoplakia.

urgent need for total excision of all these lesions is self-evident. However, the term leukoplakia with dyskeratosis does not mean *any* white lesion but refers only to those that show dyskeratosis (dysplasia).

Verrucous leukoplakia. This type of leukoplakia is a verrucous (papillary) lesion of the oral mucous membrane that is usually seen on the lip, alveolar ridge, floor of the mouth, or palate (Fig. 13-7). Except for its papillary appearance, it resembles leukoplakia in all other aspects.

Carcinoma in situ. The term carcinoma in situ is applied to mucosal lesions that resemble leukoplakia in all respects except that the dyskeratosis is very pronounced and involves almost all epithelial strata (Fig. 13-8 and 13-9). It constitutes about 2.5% of all white lesions of the oral mucosa.

Clinically carcinoma in situ, like leukoplakia, may appear as a white plaque or as an ulcer, erosion, or reddened area (Fig. 13-8). It is, of course, a premalignant lesion and requires wide and complete excision. The prognosis depends on its location. Lesions of the floor of the mouth, tongue, and lip are most aggressive.

Erythroplakia. This term is applied to bright red velvety plaques on the oral mucosa that are irregular in outline but well defined. They may have a nodular surface and may have white or yellow spots on a red background. In other instances the lesion may consist of intermingled red and white patches. Microscopically erythroplakia shows epithelial atrophy and varying degrees of epithelial dyskeratosis. Thus this condition is similar to leukoplakia with dyskeratosis or to carcinoma in situ. A similar lesion occurs on other mucous membranes, where it is called *erythroplasia of Queyrat,* and on skin, where it is called *Bowen's disease*.

Squamous cell carcinoma. From 3% to 5% of squamous cell carcinomas appear as a white patch. Squamous cell carcinoma is discussed in detail in Chapter 16 (p. 539).

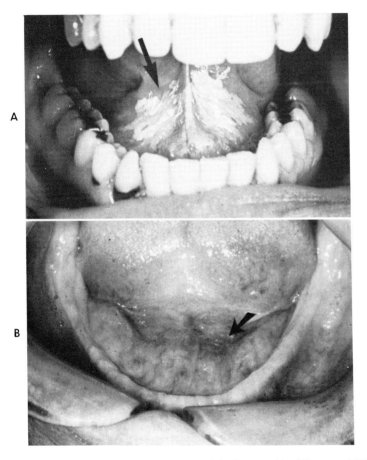

Fig. 13-8. Carcinoma-in-situ may appear clinically as a white **(A)** or a red **(B)** lesion.

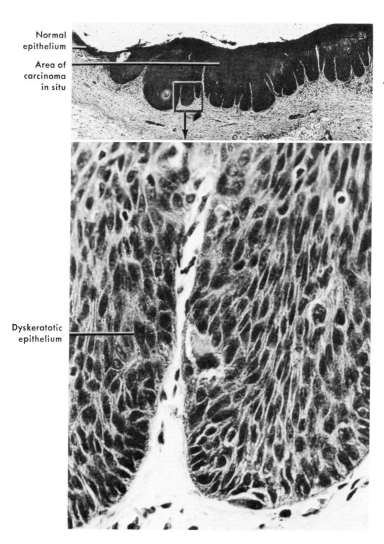

Normal
epithelium

Area of
carcinoma
in situ

A

Dyskeratotic
epithelium

Fig. 13-9. Carcinoma in situ. **A,** Low-power view. Note the transition from the normal to the abnormal oral epithelium. **B,** High-power view of area from **A** (inset). Note that the epithelium of all layers is dyskeratotic.

White sponge nevus (naevus spongiosis albus mucosae; white folded gingivostomatitis; congenital leukokeratosis mucosae oris; leukoedema exfoliativum mucosae oris). White sponge nevus is a hereditary or familial disease. It may be congenital, or it may appear in childhood and the lesions reach their maximum severity in adolescence. After this time no further changes occur during the patient's life. Other members of the patient's family may have the disease.

The mucosa appears white, thickened, and parboiled and is soft and spongy to touch (Fig. 13-10). Its surface may be folded and may show areas of desquamation. The lesion, which is asymptomatic, may involve the entire oral mucosa or be distributed in patches, and may be associated with similar lesions on the vaginal and rectal mucosae. The cheek mucosa is always involved, and the gingival margin almost never.

Microscopically the epithelium is thickened and shows acan-

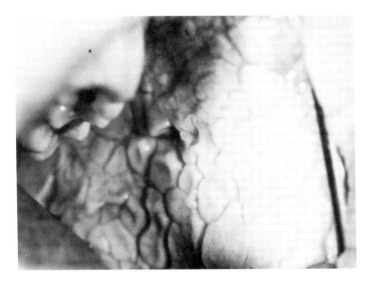

Fig. 13-10. White sponge nevus. The mucosa is folded and white and looks parboiled but is asymptomatic.

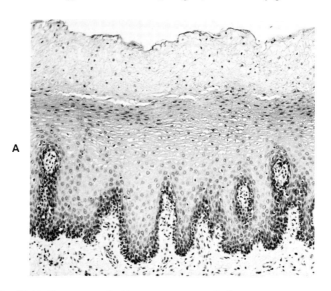

Fig. 13-11. Two cases of white sponge nevus. A characteristic feature is the inability of superficial cells to stain **(A)**. In **B** and **C** the histologic sections show hyperkeratosis (right) and white sponge nevus (left).

thosis, but the most striking feature is that the epithelial cells fail to take any stain and have a washed-out appearance (Fig. 13-11).

Ultrastructure studies reveal that the epithelial cells in white sponge nevus have an atypical aggregation of tonofilaments. The tonofilaments do not form tonofibrils and do not contribute to the formation of keratohyalin. Odland bodies are formed, but they are not extruded into the intercellular spaces and they are unable to perform their extracellular enzymatic function. This is believed to lead to an increased intercellular attachment and the piling up of surface cells.

The connective tissue underneath the epithelium may be infiltrated by plasma cells and lymphocytes.

The lesion is benign and should be left untreated.

Hereditary benign intraepithelial dyskeratosis (red eye). Similar to the white sponge nevus, hereditary benign intraepithelial

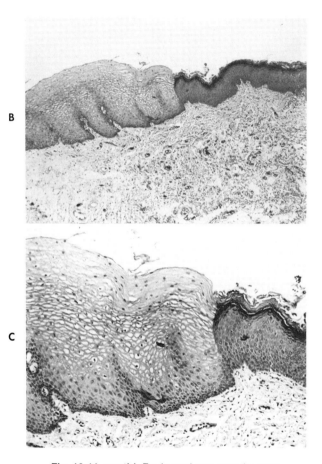

Fig. 13-11, cont'd. For legend see opposite page.

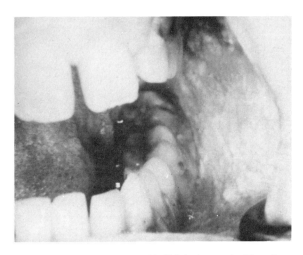

Fig. 13-12. Benign hereditary intraepithelial dyskeratosis. Note the presence of numerous white plaques on the cheek. This is a hereditary benign disorder.

dyskeratosis represents a mutation that has been observed in a mixed racial group of white, Indian, and black lineage.

The oral mucosa shows extensive white folded or smooth lesions that occur in the form of plaques. The lesions are asymptomatic (Fig. 13-12). Besides the oral lesions, there are gelatinous plaques in the eye and a red conjunctiva. Because of the latter feature, the disease is called *red eye*. Lesions undergo exacerbation in spring and improve in late summer and fall. If the cornea is involved, blindness may follow.

Microscopically the mucosal lesions resemble those of the white sponge nevus. However, the epithelium also shows small eosinophilic bodies that are derived from single epithelial cells and have been described to represent "benign dyskeratosis" (Fig. 13-13). These cells are also called "tobacco cells" or "cells within cells."

Studies with a transmission electron microscope show numerous vesicular bodies in immature dyskeratotic cells, densely packed tonofilaments in the cytoplasm of mature dyskeratotic

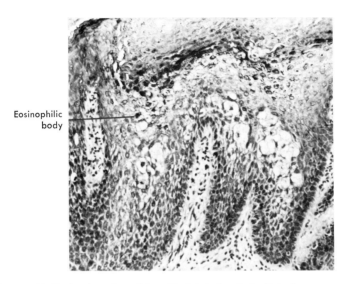

Eosinophilic
body

Fig. 13-13. Benign hereditary intraepithelial dyskeratosis. Note the presence of clear epitheliial cells, which fail to take stain, and the dark spots, which represent eosinophilic bodies.

cells, an absence of cell interdigitations and desmosomes, and nuclear degeneration.

The disease requires no treatment.

Lichen planus. This lesion involves the skin and mucous membrane. Although emotional stress may precede its appearance, the exact cause of the lesion is unknown.

On the skin lichen planus appears as multiple red or violaceous scaly lesions that are pruritic and occur anywhere on the body. However, the most common sites are the flexor aspects of the wrists and lower legs. The lesions are symmetrically distributed.

Lesions of lichen planus are more common in the oral cavity than on the skin, and less than 50% of patients with oral manifestations show dermal lesions.

Lichen planus constitutes about 9% of all white lesions of

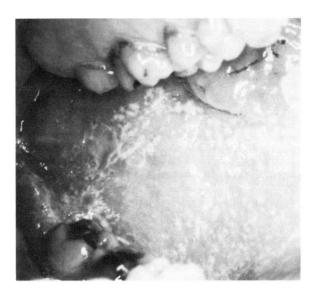

Fig. 13-14. Lichen planus is characterized by a lacelike arrangement of white lines.

the oral mucosa, occurring more frequently in females than in males, and has an average duration of 45 months. It occurs between the ages of 20 and 80 years, with the average age being 49 years. The highest incidence is during the fifth and sixth decades. About 70% of the lesions occur on the cheek mucosa, 9% on the palate, 9% on the tongue, and the remainder on the lip, alveolar mucosa, gingiva, and floor of the mouth.

Clinically, mucosal lesions appear as minute white papules that coalesce to form a reticular, annular, or plaque pattern. Slender white lines (Wickham's striae) that radiate from the papules are a characteristic feature (Fig. 13-14). The lesions are asymptomatic, although the patient may complain of a burning sensation, and they may spontaneously disappear in a few months.

Microscopic sections show thickening of the keratin layer (a feature that may be absent in mucosal lesions), formation of "sawtooth" ridges in the epithelium, edema of the basal layer of

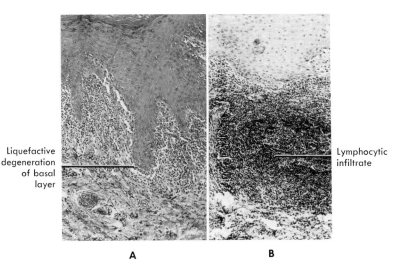

Liquefactive
degeneration
of basal
layer

Lymphocytic
infiltrate

A   B

Fig. 13-15. Lichen planus. **A,** Note the sawtooth ridges of the epithelium. **B,** A dense lymphocytic infiltrate lies immediately below the basement membrane.

the epithelium (Fig. 13-15), and an infiltrate in the subepithelial connective tissues that consists almost exclusively of lymphocytes and closely hugs the epithelium (Fig. 13-15).

By scanning electron microscopic and immunologic studies these lymphocytes have been shown to be almost exclusively T lymphocytes, indicating a cell-mediated (rather than a humoral mediated) system in the pathogenesis of the disease and suggesting a delayed hypersensitivity reaction as the basis of the disease.

Lichen planus requires only symptomatic therapy. Lesions may disappear spontaneously, and those that are rapid in onset disappear promptly. They do not undergo malignant transformation.

Besides the usual form of lichen planus—*bullous or vesicular, erosive* (Fig. 13-16), *atrophic,* and *hypertrophic* forms are recognized but are rare. In all these varieties the characteristic white lines or papules of lichen planus are seen on the periph-

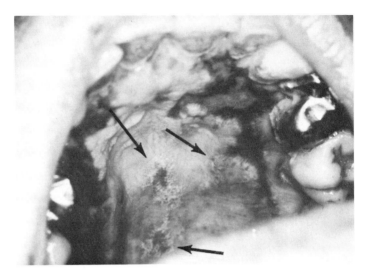

Fig. 13-16. Erosive lichen planus. Arrows denote areas of ulceration with surrounding white lines or patches.

ery of the vesicle, in the erosion area, in the area of atrophy, and in the area of hypertrophy respectively.

The bullous or vesicular form is usually seen on the lateral border or ventral surface of the tongue. The erosive form usually occurs on the cheek and the tongue. The atrophic form is seen on the dorsum of the tongue, and its striking feature is the disappearance of the lingual papillae. The hypertrophic form is accompanied by thick white plaques, and these are seen usually on the tongue or retromolar pad.

In addition to the usual microscopic picture of lichen planus, these lesions may reveal the formation of a subepithelial vesicle (bullous type), an ulcer (erosive type), thinning of the epithelium (atrophic type), or marked thickening of the epithelial layer (hypertrophic type). A symptom complex consisting of lichen planus, diabetes mellitus, and vascular hypertension is called the *Grinspan syndrome*.

Stomatitis nicotina (leukokeratosis nicotini palati, nicotinic

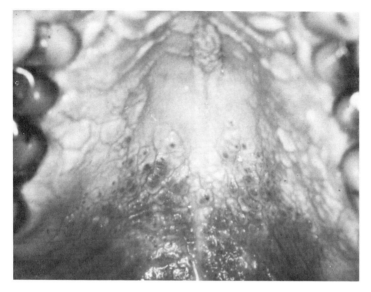

Fig. 13-17. Nicotinic stomatitis. The palate is covered by small raised lesions as well as white plaques.

stomatitis). This condition is related to smoking and usually occurs on the palate.

Stomatitis nicotina constitutes about 3.5% of all white lesions of the oral mucous membrane. On the palate it appears as a number of umbilicated papules that in the early stages are dispersed on a background of red mucosa, but soon the mucosa becomes gray or white (Fig. 13-17). The papules and the central depressions correspond to the orifices of salivary gland ducts.

Microscopically the palatal lesions show hyperkeratosis and parakeratosis, but dyskeratosis is absent (Fig. 13-18). In the connective tissue underneath the epithelium, around the salivary gland ducts, and in the interstitial tissue of the palatal salivary glands, there is edema and infiltration by plasma cells and lymphocytes. The ducts of the salivary glands show intraductal epithelial proliferation and plugging of the lumina. The plugging and inflammatory exudate produce the characteristic

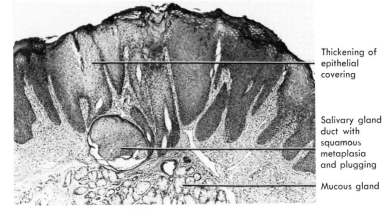

Thickening of epithelial covering

Salivary gland duct with squamous metaplasia and plugging

Mucous gland

Fig. 13-18. Nicotinic stomatitis of the palate. Note the thickening of the epithelium and the plugging of the salivary gland duct.

bumps, and the hyperkeratinization produces the characteristic white appearance of the lesion. In other areas of the palate, the lesions appear as benign hyperkeratosis.

Treatment consists of the elimination of smoking. If the cause is removed, the condition regresses. Very rarely lesions show dyskeratosis. These are premalignant and should be classified as leukoplakia or carcinoma in situ, as the case may be.

White hairy tongue (lingua villosa alba). Although a fungous origin and an allergic origin have been suggested, white hairy tongue is probably caused by dehydration, poor oral hygiene, and physiologic xerostomia of old age.

The condition is characterized by elongation of the filiform papillae and a white hairy appearance of the dorsal surface of the tongue (Fig. 13-19). Food debris collects between the "hairs," and secondary inflammation may follow. The condition is usually asymptomatic. In some instances there is brown or black discoloration of the "hair." This is usually due to some exogenous pigment in foods and medicaments (black hairy tongue).

Microscopic sections show hyperplasia of the filiform papillae (i.e., thickening and accumulation of epithelium), but the

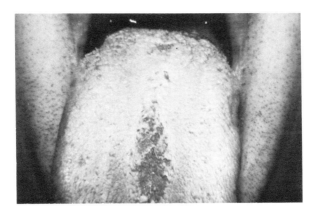

Fig. 13-19. White hairy tongue. Note the presence of numerous white "hairs" on the dorsum of the tongue.

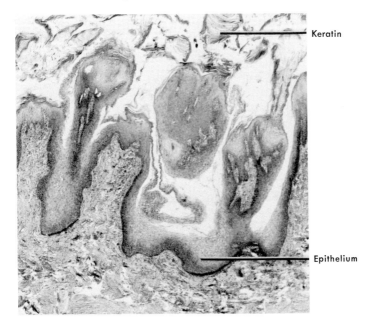

Fig. 13-20. White hairy tongue. There is marked accumulation of keratin on the surface of the tongue and elongation of the filiform papillae.

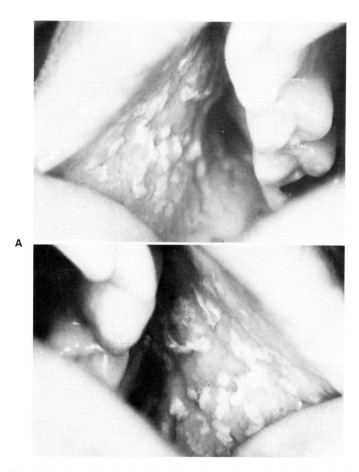

A

Fig. 13-21. Candidiasis (thrush) of the cheek **(A)**, vestibule **(B)**, and palate **(C)**. These white patches can be wiped off with a piece of gauze—an important diagnostic feature.

B

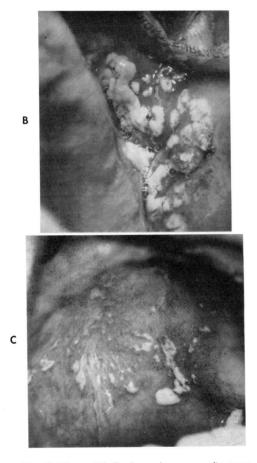

C

Fig. 13-21, cont'd. For legend see opposite page.

epithelial cells are all normal (Fig. 13-20). The connective tissue underneath the epithelium may be infiltrated by plasma cells and lymphocytes.

The lesion is benign and needs no treatment. Daily brushing or scraping of the tongue is curative.

Candidiasis (moniliasis; thrush). Candidiasis is a fungous infection caused by *Candida (Monilia) albicans* and most commonly affects the mucous membranes of the mouth, gastrointestinal tract, and vagina. Lesions of the mucous membranes of the mouth are called thrush.

Candidiasis is a surface infection. Oral lesions occur either at the two extremes of life, infancy and old age, or in patients who are debilitated due to some other cause such as alcoholism, leukemia, or diabetes. Also, lesions may occur in patients who are on prolonged therapy with antibiotics or corticosteroids.

Clinically the lesions can be seen anywhere on the oral mucosa and appear as white or gray-white patches that sometimes resemble curdled milk (Fig. 13-21). The fact that lesions are multiple aids in differential diagnosis. Unlike many other white lesions, patches of thrush can be wiped off or stripped, leaving raw, painful, bleeding surfaces. The patches vary in location and size from time to time.

Microscopic sections through a patch of thrush show necrotic cells, keratin, and a dense network of *Candida* organisms in the form of hyphae and spores (mycelium) (Fig. 13-22). The epithelium in the area of the patch is destroyed or densely infiltrated by the fungi, and the connective tissue underneath the lesion shows edema and infiltration by plasma cells, neutrophils, and lymphocytes.

The fungus *Candida albicans* is present in all mouths but becomes pathogenic in persons in whom tissue resistance is lowered (e.g., due to diabetes or leukemia), in persons in whom the "balance" of oral flora is altered so that the growth of the *Candida* is favored (e.g., by the prolonged use of antibiotics), and in newborn infants (in whom the oral bacteria have not as yet established themselves).

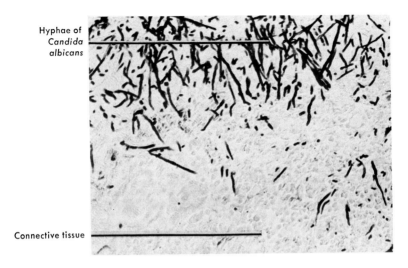

Fig. 13-22. Hyphae of *Candida (Monilia) albicans* in a lesion that clinically appeared as a white patch.

Treatment of thrush consists of controlling the cause of debilitation (e.g., diabetes) whenever possible, discontinuing the use of antibiotics if such a course is not incompatible with the patient's health, swabbing the newborn infant's mouth with the mother's saliva to promote the growth of organisms other than *Candida*, and administering nystatin (100,000 units four times a day).

Although not confirmed, it is believed that chronic lesions of candidiasis predispose the area to malignant change.

Fordyce's disease. This developmental anomaly affects the oral mucosa and is characterized by the presence of multiple small yellowish white granules that may occur in clusters or form plaquelike areas (Fig. 13-23).

Fordyce's disease is seen in almost 80% of the population; and the most common sites are the buccal mucosa at the level of the occlusal plane, the lip, and the retromolar area. Micro-

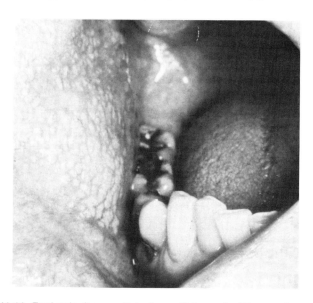

Fig. 13-23. Fordyce's disease. Note the multiple small white granules on the cheek mucosa.

scopic sections show normal sebaceous glands in the lamina propria and submucosa of the mucous membrane (Fig. 13-24).

The cheeks develop by the posteroanterior fusion of the maxillary and mandibular processes of the face. These processes are covered by ectoderm that gives rise not only to the skin and its appendages but also to the vestibular mucosa. The ectoderm along the line of fusion of the maxillary and mandibular processes forms the sebaceous glands, which appear as granules on the mucosal surface. Although these glands are present in the mucosa from birth, hypertrophy does not occur until after sexual maturity. For this reason the incidence of Fordyce's disease increases with age. The use of oral contraceptives has produced an increased incidence of Fordyce granules in females.

The condition is harmless, and it should be left untreated.

Chemical burn. Certain chemicals used in self-medication

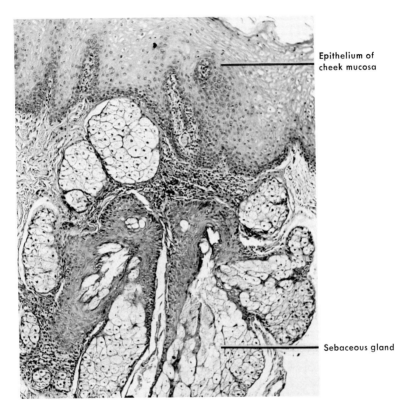

Epithelium of cheek mucosa

Sebaceous gland

Fig. 13-24. Fordyce's disease. Section through a single granule.

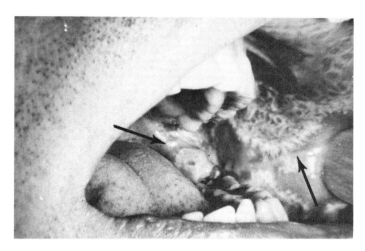

Fig. 13-25. Aspirin burn (arrows). To find relief from pericoronitis, the patient held an aspirin tablet in the area.

can produce a burn of the oral mucosa that presents as a white lesion.

Aspirin tablets are often held locally against a painful tooth or pericoronitis and allowed to dissolve slowly in the area. This leads to a white irregular patch of tissue coagulation that because of its history is easily distinguished from other white lesions of the oral mucosa (Fig. 13-25). After the necrotic surface sloughs off, it leaves a raw, red, bleeding area. Microscopic sections show areas of necrosis.

Geographic tongue. This condition is discussed in detail later in the chapter (p. 443).

Epstein's pearl (Bohn's nodule). Multiple or single white lesions are seen on the alveolar ridges of almost 85% of newborn infants. These are called Epstein's pearls and are discussed later in the book (p. 639).

VESICULAR LESIONS

The lesions to be described in the following paragraphs share in common the fact that they pass through a vesicular stage during their development.

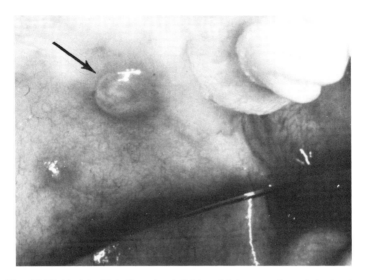

Fig. 13-26. Vesicle. Note the raised, fluid-containing area (arrow). Its border is red.

A *vesicle* is a circumscribed, superficial elevation on the skin or mucous membrane—a subepithelial or intraepithelial collection of serum, plasma, or blood (Fig. 13-26). Because of the attendant trauma in the oral cavity, it is short-lived. It quickly ruptures and leaves a superficial, painful ulcer. Most vesicular lesions are either viral or allergic in origin and microscopically resemble each other so markedly that they cannot be positively identified from biopsy. Identification of the disease process depends entirely on clinical features and laboratory tests (e.g., sensitivity, complement fixation, animal inoculation).

Since vesicles are similar if not identical microscopically, the description of their development and histology is applicable to all vesicular lesions discussed herewith.

The earliest change is an area of hyperemia and edema in the subepithelial tissue. Fluid begins to accumulate either in the epithelium or between the epithelium and connective tissue (Fig. 13-27). Small pockets of fluid coalesce to form a single sac that appears clinically as an elevation (vesicle).

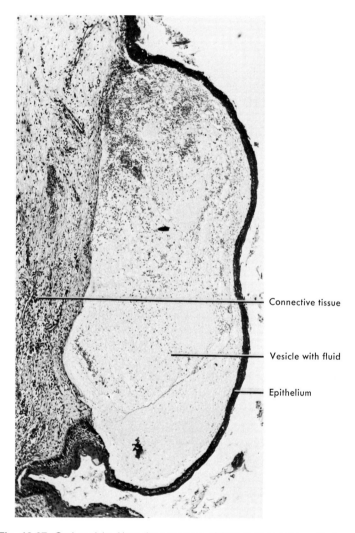

Connective tissue

Vesicle with fluid

Epithelium

Fig. 13-27. Oral vesicle. Note the presence of fluid between the epithelium and the connective tissue.

In vesicles of viral origin, some of the epithelial cells are washed off the vesicle wall and swell up. Their nuclei undergo division, and the cell may float in the fluid of the vesicle. This is called ballooning degeneration. Some of the viral vesicles show intranuclear and/or intracytoplasmic inclusion bodies. These are homogeneous eosinophilic structures that represent viruses or viral products. Examples of inclusion bodies are the Guarnieri bodies of smallpox and the Lipschütz bodies of the herpesvirus. Vesicles soon rupture, leaving an ulcer that becomes secondarily infected. Microscopic sections show a topmost layer of fibrin and necrotic debris and an underlying dense infiltrate of neutrophils and lymphocytes.

Treatment of most vesicular lesions is identical and is only symptomatic. Its rationale is to relieve pain, which is especially annoying during meals, and to alleviate excessive secondary inflammation. Toward these ends, the use of corticoids and sparingly applied topical anesthetics, a regimen of fluid diet, and the application of Orabase or other surface adhesives are all of some value.

Primary herpetic gingivostomatitis and secondary herpetic lesions (herpes labialis). The herpes simplex virus belongs to the herpes family of viruses, which are a group of DNA viruses.

These viruses replicate themselves in the cell nucleus and share a number of similar properties. There are four major herpesviruses that afflict man: the herpes simplex virus (HSV), the herpes zoster or varicella zoster virus (VZV), the cytomegalovirus (CMV), and the Epstein-Barr virus (EBV). HSV causes oral and genital infections; VZV causes herpes zoster (p. 413); CMV infects the salivary glands and the vital organs of infants; and EBV is believed to produce infectious mononucleosis. In addition to acute infections caused by all of these viruses, EBV, CMV, and HSV have been implicated in certain malignant lesions as well. EBV is the cause of Burkitt's lymphoma (p. 328); CMV causes Kaposi's sarcoma (p. 568); and HSV is believed to be related to carcinoma of the cervix (HSV type 2), and probably with carcinoma of the oral cavity (HSV type 1).

As indicated in the preceding sentence, the herpes simplex virus is of two types: type 1 and type 2. In general *type 1 virus* affects nongenital areas such as the mouth, eyes, central nervous system, and skin above the waist and is most common in patients after the newborn period. Type 2 virus is associated with lesions of the genital areas or skin below the waist in adults and with any site in neonates. Although as a rule HSV type 1 primarily involves the oral and perioral tissues while HSV type 2 involves the genital areas, oral infections with HSV type 2 and genital lesions of HSV type 1 are becoming more common.

The portal of entry for the herpes simplex virus may be the respiratory tract, sexual contact, the abrasion of skin or mucous membrane, or the placenta.

Primary herpetic gingivostomatitis is caused by HSV type 1. The highest incidence is between 1 and 3 years of age, but the disease does occur in adults. Lesions may be preceded by some

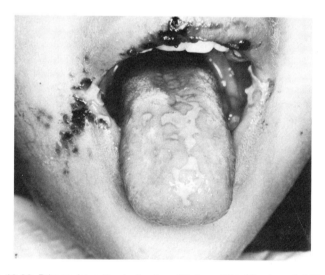

Fig. 13-28. Primary herpetic gingivostomatitis in a child. (Courtesy Sol Silverman, D.D.S., San Francisco.)

other infectious process (e.g., upper respiratory tract infection). The disease may be subclinical or may be associated with headache, pain, and sore mouth accompanied by irritability, drooling, and refusal of food.

Oral lesions are often preceded by enlargement of the cervical nodes and a high temperature. Symptoms consist of reddening of the oral mucosa, followed by the appearance of numerous vesicles on the mucous membrane. Vesicles soon rupture, leaving clear ulcers (Fig. 13-28). A little later, secondary infection supervenes and a red ring of inflammation (halo) appears around the ulcer. The ulcers are painful, but healing begins in about 3 days; and within 7 to 14 days the lesions completely heal without leaving any scar. In less severe forms of the disease, the lesions may go unnoticed and the child recovers without the parents' ever having been aware that the condition existed.

Many cases of so-called teething problems in children are probably primary herpes simplex infections. Primary herpes infections in adults have the same features as in children (Figs. 13-29 and 13-30).

It was previously believed that after *primary infection* the herpesvirus remained dormant in the local cells. However, it is now believed that the virus probably retreats to the sensory ganglia, where it lies dormant in a latent form (e.g., the trigeminal ganglion for oral lesions). Under appropriate stress the virus becomes activated in the trigeminal ganglion and proceeds centrifugally down the axon of the sensory nerve to the epithelium, where it may produce the typical herpetic vesicles (*secondary herpetic lesions*). Reactivation of the virus is not always accompanied by lesions. The epithelial cells of the area exposed to HSV-type 1 may survive, and the virus is shed without symptoms. When the secondary lesions occur, they are usually restricted to the bound-down areas of the oral mucosa (attached gingiva and hard palate) or to the lip (on or near the vermilion border). Multiple intraoral herpetic attacks are rare, however, and secondary lesions are usually confined to the lip. On the lips they are referred to as *herpes labialis* or *cold sores*.

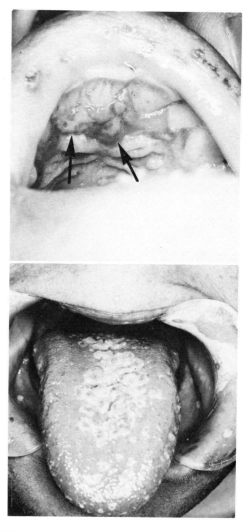

Fig. 13-29. Primary herpetic gingivostomatitis lesions in an adult. Note the ulcerations and necrosis. (Courtesy Sol Silverman, D.D.S., San Francisco.)

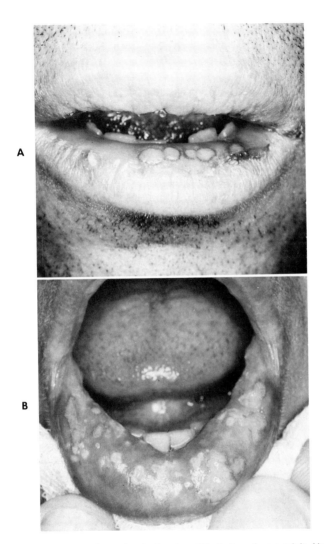

Fig. 13-30. Primary herpetic gingivostomatitis lesions in an adult. Note the vesicles **(A)** and the ulcers and vesicles **(B)**. (Courtesy Sol Silverman, D.D.S., San Francisco.)

Secondary herpetic lesions occur in about 40% of the population. They may follow fever (fever blister), upper respiratory tract infection, trauma, stress, dental appointments, etc. The relationship of lesions to the onset of menstruation is not proved. Lesions start as an area of burning, itching, tingling, dysesthesia, and erythema. These prodromal symptoms may or may not be followed in 24 to 48 hours by the appearance of a single vesicle or cluster of vesicles (Fig. 13-31). The vesicles soon ulcerate. They begin to form scabs in 4 or 5 days and heal within a week to 10 days without leaving scars. Topical application of 5-iodo-2-deoxy uridine (IDU) is effective in the management of herpes simplex virus lesions.

The microscopic features of primary and secondary herpetic gingivostomatitis are identical and have been described on p. 401. The herpesvirus can be cultured from the vesicular fluid. This fluid, if swab-streaked on a rabbit's eye, produces a severe infection in 24 hours (Paul's test). Cytologic smears from the herpes lesions show pseudogiant squamous cells. The antibody titer for the herpesvirus increases fourfold to eightfold within 9

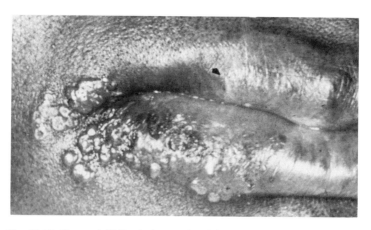

Fig. 13-31. Herpes labialis. A cluster of vesicles on the lip of an adult represents secondary herpetic lesions.

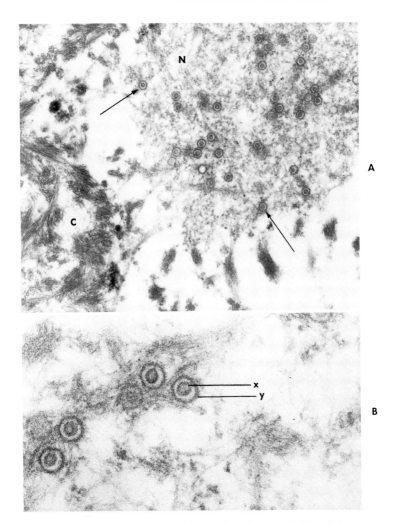

A

B

Fig. 13-32. Transmission electron micrographs of an epithelial cell from a herpetic lesion. In **A** (×32,000) the nucleus *(N)* shows a number of viruses (arrows). *C* is the cytoplasm. In **B** (×97,500) five viruses can be identified. *x* is the core of the virus, and *y* the capsid. (Courtesy Sol Silverman, D.D.S., San Francisco.)

to 14 days after the initial attack, and the electron microscopic examination may reveal the virus in the epithelial cells of the lesion (Fig. 13-32).

Herpes infection of the hand and fingernails can occur in dentists or other health personnel who treat patients with the disease. It has also been observed in nail and cuticle biters who, during an oral episode, can reinfect themselves (Fig. 13-33). Lesions of the nail bed are persistent and take many months to heal.

HSV type 1 is probably related to trigeminal neuralgia and some cases of facial paralysis.

Aphthous ulcers. These are not vesicular lesions but for convenience are described in this section.

It was previously believed that recurrent aphthae (canker sores) or recurrent habitual aphthae were a manifestation of the herpes simplex virus. However, the virus cannot be cultured from the lesions, and the causative organism is now considered

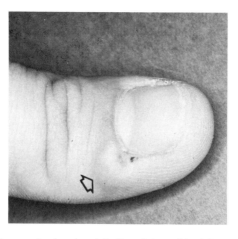

Fig. 13-33. Herpes simplex virus infection of the nail bed (herpetic paronychia) in a patient who had oral lesions and was a nail biter. (Courtesy Sol Silverman, D.D.S., San Francisco.)

to be an L form of the alpha hemolytic *Streptococcus*. It is believed that the L form is seen in the ducts of mucous glands of the oral cavity and that under certain circumstances the bacterium undergoes transition into a mature form. During this transition the organism produces a mucopolysaccharide capsule. The formation of an aphthous ulcer results from an allergic response (delayed hypersensitivity) to the mucopolysaccharide. Aphthous ulcers therefore are usually seen in the mucous gland–bearing areas of the oral mucosa.

The disease is characterized by repeated episodes of oval or round superficial ulcerations on the mucous membrane of the inside of the lip, cheek, tongue, floor of the mouth, soft palate, and sometimes the gingiva (Fig. 13-34). Lesions are from 2 to 20 mm in diameter and are painful. They start as a small white area or raised red papule on the mucosa that expands in size and then undergoes central necrosis to form an ulcer. Patients usually do not have fever or lymphadenopathy. The disease is

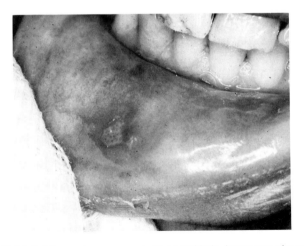

Fig. 13-34. Aphthous ulcer surrounded by a red halo. It was one of a number in this patient's mouth.

estimated to occur in 20% to 50% of the population; in about 2% it presents a severe and very painful form. In children its incidence is about 40%, and it has a strong familial tendency. It is slightly more common in females than in males (3:2) and has greatest prevalence during the winter and spring months. Its incidence appears to decrease with age.

More than 90% of patients with recurrent aphthae are non-smokers. It is believed that increased keratinization of the oral mucosa in smokers offers protection against the disease. The fact that the lesions often occur in women during the premenstrual period, when the degree of keratinization of the oral mucosa is low, may further attest to this phenomenon. There is a definite correlation between physical and emotional stress and the onset of lesions.

The lesions are self-limiting and heal spontaneously within 1 to 2 weeks. However, recurrences are common and are more frequent than recurrences of the herpetic lesion, or cold sores.

Treatment of recurrent aphthae is symptomatic. In persistent and especially painful ulcers, tetracycline has been tried with success (250 mg in 5 ml of water used as a rinse followed by swallowing, three to four times a day). A mouthwash containing equal parts of Benadryl (diphenhydramine) and Kaopectate is also helpful for reducing pain and discomfort. Application of triamcinolone acetonide in an emollient paste may help relieve acute symptoms. Vitamin B, smallpox vaccine, and *Lactobacillus* tablets are of questionable value.

In summary, primary herpetic gingivostomatitis and herpes labialis (cold sores) are caused by the herpes simplex virus, but recurrent aphthae (canker sores) are caused by the L form of alpha hemolytic *Streptococcus*.

Periadenitis mucosa necrotica recurrens (Sutton's disease; Mikulicz's ulcer; periadenitis aphthae; aphthous major). Like recurrent aphthae, periadenitis mucosa necrotica recurrens is caused by the L form of alpha hemolytic *Streptococcus*.

This condition occurs exclusively on the salivary gland–bearing areas of the oral and laryngeal mucosa and may

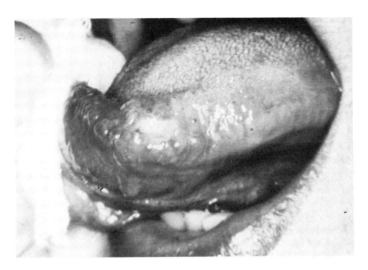

Fig. 13-35. Periadenitis mucosa necrotica recurrens. The ulcer on the lateral border of the tongue is deeper than an aphthous ulcer. These lesions heal with scar formation.

be considered a more severe form of the aphthous ulcer. It begins as small smooth, painful red nodules or plaques that soon ulcerate. The craterlike, painful ulcers are much larger and deeper and heal much more slowly than do aphthous ulcers (Fig. 13-35). The lesions heal in 3 to 6 weeks but leave scars. While one lesion heals, another appears in another area of the oral mucosa.

Microscopic features are those of a nonspecific ulcer over a salivary gland–bearing mucosa. The connective tissue under the ulcer shows edema and infiltration by neutrophils, plasma cells, and lymphocytes.

Treatment is the same as that described for aphthous lesions.

Herpes zoster (shingles). This disease is caused by a neurotropic virus that is believed to be identical with the virus of varicella (chickenpox). Whereas the poliomyelitis virus affects the motor neurons, the herpes zoster virus affects the sensory neurons. Usually the nerve cells in the dorsal root ganglion are involved. Therefore, the symptoms occur along the course of one of the spinal nerves.

Clinical symptoms are fever, malaise, pain, and the appearance of vesicles in the area of the skin supplied by the involved sensory nerve. Vesicles rupture, leave ulcers, crust, and heal.

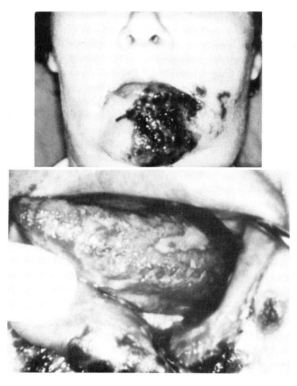

Fig. 13-36. Skin and oral lesion in a patient with herpes zoster (shingles). Note that the lesions do not cross the midline. The disease follows the distribution of a sensory nerve.

The disease may involve the sensory neurons in the trigeminal nerve ganglion (Fig. 13-36). In such cases oral vesicles may form that are preceded by toothache or pain in the area by 2 to 3 days. The vesicles rupture and leave painful ulcers but heal in a few days without scars. Lesions usually are seen on the cheek, soft palate, buccal mucosa, and tongue (Fig. 13-36). In older patients herpes zoster may spread from a segmental distribution and become generalized. This usually implies a malignant lymphoma or metatasizing carcinoma of some internal organ.

Erythema multiforme. The cause of this self-limiting disease of the skin and mucous membrane is unknown, but a viral or allergic origin has been suggested.

In many instances the disease has been shown to be an allergic response to foods, infectious agents, or drugs (e.g., sulfonamides, penicillin, salicylates). Lesions can occur anywhere on the skin, oral mucosa, conjunctiva, and genital mucous membrane. Patients are usually young adults.

The lesions consist of red macules (erythema) that change to vesicles, bullae, and ulcers (multiforme) (Fig. 13-37). Skin lesions may be concentric with rings of varying degree of erythema and have been termed "target," "iris," or "bull's eye" in appearance. The oral vesicles soon break, leaving ulcers with red borders (like other viral lesions) (Fig. 13-37). Oral lesions can be seen anywhere on the mucosa, and they heal without a scar.

Treatment is only palliative. Maintaining fluids and proper nutrition is important. In cases of secondary infection, antibiotics are necessary. The administration of corticosteriods causes remission but not cure.

Microscopic features have already been described (p. 401). For a diagnosis of erythema multiforme and other vesicular oral lesions, however, the history and clinical features are of utmost importance.

Since the dermal, oral, conjunctival, and genital lesions of erythema multiforme may occur in many combinations, a number of symptom complexes or syndromes have been described:

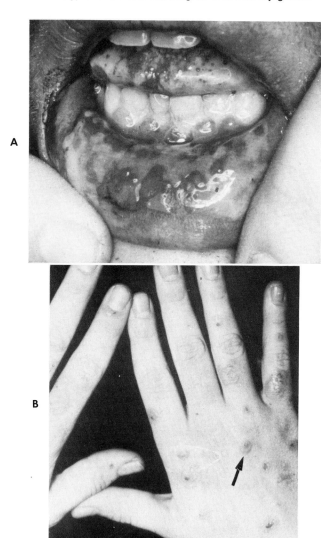

Fig. 13-37. Erythema multiforme. **A,** Note the presence of numerous ulcerations on the oral mucous membrane. **B,** The skin lesions have a targetlike appearance (arrow).

Behçet's syndrome, Stevens-Johnson syndrome, ectodermosis erosiva pluriorificialis. Although the differences between these are often described more precisely, the information necessary for our purposes is given in Table 16.

It has been suggested that *Behçet's syndrome* is of viral origin. The syndrome consists of ulcers on the oral and genital mucosae and eye lesions (Fig. 13-38). The presence of lesions in only two of the three sites may be sufficient for the diagnosis of this syndrome. Patients are most often males between 10 and

Table 16. Variations of erythema multiforme

Syndrome	Oral lesions	Eye lesions	Genital lesions	Skin lesions
Behçet's syndrome	x	x	x	
Stevens-Johnson syndrome	x	x		x
Ectodermosis erosiva pluriorificialis	x	x		x

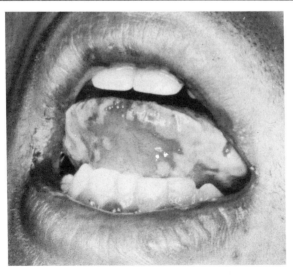

Fig. 13-38. Oral lesions of Behçet's syndrome are similar to those seen in erythema multiforme and consist of multiple ulcers.

418 Pathology of oral mucosa, tongue, and salivary glands

30 years of age. Oral lesions and genital lesions (on the labia majora, root of penis, or scrotum) are ulcers, whereas eye lesions consist of photophobia, conjunctivitis, uvetis, and hypopyon.

Reiter's syndrome. This symptom complex occurs usually in males between the ages of 20 and 30 years and is characterized by urethritis, arthritis, conjunctivitis, and lesions on the skin and mucous membrane.

The skin lesions are keratinized papules that occur on the palms and soles. Oral and penile mucous membranes show ves icles and ulcers with a white border. Lesions on the tongue resemble those seen in glossitis migrans (p. 443). The cause of this disease is not known; but viruses, allergy, and mycoplasma have been implicated.

Microscopic features are not diagnostic and consist of ulcers with dense neutrophilic infiltrate. Reiter's syndrome has a good prognosis. However, remissions may be followed by recurrences. Treatment is symptomatic.

Pemphigus. This disease affects the skin and mucous membrane and occurs in a number of different forms: vulgaris, vegetans, foliaceus, and erythematosus.

Pemphigus vulgaris is by far the most common type and is believed to be an autoimmune disease. It usually occurs between the ages of 40 and 70 years, shows a predilection for Jewish and Mediterranean peoples, and affects males and females equally. Although worldwide in distribution, it is endemic in certain parts of Brazil. The characteristic lesion is a bulla (large vesicle) on areas of the skin and oral mucosa. Oral lesions occur more frequently on the buccal mucosa, palate, and gingiva than elsewhere. The epithelial covering of the involved areas of the skin and oral mucosa can be rubbed off with thumb or finger pressure (Nikolsky's sign). In about 55% of patients, oral lesions precede skin lesions; and in 20%, oral lesions are the only manifestation. The bullae rupture rapidly and leave large painful superficial ulcers (Fig. 13-39). In more than 50% of patients, the disease is rapidly fatal. There is no known cure, but local and systemic administration of cortisone is of value.

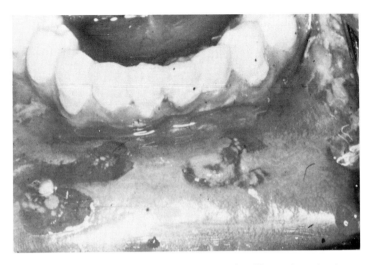

Fig. 13-39. Pemphigus vulgaris. The lesions consist of large ulcers that began as bullae.

The microscopic picture of a pemphigus bulla is essentially the same as that described for vesicles in general. However, some other features of pemphigus deserve attention. The epithelium of the prickle cell layer shows loss of intercellular brides (desmosomes), collection of fluid between them, and the formation of a bulla. The bulla is intraepithelial, so its base is lined by a layer of epithelium. Furthermore, in a ruptured bulla this basal layer can be seen to be adherent to the mucosa. Within the vesicle or bulla of pemphigus, round degenerating epithelial cells with hyperchromatic nuclei can be seen. These are called *Tzanck cells*.

Electron microscopic studies have shown that the bulla results from dissolution of the intercellular cement. In patients with pemphigus vulgaris, antibodies to the intercellular substance have been demonstrated. These are autoantibodies, and their titer is proportional to the severity of the disease. Antibodies to the intercellular substance can be demonstrated by immunofluorescent techniques, and this test is of diagnostic significance.

One of the less common forms of pemphigus is *pemphigus vegetans*. It resembles pemphigus vulgaris in all aspects except that after the rupture of the bulla a papillomatous hyperplasia of the epithelium occurs. Oral lesions are present in about 50% of

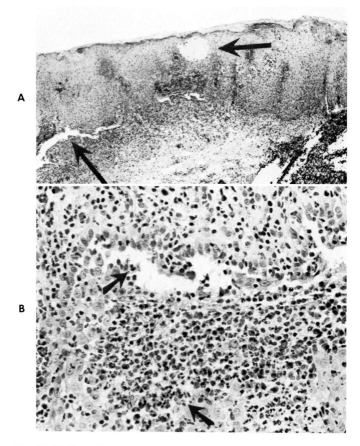

Fig. 13-40. Pemphigus vegetans. **A,** Arrows indicate separation of epithelium and connective tissue and vesicle formation. **B,** Note the dense eosinophilic inflitrate (lower arrow) and the separation of epithelium from connective tissue (upper arrow).

cases. Microscopically this type shows many eosinophils (Fig. 13-40).

In *pemphigus foliaceus* and *pemphigus erythematosus,* which are rare forms, the bullae are associated with marked erythema. The erythematosus is a mild form of the foliaceus. Oral lesions are rare.

Benign mucous membrane pemphigus (pemphigoid). A rare disease of the oral mucosa, benign mucous membrane pemphi-

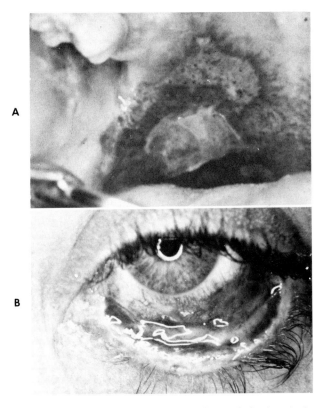

Fig. 13-41. Benign mucous membrane pemphigus. **A,** Lesions in the palate consist of an ulcer with a wide red halo. **B,** Ulceration of the conjunctiva and a necrotic slough can be seen.

gus is characterized by bullous lesions of the oral mucosa and conjunctiva (Fig. 13-41).

Because of consistent involvement of the conjunctiva, the disease is also called *pemphigus conjunctivae*. In the conjunctiva, scarring is frequent and blindness may follow. Skin and mucous membranes of the nose, larynx, esophagus, penis, and vulva are sometimes involved. Oral vesicles and bullae heal in about 2 weeks.

Pemphigoid affects elderly persons, with the average age being 60 years. The disease is chronic but not fatal. Patients are in good health. In severe cases corticosteroids produce remission of symptoms.

Smallpox and chickenpox (variola and varicella). Oral lesions may occur in smallpox and chickenpox, which are viral diseases of the skin. The lesions consist of vesicles that change to ulcers.

Microscopically the vesicles of smallpox and chickenpox present the features described for vesicles in general. Since the skin lesions form the predominant part of the disease, the oral lesions do not have any diagnostic significance and present no serious problem.

Measles (rubeola). Measles (rubeola) also a viral disease of the skin, is of interest because its oral manifestation occurs from 2 to 4 days before its general symptoms. Although the oral lesions, called *Koplik's spots*, do not consist of vesicles, for convenience a discussion of measles is included in this chapter.

Koplik's spots consist of a few or a cluster of white or yellow-white pinpoint papules on an inflamed, red background on the buccal mucosa (Fig. 13-42). Microscopic sections through the spots show necrosis of epithelial cells and dense neutrophilic infiltration.

Oral lesions of measles other than Koplik's spots are rare but may occur as red macules. These appear simultaneously with the skin eruption (Fig. 13-43).

German measles (rubella) is not associated with Koplik's spots. Oral lesions, when present, consist of erythema of the mucosa or a few macules in the posterior part of the mouth.

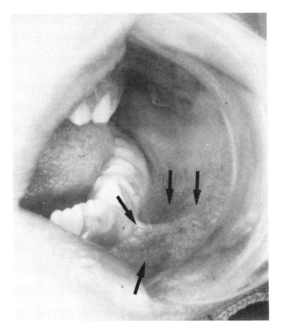

Fig. 13-42. Oral lesions of measles. The cheek mucosa contains numerous Koplik's spots (arrows).

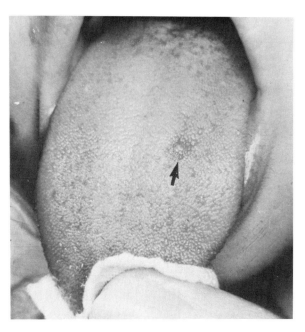

Fig. 13-43. Oral lesion of measles other than Koplik's spots are rare but may appear as red macules with the skin eruption.

Herpangina. This disease of childhood occurs in the summer months. It is caused by one of the coxsackieviruses (first discovered in Coxsackie County, New York).

The incubation period is from 3 to 7 days. The disease is characterized by fever, malaise, dysphagia, anorexia, and the appearance of vesicles on the soft palate, tonsils, uvula, and pharynx. The vesicles soon change to ulcers.

Microscopic features are the same as those described for vesicles in general. Treatment is symptomatic, the disease is self-limiting, and the ulcers heal spontaneously.

Hand-foot-and-mouth disease. This disease, caused by a coxsackievirus (A-16), should not be confused with foot-and-mouth disease (aphthous fever, hoof-and-mouth disease), which is also caused by a virus but which rarely affects man.

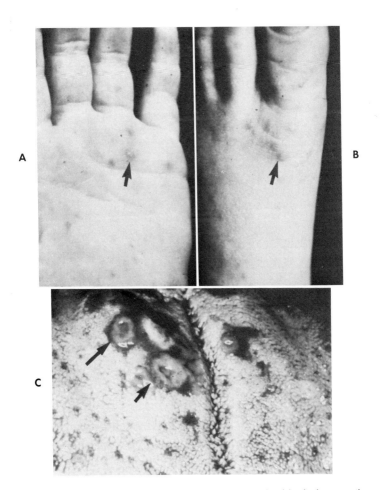

Fig. 13-44. Hand-foot-and-mouth disease is characterized by lesions on the hand **(A)**, foot **(B)**, and mouth **(C)**. (Courtesy James Adrian, D.D.S. Washington, D.C.)

Hand-foot-and-mouth disease affects children under 5 years of age. Skin lesions consist of vesicles, ulcers, and papules that especially involve the feet and hands but can occur anywhere (Fig. 13-44). Patients have fever, anorexia, diarrhea, vomiting, and lymphadenopathy. Oral lesions consist of vesicles and ulcers on the hard palate, tongue, and buccal mucosa. However, lesions can occur elsewhere on the oral mucosa.

Histologic features are similar to those seen in herpes simplex lesions. In some cases intracytoplasmic viral inclusion bodies can be demonstrated.

Foot-and-mouth disease, primarily a disease of cattle, rarely affects humans. Oral lesions occur anywhere and are indistinguishable from those of hand-foot-and-mouth disease.

Epidermolysis bullosa. Primarily a hereditary disease of the skin, epidermolysis bullosa occurs in three forms: *simple, dystrophic,* and *lethal*. All forms are characterized by vesicles and bullae on the pressure areas of the skin that rupture and leave raw, painful ulcers (Fig. 13-45).

In the *simple* form there is no scarring, the patient develops normally, and at puberty the disease often resolves itself. In the *dystrophic* form mental retardation, retarded growth, and ectodermal dysplasia may be present. Skin lesions heal with scarring, and the patient may die in childhood. In the *lethal* form most patients die before 3 months of age.

Oral lesions are rare in the simple form but are common in the dystrophic and lethal forms, consisting of multiple bullae that occur rapidly in areas of trauma (Fig. 13-45). Bullae may be preceded by white patches, but they soon rupture and leave ulcers. Oral lesions may develop into squamous cell carcinoma. The microscopic features are the same as those of the typical vesicle. Vesicles have been described in the enamel organs of developing teeth. There is no known cure for the disease.

Allergic reactions (stomatitis venenata; stomatitis medicamentosa). Vesicular or bullous lesions of the oral mucous membrane may follow either local contact with or the ingestion of a foreign substance (allergen). When the allergic reaction follows

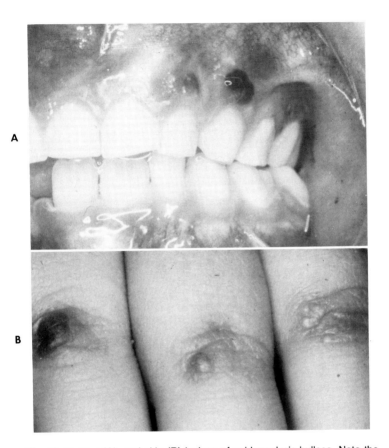

Fig. 13-45. Oral **(A)**, and skin **(B)** lesions of epidermolysis bullosa. Note the hemorrhagic bullae on the mucous membrane and the fingers.

local contact, it is called *stomatitis venenata*. When it follows systemic administration, it is called *stomatitis medicamentosa*.

In either instance lesions are varied. They may be erythematous patches, vesicles, and later ulcers (Fig. 13-46). The onset is sudden and usually can be related to the offending agent.

The microscopic appearance of the lesion depends on its clinical appearance. Generally the microscopic features of a vesicle or an ulcer can be seen. The histology of the vesicle has been described previously. The ulcers show a loss of epithelial covering, the presence of edema, and infiltration of the underlying connective tissue by neutrophils and lymphocytes.

Although almost any foreign substance may act as an aller-

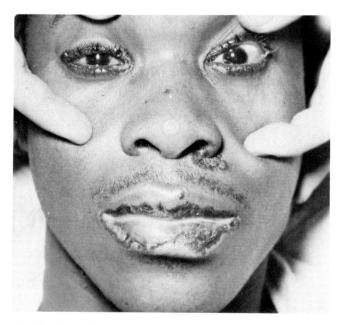

Fig. 13-46. Stomatitis medicamentosa. Lesions also were present in the mouth and on the genital mucosa.

gen, drugs such as the sulfonamides, aminopyrine, quinine, and arsphenamine most frequently produce stomatitis medicamentosa. By contrast, stomatitis venenata is associated most frequently with the use of certain toothpowders, toothpastes, lipsticks, lozenges, mouthwashes, and denture materials.

Treatment of the condition consists of discontinuing the use of the medication or product that contains the allergen. Delayed allergic reactions to local injections of anesthetic solutions can occur and consist of a crop of vesicles or ulcers at the site of injection (Fig. 13-47). These lesions are self-limiting.

Mucocele. This vesicular lesion of the oral mucosa is described in Chapter 14 (p. 461).

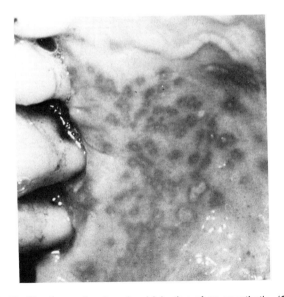

Fig. 13-47. Allergic reaction to a local injection of an anesthetic. (Courtesy Milton Knapp, D.D.S., Portland, Ore.)

PIGMENTED LESIONS

Amalgam tattoo. An area of brown to black pigmentation of the oral mucosa may be caused either by accidental implantation of silver or copper amalgam or by prolonged contact of the oral mucosa with an amalgam restoration (Fig. 13-48). Gingiva and alveolar mucosa are the most common sites.

Microscopic sections show pieces of amalgam and/or the presence of brown or black granular pigment in the basement membrane, along collagen bundles, striated muscle, and acini of glands, and in giant cell fibroblasts, macrophages, and perivascular areas (Fig. 13-49). In about 45% of cases there is no tissue reaction to amalgam, while in the remainder chronic inflammatory response can be seen. Usually the condition requires no treatment.

Addison's disease. Brown to black pigmentation may develop on the buccal mucosa, tongue, lip, and gingiva in Addi-

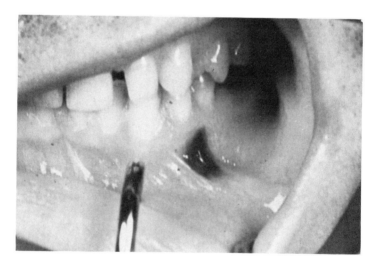

Fig. 13-48. Amalgam tattoo. The black area was produced by accidental implantation of amalgam in the oral mucosa.

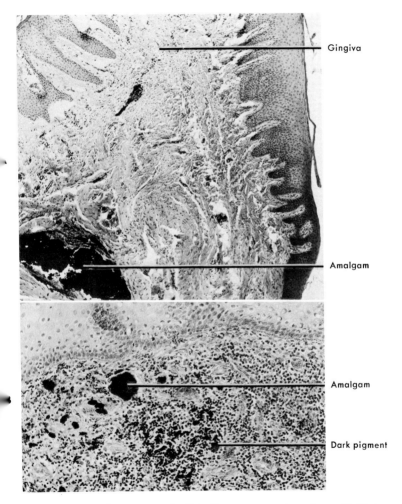

Gingiva

Amalgam

Amalgam

Dark pigment

Fig. 13-49. Amalgam tattoo. **A,** Note the presence of amalgam. **B,** Dark granules of amalgam can be seen in the connective tissue.

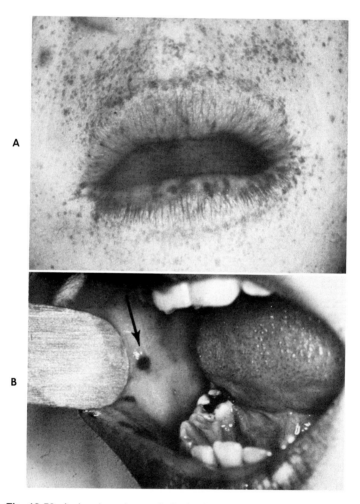

A

B

Fig. 13-50. Jeghers' syndrome. **A,** Perioral pigmentation. **B,** Buccal pigmentation.

son's disease and is due to melanin that is deposited in the basal layer of the epithelium (p. 671).

Normal pigmented patches. The gingiva or buccal mucosa may show pigmented patches in any person of any race. These patches are caused by melanin; are asymptomatic, benign, and harmless; and should be left untreated.

Jeghers' syndrome. Also known as Peutz-Jeghers syndrome, this is characterized by hereditary intestinal polyps and pigmentation of the oral mucous membrane.

Oral pigmentation is due to melanin and consists of patches of 1 to 10 mm in diameter. Lesions are prominent on the lips and buccal mucosa but may also be seen on the gingiva, hard palate, soft palate, and tongue (Fig. 13-50).

Pigmented spots may be present on the face, particularly around the mouth, nose, and eyes. Polyps are seen in the small intestines or may involve the entire intestinal tract and produce intestinal obstruction with obdominal pain and bleeding, leading to anemia and melena.

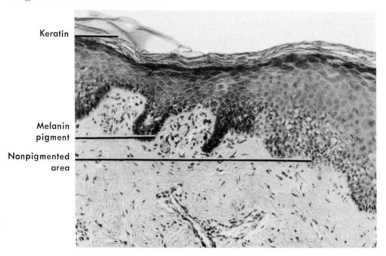

Keratin

Melanin pigment

Nonpigmented area

Fig. 13-51. Jeghers' syndrome. The basal layer of the epithelium shows melanin pigmentation.

Microscopic sections of an oral lesion show normal mucous membrane with melanin pigment in the basal layer of the epithelium (Fig. 13-51). Oral lesions are harmless and need no treatment. Skin lesions may disappear after puberty, but the oral lesions persist through life.

Melanotic macule. This is a recently identified oral mucosal pigmented lesion that is similar to the freckle (ephelis) and lentigo of the skin (Fig. 13-52). These are solitary, discrete, gray, brown, blue, or black, nonelevated lesions that range from 0.1 to 2.0 cm in size. They are of long duration, and occur most often on the vermilion border of the lip, followed by the gingiva, buccal mucosa, and palate. They can, however be seen in any area of the oral mucosal surface. Patients are usually adult (mean age 40 years) and usually male (2:1). More than 80% of patients are white. Histologic examination reveals melanin pigmentation of the basal layer of oral epithelium and/or the upper portions of the lamina propria (Figs. 13-53 and 13-54). The melanotic macule is benign, and local excision is curative.

Focal melanosis. The term focal melanosis is sometimes applied to lesions that have been described above as melanotic macule. However, it is more appropriate to reserve this term for those lesions of the oral mucosa which, though microscopically resembling the melanotic macule, do not have a discrete,

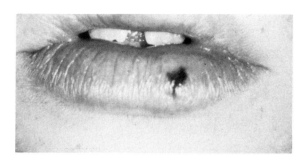

Fig. 13-52. Melanotic macule of the lower lip in a child. This is a smooth black or brown melanin-containing lesion. (Compare with Fig. 13-54.)

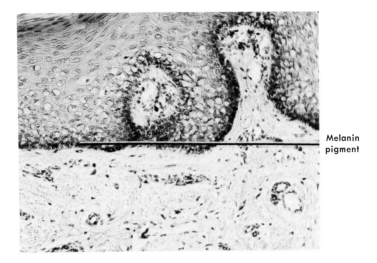

Melanin
pigment

Fig. 13-53. Melanotic macule. Note the presence of melanin in the basal layer of otherwise normal epithelium.

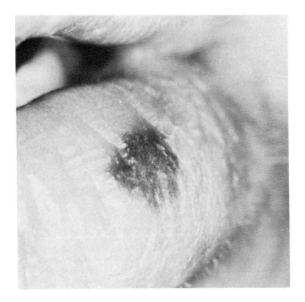

Fig. 13-54. Melanotic macule of the lower lip in a child. This is a smooth black melanin-containing lesion. (Compare with Fig. 13-52.)

pigmented clinical appearance. Focal melanosis may be associated with trauma or other mucosal lesions such as lichen planus, hyperkeratosis, or mucosal scars.

Nevi. Primarily lesions of the skin, nevi are occasionally seen in the oral cavity and are therefore of interest to the dentist. A nevus (Latin, "birthmark") can be of many types (e.g., vascular, sebaceous), but the term is usually used in connection with the pigmented lesions.

Pigmented nevi are of four types: *junctional, compound, intramucosal,* and *blue*. Clinically they are usually pigmented (about 85%), raised (more than 80%) lesions that range from 0.1 to 0.5 cm in size. Lesions are asymptomatic, patients are usually between 20 to 40 years of age (mean age, 35 years), and the female to male ratio is about 2:1. More than half of the patients are white. About 40% of the lesions occur on the hard palate, 25% on the lip, 16% on the buccal mucosa, and the remainder on the gingiva, retromolar area, soft palate, and elsewhere (Figs. 13-55 and 13-56). They may be nonpigmented (about 15%). The intramucosal type is the most common (55%); about

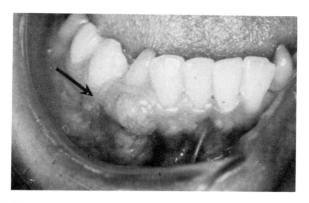

Fig. 13-55. Intramucosal nevus of the gingiva (arrow). Clinically it appeared as a growth of the interdental papilla and was not pigmented. (Courtesy Alejendro Acevedo, D.D.S., Iowa City.)

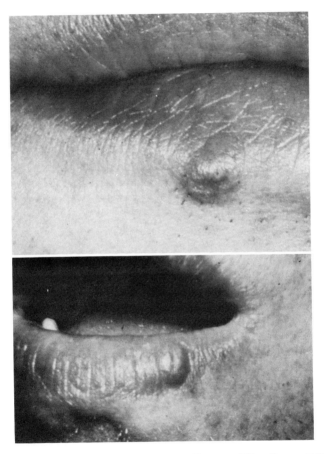

Fig. 13-56. Two compound nevi of the lip. (Courtesy Milton Knapp, D.D.S., Portland, Ore.)

36% are blue nevi; 6% are of the compound type; and 3% are of the junctional type.

The essential component of the *junctional, compound,* and *intramucosal* types is the nevus cell; and upon its location is based the distinction between these three types. The nevus cell is a small round or polyhedral cell with distinctly outlined homogeneous or clear cytoplasm and a centrally located nucleus (Fig. 13-57). The cells are usually found in clusters or groups, and some or many of them contain melanin.

In the *junctional* type the nevus cells are limited to the lower layers of the mucosal epithelium, which usually shows long epithelial ridges. In the *intramucosal* type the epithelium covering the lesion is normal, and the nevus cells and clusters are seen only in the connective tissue of the mucous membrane (Fig. 13-57). In the *compound* type the nevus cells and clusters are seen in both the connective tissue and the lower layers of the mucosal epithelium.

It has been suggested, but not proved, that the nevi progress or age from the junctional to the compound to the intramucosal type. Active nevi of the oral regions (i.e., the lesions that show junctional activity—junctional and compound types) deserve wide and careful excision. An increase in size or intensity of pigmentation of a nevus and the appearance of an inflammatory border around it are danger signs and require immediate attention.

The *blue* nevus is a rare type of pigmented lesion that occurs as a single smooth, firm, round or oval, bluish black or blue area less than 1 cm in size (Fig. 13-58). Most of the reported cases have been on the palate. The blue nevus is composed of fusiform cells that contain melanin and form a dense, circumscribed mass or masses (Fig. 13-59). On rare occasion, it may undergo malignant tranformation. The prognosis of the malignant blue nevus, however, is better than that of the melanoma.

A cellular variant of the blue nevus, called the *cellular blue nevus,* is composed of larger plump melanoblasts, may metastasize to a lymph node, and may be misdiagnosed as a melanoma. However, it is benign.

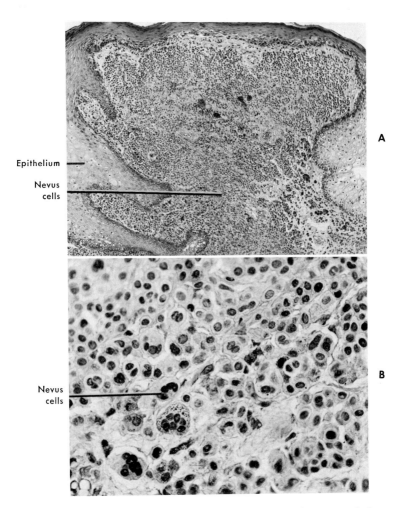

Epithelium

Nevus
cells

A

Nevus
cells

B

Fig. 13-57. Intramucosal nevus. **A,** The entire raised lesion is composed of
a solid mass of nevus cells. **B,** Note the nevus cells, many of which contain
melanin granules.

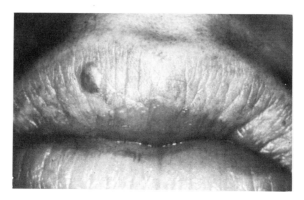

Fig. 13-58. Blue nevus of the upper lip. The most common site of this rare lesion, however, is the palate.

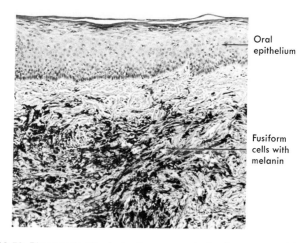

Oral
epithelium

Fusiform
cells with
melanin

Fig. 13-59. Blue nevus. The lesion is composed of a dense mass of fusiform cells that contain melanin.

Melanoma. This malignant lesion of the skin and mucous membranes is discussed in detail later in the book (p. 550).

Miscellaneous pigmentations. In addition to the conditions described, pigmentation of the oral mucosa may occur in *multiple neurofibromatosis, Albright's syndrome, malnutrition, chronic intestinal disorders* (due to deposition of melanin), and *poisoning with heavy metals* (due to deposition of metallic salts in the connective tissue of the oral mucosa).

White hairy tongue may accumulate foreign pigment and appear as *black hairy tongue*. Pigmentation of the attached gingiva has been observed in the *postmenopausal state* and following the use of *tranquilizers, oral contraceptives, antimalaria drugs* (e.g., Aralen, Plaquenil), and the *anticonvulsant drug mephenytoin*.

Pigmentation of the soft palate has been reported in patients with lung cancer or other lung diseases.

Varicosities of the oral vessels are seen in more than 80% of patients past 50 years of age. They appear as bluish areas on the ventral surface of the tongue and sometimes on the lip and cheek (Fig. 13-60). Since these areas can be blanched on pres-

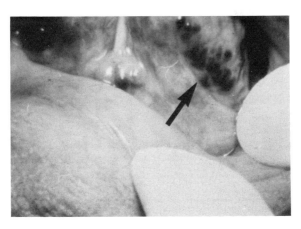

Fig. 13-60. Varicosities on the ventral surface of the tongue (arrow) in an elderly patient.

sure, they are not difficult to diagnose. A varicosity usually requires no therapy and is not always related to liver disease. Hematomas in the oral mucosa appear as bluish areas of discoloration.

Pigmentation of the oral mucosa also occurs in about 25% of cases of *hemochromatosis*. This is a disturbance of iron metabolism in which ferritin and hemosiderin are deposited in the body tissues, leading to fibrosis of the involved organs. It may be idiopathic, due to blood transfusions, or caused by dietary abnormalities. It is characterized by cirrhosis of the liver, cardiac failure, diabetes, and skin pigmentation. The pigmented skin, called bronzed skin, occurs in almost 90% of cases; and the oral mucous membrane is pigmented in about 25% of cases. The pigmentation of the skin and mucous membrane is caused by melanin (in the epithelium) and hemosiderin (in the connective tissue).

MISCELLANEOUS SURFACE LESIONS

Submucosal fibrosis. This oral disease is seen most frequently in people of Southeast Asia, but cases have been reported in people of other countries.

It involves any part of the oral mucosa and sometimes the pharynx and produces stiffening and restricted mobility of the oral mucous membrane; in severe cases it makes opening the mouth and eating difficult.

The disease may be preceded by vesicle formation, but ultimately the fibrous strands bind the mucosa to the underlying tissues, and the mucosa appears pale, opaque, and white in some areas. It is slightly more common in females; most cases have been reported from India; and the majority of patients are between 20 and 40 years of age. The cause of the disease is not known, although an allergic reaction to spices has been suggested. The lesion is premalignant.

Microscopic features consist of atrophy of the epithelium, loss of rete pegs, hyperparakeratosis, reduction in thickness of the stratum spinosum, and cellular atypia that at times can be classified as dyskeratosis. The connective tissue under the epithelium shows inflammatory infiltrate, loss of elastic fibers, and hyalinization of collagen. There is no known treatment of this disease.

Geographic tongue (wandering rash; glossitis migrans; migratory glossitis; glossitis areata exfoliativa). Of unknown cause, geographic tongue is characterized by one or more irregular areas of desquamation (bald spots) on the tongue.

The condition is slightly more common in females than in males, and emotional stress is often an associated factor. The filiform papillae in the bald spots are missing, but fungiform papillae remain (Fig. 13-61). The bald spots are surrounded by normal filiform papillae that, either by comparison or due to

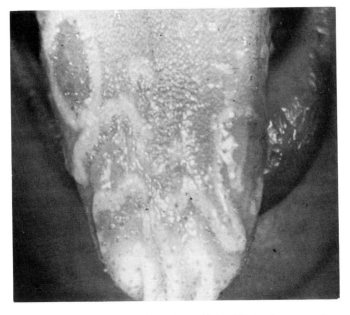

Fig. 13-61. Geographic tongue. Note the multiple white borders around areas of desquamation.

accumulation of keratin, appear to be hypertrophied. These areas are white. They heal, but new areas appear in another part of the tongue—thus the name wandering rash.

Glossitis migrans affects about 0.5% of the population. The bald spots on the tongue may change size and shape within a 2-hour period. In many cases (up to 50%) the condition is associated with fissured tongue.

The lesions usually do not respond to treatment but disappear spontaneously. However, recurrences are not uncommon. Microscopic sections show absence of filiform papillae, loss of keratin, thinning of the epithelium, and varying amounts of inflammatory exudate in the subepithelial connective tissue. No treatment is necessary, but vitamin B complex is frequently administered.

Perlèche. Also called *angular cheilitis* and *angular cheilosis,* perlèche is characterized by fissuring, cracking, burning, and dryness at the angles of the mouth. Saliva seeps into these cracks, leading to maceration of the skin.

The lesions are found in children as well as in adults and edentulous patients. The patients lick the corners of the mouth.

Among the causes of perlèche are loss of vertical dimension, riboflavin deficiency (p. 645), and fungus infection *(Candida albicans).*

Treatment depends on removal of the cause if such is apparent (e.g., the loss of vertical dimension). The use of nystatin ointment (100,000 units per gram) has been beneficial in many instances.

Denture stomatitis. Denture stomatitis, or denture-sore mouth, is an inflammatory lesion in which the mucosa underneath a denture becomes red and painful (Fig. 13-62). This lesion is more common under an upper than a lower denture. The most common cause of this lesion is poor oral hygiene and unclean dentures. In some patients, lesions are produced by *Candida albicans* and a hundred fold increase in the number of these organisms can be demonstrated (from about 100 organisms per square centimeter on the normal palate surface to

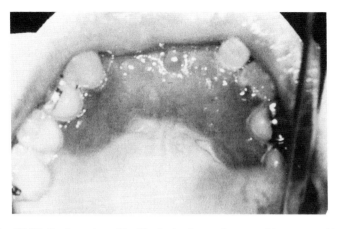

Fig. 13-62. Denture stomatitis. The lesion is usually caused by poor oral hygiene. It appears as a very red area of oral mucosa that corresponds to the denture outline.

10,000 organisms per square centimeter on the surface of the lesion). In very rare circumstances, denture stomatitis may be caused by contact allergy to the denture material.

Microscopic sections reveal thinning of the epithelial covering, edema, and infiltration of the subepithelial tissue by neutrophils and eosinophils. In lesions caused by *C. albicans* the organisms can be seen in the superficial layers of the stratified squamous epithelium.

Treatment of denture stomatitis consists of rigid attention to oral hygiene and removal of the dentures at night. In lesions produced by *C. albicans,* nystatin ointment or oral suspension is curative.

Leukoedema. In a small number of white adults, 50% of black children, and 90% of black adults, the buccal mucosa has a white or grayish white appearance. This condition is bilateral, cannot be wiped off, and is called leukoedema. Its intensity is directly related to the melanin pigmentation of the buccal mucosa. In patients with poor oral hygiene, the condition is more

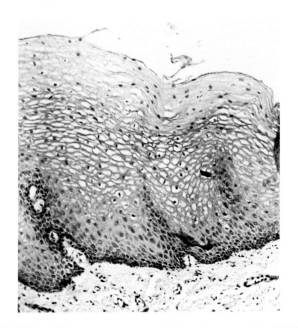

Fig. 13-63. The histologic appearance of leukoedema consists of thickening of the epithelium, parakeratosis, edema of the spinous layer (clear areas in cells), and thick rete pegs.

prominent; but its cause is not known. Microscopically the epithelium shows increased thickness, edema of the spinous layer, parakeratosis, and broad rete pegs. There is no evidence of dyskeratosis (Fig. 13-63). The condition requires no treatment.

Palatal erythema, ecchymoses, and petechiae. These disorders of the soft palate have been reported in fellatio and early stages of infectious mononucleosis (Fig. 13-64). They require no treatment.

Mucocutaneous lymph node syndrome. A newly described symptom complex called the mucocutaneous lymph node syndrome (MLNS) occurs in patients under 5 years of age and is characterized by erythema of oral and pharyngeal mucosa, dry

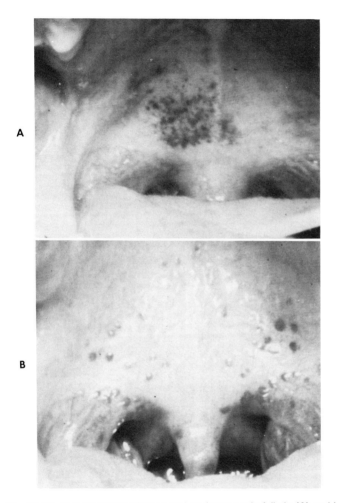

Fig. 13-64. Petechial hemorrhages and ecchymoses in fellatio **(A)** and infectious mononucleosis **(B)**.

and fissured lips, prominent red lingual papillae producing a strawberry-like tongue, conjunctivitis, fever, reddening of the skin of the hands and feet, and desquamation of nails as well as cervical lymphadenopathy. The disease was originally reported in Japan, resolves in about 2 weeks, and is of unknown etiology.

Hereditary mucoepithelial dysplasia. This is a recently described autosomal, dominantly inherited disorder affecting the oral mucosa, eyes (cataracts), skin (follicular keratosis alopecia), lungs (pneumonia, pneumothorax), and heart (cor pulmonale). Oral lesions consist of fiery red, flat or micropapillary-appearing mucosa of the gingiva and hard palate. However, lesions may occur anywhere in the oral mucosa and pharynx. The tongue has a red "scrotal" appearance. Oral lesions are usually asymptomatic. Histologic sections show a lack of keratinization, reduction in thickness of the epithelium, a lack of cohesion of cells, and benign dyskeratosis of individual cells. Ultrastructure studies of the epithelial cells reveal a lack of desmosome formation and intercellular accumulation of amorphous material.

REFERENCES

Abbey, L., and Shklar, G.: A histochemical study of oral lichen planus, Oral Surg. **31:**226,1971.

Alario, A., Ortonne, J. P., Schmitt, D., and Thivolet, J.: Lichen planus: study with anti-human T lymphocyte antigen (anti-HTLA) serum on frozen tissue sections Br. J. Dermatol. **98:**601, 1978.

Album, M. M., Gaisin, A., Lee, K. W. T., Buck, B. E., Sharrar, W. G., and Gill, F. M.: Epidermolysis bullosa dystrophica polydysplastica, Oral Surg. **43:**859, 1977.

Al-Ubaidy, S. S., and Nally, F. F.: Erythema multiforme, Oral Surg. **41:**601, 1976.

Anderson, H. J., Newcomer, V. D., Landau, J. W., and Rosenthal, L. H.: Pemphigus and other diseases, Arch. Dermatol. **101:**538, 1970.

Andreasen, J. O.: Oral lichèn planus. I. A. clinical evaluation of 115 cases. II. A histologic evaluation of 97 cases, Oral Surg. **25:**31, 158, 1968.

Arwill, T., Bergenholtz, A., and Olsson, O.: Epidermolysis bullosa hereditaria, Oral Surg. **19:**723, 1965.

Aufdemorte, T. B., and McPherson, M. A.: Refractory oral candidiasis, Oral Surg. **46:**776, 1978.

Banoczy, J., and Csiba, A.: Migratory glossitis, Oral Surg. **39:**113, 1975.

Banoczy, J., and Csiba, A.: Occurrence of epithelial dysplasia in oral leuko-
plakia, Oral Surg. **42:**766, 1976.
Banoczy, J., Roed-Petersen, B., Pindborg, J. J., and Inovay, J.: Clinical and
histologic studies on electrogalvanically induced oral white lesions, Oral
Surg. **48:**319, 1979.
Banoczy, J., Szabo, L., and Csiba, A.: Migratory glossitis: a clinical-histologic
review of seventy cases, Oral Surg. **39:**113, 1975.
Baringer, J. R., and Swoveland, P.: Recovery of herpes-simplex virus from hu-
man trigeminal ganglions, N. Engl. J. Med. **288:**648, 1973.
Bean, S. F., Alt, T. H., and Katz, H. I.: Oral pemphigus and bullous pemphi-
goid; immunofluorescent studies of two patients, J.A.M.A. **216:**673, 1971.
Becker, M. H., and Swinyard, C. A.: Epidermolysis bullosa dystrophica in chil-
dren, Radiology **90:**124, 1968.
Ben-Aryeh, H. Malberger, E., Gutman, D., Szargel, R., and Anavi, Y.: Salivary
IgA and serum IgG and IgA in recurrent aphthous stomatitis, Oral Surg.
42:746, 1976.
Bernstein, M. L.: Oral mucosal white lesions associated with excessive use of
Listerine mouthwash, Oral Surg. **46:**781, 1978.
Bernstein, M. L., and Carlish, R.: The induction of hyperkeratotic white lesions
in hamster cheek pouches with mouthwash, Oral Surg. **48:**517, 1979.
Bhaskar, S. N.: Oral pathology in the dental office; survey of 20,575 biopsy
specimens, J. Am. Dent. Assoc. **76:**761, 1968.
Bhaskar, S. N., and Bell, W. B.: Benign mucous membrane pemphigus, Oral
Surg. **20:**392, 1965.
Bhaskar, S. N., and Jacoway, F. R.: Blue nevus of the oral mucosa, Oral Surg.
19:678, 1965.
Boozer, C. H., Langeland, O. E., and Cuillory, M. B.: Benign migratory glos-
sitis associated with lichen planus, J. Oral Med. **29:**58, 1974.
Brabant, H., and Ketelbant, R.: Nouvelle contribution à l'étude du psoriasis
buccal, Rev. Stomatol. **68:**613, 1967.
Brener, M. D., and Harrison, B. D.: Intraoral blue nevus, Oral Surg. **28:**326,
1969.
Brightman, V. J., and Guggenheimer, J. G.: Herpetic paronychia—primary
herpes simplex infection of the finer, J. Am. Dent. Assoc. **80:**112, 1970.
Brody, H. A., and Silverman, S., Jr.: Studies on recurrent oral aphthae, Oral
Surg. **27:**27, 1969.
Brooke, R. I.: The oral lesions of bullous pemphigoid, J. Oral Med. **28:**36, 1973.
Bruggenkate, C. M., Cardozo, E. L., Maaskant, P., and van der Waal, I.: Lead
poisoning with pigmentation of the oral mucosa, Oral Surg. **39:**747, 1975.
Buchner, A.: Hand, foot, and mouth disease, Oral Surg. **41:**333, 1976.
Buchner, A., and Begleiter, A.: Oral lesions in psoriatic patients, Oral Surg.
41:327, 1976.
Buchner, A., and Hansen, L. S.: Pigmented nevi of the oral mucosa: a clinico-

pathologic study of 32 new cases and review of 75 cases from the literature. I. A. clinicopathologic study of 32 new cases, Oral Surg. **48**:131, 1979.

Buchner, A., and Hansen, L. S.: Melanotic macule of the oral mucosa, Oral Surg.: **48**:244, 1979.

Buchner, A., and Hansen, L. S.: Pigmented nevi of the oral mucosa: a clinico-pathologic study of 32 cases and a review of 75 cases from the literature. II. Analysis of 107 cases, Oral Surg. **49**:55, 1980.

Buchner, A., and Hansen, L. S.: Amalgam pigmentation (amalgam tattoo) of the oral mucosa, Oral Surg. **49**:139, 1980.

Buchner, A., Lozada, F., and Silverman, S., Jr.: Histopathologic spectrum of oral erythema multiforme, Oral Surg. **49**:221, 1980.

Buchner, A., and Ramon, Y.: Ultrastructural study of focal epilhelial hyperplasia, Oral Surg. **39**:622, 1975.

Budtz-Jorgensen, E.: Clinical aspects of candida infection in denture wearers, J. Am. Dent. Assoc. **96**:474, 1978.

Budtz-Jorgensen, E., and Bertram, U.: Denture stomatitis. I. The etiology in relation to trauma and infection II. The effect of antifungal and prosthetic treatment, Acta Odontol. Scand. **28**:71, 283, 1970.

Burdick, D., Prior, J. T., and Scanlon, G. T.: Peutz-Jeghers syndrome: a clinical-pathological study of a large family with 10 years follow-up, CA **16**:854, 1963.

Cannon, A. B.: White sponge nevus of the mucosa (naevus spongiosus albus mucosae), Arch. Dermatol. Syph. **31**:365, 1935.

Chang, T. W.: Genital herpes and Type 1 herpesvirus hominis, J.A.M.A. **238**:155, 1977.

Chellemi, S. J., and Biddix, J. C.: Desquamative gingivitis; summary of the literature and report of a case, Oral Surg. **29**:201, 1970.

Chellemi, S. J., and Shapiro, S.: The association between smoking and aphthous ulcers: a preliminary report, Oral Surg. **29**:832, 1970.

Chenitz, J. E.: Herpes zoster in Hodgkin's disease: unusual oral sequelae, J. Dent. Child. **43**:184, 1976.

Christenson, B. and Espmark, A.: Long-term follow-up studies on herpes simplex antibodies in the course of cervical cancer: patterns of neutralizing antibodies Am. J. Epidemiol. **105**:296, 1977.

Cohen, L., and Young, A. H.: The white sponge nevus, Br. J. Oral Surg. **5**:206, 1968.

Cooke, B. E. D.: Keratinizing lesions affecting the oral mucosa, Proc. R. Soc. Med. **60**:819, 1967.

Cooke, B. E. D.: Recurrent oral ulceration, Br. J. Dermatol. **81**:159, 1969.

Crawford, E. G., Jr., Burkes, E. J., Jr., and Briggaman, R. A.: Hereditary epidermolysis bullosa: oral manifestations and dental therapy, Oral Surg. **42**:490, 1976.

Cunliffe, W. J., and Menon, I. S.: Treatment of Behçet's syndrome with performin and ethyloesterenol, Lancet **1**:1239, 1969.

Dabelsteen, E., Ullman, S., Thomsen, K., and others: Demonstration of basement membrane autoantibodies in patients with benign mucous membrane pemphigoid, Acta Derm. Veneral (Stockh.) **54**:189, 1974.

Davenport, J. C.: The oral distribution of candida in denture stomatitis, Br. Dent. J. **129**:151, 1970.

Davies, R. M.: Herpetic infection in adults, Oral Surg. **30**:41, 1970.

Dean, A. G., Williams, E. H., Attobua, G., Gadi, A. Omeda, J., Amuti, A., and Atima, S. B.: Clinical events suggesting herpes-simplex infection before onset of Burkitt's lymphoma, Lancet **2**:1225, 1973.

Dockrell, H. M., and Greenspan, J. S.: Histochemical indentification of T cells in oral lichen planus, Oral Surg. **48**:42, 1979.

Francis, T. C.: Recurrent aphthous stomatitis and Behçet's disease: a review, Oral Surg. **30**:476, 1970.

Frantzis, T. G., Sheridan, P. J., and Reeve, C. M.: Oral manifestations of hemochromatosis, Oral Surg. **33**:186, 1972.

Friedmann, E., Katcher, A. H., and Brightman, V. J.: Incidence of recurrent herpes labialis and upper respiratory infection: a prospective study of the influence of biologic, social, and psychologic predictors, Oral Surg. **43**:873, 1977.

Frithiof, L., and Banoczy, J.: White sponge nevus (leukoedema exfoliativum mucosae oris): ultrastructural observations, Oral Surg. **41**:607, 1976.

Furey, N., West, C., Andrews, T., Paul, P. D., and Bean, S. F., Immunofluorescent studies of ocular cicatricial pemphigoid, Am. J. Ophthalmol. **80**:825, 1975.

Gardner, D. G., and Hudson, C. D.: The disturbances in odontogenesis in epidermolysis bullosa hereditaria fetalis, Oral Surg. **40**:483, 1975.

Gardner, J. A., and Hauft, R. J.: Herpes zoster of the mandibular nerve, Oral Surg. **14**:414, 1961.

Germishuys, P. J.: Hand-foot-and mouth disease, J. Oral Med. **35**:4, 1980.

Giansanti, J. S., Cramer, J. R., and Weathers, D. R.: Palatal erythema: another etiologic factor, Oral Surg. **40**:379, 1975.

Giansanti, J. S., Drummond, J. F., and Sabes, W. R.: Intraoral melanocytic cellular nevi, Oral Surg. **44**:267, 1977.

Giansanti, J. S., Tillery, D. E., and Olansky, S.: Oral mucosal pigmentation resulting from antimalarial therapy, Oral Surg. **31**:66, 1971.

Gilmore, H. K.: Early detection of pemphigus vulgaris, Oral Surg. **46**:641, 1978.

Goebel, W. M., and Duquette, P.: Mycotic infections associated with complete dentures: report of three cases, J. Am. Dent. Assoc. **88**:842, 1974.

Goldberg, J. R., Beasley, J. D., and Andrews, J. L.: Blue nevus of the oral mucosa; report of a case, Oral Surg. **27**:697, 1969.

Goldstein, B. H., and Katz, S. M.: Immunofluorescent findings in oral bullous lichen planus, J. Oral Med. **34**:8, 1979.

Gordon, N. C., Brown, S., Khosla, V. M., and Hansen, L. S.: Lead poisoning, Oral Surg. **47:**500, 1979.

Graykowski, E. A.: Summary of workshop on recurrent aphthous stomatitis and Behçet syndrome, J. Am. Dent. Assoc. **97:**599, 1978.

Greedman, G. L., Hooley, J. R., and Redman, R. S.: Median rhomboid glossitis: an atypical variant, Oral Surg. **24:**621, 1967.

Griffin, J. W.: Recurrent intraoral herpes simplex virus infection, Oral Surg. **19:**209, 1965.

Griffin, J. W.: Induction of herpes simplex virus lesions on rabbit lip mucosa, Oral Surg. **23:**765, 1967.

Griffith, M., Kaufman, H. S., and Silverman, S., Jr.: Studies on oral lichen planus, Oral Surg. **37:**239, 1974.

Guggenheimer, J., and Fletcher, R. D.: Traumatic induction of an intraoral reinfection with herpes simplex virus, Oral Surg. **38:**546, 1974.

Gutman, J., Cifuentes, C., Gondulfo, P., and Guesalaga, F.: Intradermal nevus associated with epidermoid cyst in the mucous membrane of the cheek, Oral Surg. **45:**76, 1978.

Halperin, V., Kolas, S., Jefferis, K. R., Huddleston, S. D., and Robinson, H. B. G.: The occurrence of Fordyce spots, benign migratory glossitis, median rhomboid glossitis, and fissured tongue in 2,478 dental patients, Oral Surg. **6:**1072, 1953.

Hamner, J. E., Looney, P. D., and Chused, T. M.: Submucous fibrosis, Oral Surg. **37:**412, 1974.

Hardwick, J. L., Lajtha, L. G., Beswick, I. S. L., and Longston, M.: Treatment of herpetic stomatitis with idoxuridine, Br. Dent. J. **126:**247, 1969.

Harrison, J. D., Rowley, P. S. A., and Peters, P. D.: Amalgam tattoos: light and electron microscopy and electron-probe micro-analysis, J. Pathol. **121:**83, 1977.

Haselden, F. G.: Bullous lichen planus, Oral Surg. **24:**472, 1967.

Hashimoto, K.: Paramyxovirus-like inclusions in several skin diseases of unknown etiology, Clin. Res. **18:**349, 1970.

Hashimoto, K.: Electron microscopy and histochemistry of pemphigus and pemphigoid, Oral Surg. **33:**206, 1972.

Hasler, J. F.: The role of immunofluorescence in the diagnosis of oral vesiculobullous disorders, Oral Surg. **33:**362, 1972.

Hazen, P. G., and Eppes, R. B.: Eczema herpeticum caused by herpesvirus type 2: a case in a patient with Darier Disease, Arch. Dermatol. **113:**1085, 1977.

Helander, I., and Hopsu-Havu, V. K.: Cell-mediated immunity in lichen planus: in vitro tests with extracts from lichen panus lesions, Arch. Dermatol. Res. **258:**1, 1977.

Herron, B. E.: Immunological aspects of cicatricial pemphigoid, Am. J. Opthalmol. **79:**271, 1975.

Hertz, R. S., Beckstead, P. C., and Brown, W. J.: Epithelial melanosis of the gingiva possibly resulting from the use of oral contraceptives, J. Am. Dent. Assoc. **100:**713, 1980.

Heyden, G., Arwill, T., and Gisslen, H.: Histochemical studies on lichen planus, Oral Surg. **37:**239, 1974.

Hicks, M. L., and Terezhalmy, G. T.: Herpesvirus hominis type 1: a summary of structure, composition, growth cycle, and cytopathogenic effects, Oral Surg. **48:**311, 1979.

Holbrook, W. P., and Rodgers, G. D.: Candidal infections: experience in a British dental hospital, Oral Surg. **49:**122, 1980.

Hurt, W. C.: Periadenitis mucosa necrotica recurrens, Oral Surg. **13:**750, 1960.

Hurt, W. C.: Observation on pemphigus vegetans, Oral Surg. **20:**481, 1965.

Jaffe, E. G., and Lehner, T.: Treatment of herpetic stomatitis with idoxuridine, Br. Dent. J. **126:**248, 1969.

Juel-Jensen, B. E.: Herpes simplex and zoster, Br. Med. J. **1:**406, 1973.

Kanaar, P.: Primary herpes simplex infection of fingers in nurses, Dermatologica **134:**346, 1967.

Kawana, T. Yoshino, K., and Kasamatsu, T.: Estimation of specific antibody to type 2 herpes simplex virus among patients with carcinoma of the uterine cervix, Gann. **65:**439, 1974.

Kennett, S.: Stomatitis medicamentosa due to barbiturates, Oral Surg. **25:**351, 1968.

Kennett, S.: Erythema multiforme affecting the oral cavity, Oral Surg. **25:**366, 1968.

Kennon, S., Tasch, E. G., and Arm, R. N.: Considerations in the management of patients taking oral contraceptives, J. Am. Dent. Assoc. **97:**641, 1978.

Kjaerheim, A., and Montes, L. F.: Blue nevus of the oral cavity (an electron microscopic study), Oral Surg. **29:**718, 1970.

Kleinman, Z.: Lingual varicosities, Oral Surg. **23:**546, 1967.

Knapp, M. J.: Lingual sebaceous glands and a possible thyroglossal duct, Oral Surg. **31:**70, 1971.

Koss, L. G., Stewart, F. W., Foote, F. W., Jordan, M. J., Bader, G. M., and Day, E.: Some histologic aspects of behavior of epidermoid carcinoma in situ and related lesions of the uterine cervix, CA **16:**1160, 1963.

Kronenbert, K., Fritzin, D., and Potter, B.: Malignant degeneration of lichen planus, Arch. Dermatol. **104:**304, 1974.

Lehner, T.: Characterization of mucosal antibody in recurrent aphthous ulceration and Behçet's syndrome, Arch. Oral Biol. **14:**843, 1969.

Lehner, T.: Pathology of recurrent oral ulceration and oral ulceration in Behçet's syndrome, J. Pathol. **97:**481, 1969.

Lehner, T.: Immunologic aspects of recurrent oral ulcers, Oral Surg. **33:**80, 1972.

Lennette, E. H., and Magoffin, R. L.: Virologic and immunologic aspects of major oral ulcerations, J. Am. Dent. Assoc. **87:**1055, 1973.

Levin, A. C.: Candida albicans and acrylic resin, J. Dent. Assoc. S. Afr. **28:**216, 1973.

Lozada, F., and Silverman, S., Jr.: Erythema multiforme, Oral Surg. **46:**628, 1978.

Luzardo-Baptista, M. J.: Aspects of the fine anatomy of aphthous stomatitis, Oral Surg. **39:**239, 1975.

Mack, L. M., and Woodward, H. W.: Blue nevus of oral mucous membrane, Oral Surg. **25:**929, 1968.

Mackie, R. M., Parratt, D., and Jenkins, W. M. M.: The relationship between immunological parameters and response to therapy in resistant oral candidosis, Br. J. Dermatol. **98:**343, 1978.

MacPhee, I. T., Sircus, W., Farmer, E. D., Harkness, R. A., and Cowley, G. C.: Use of steroids in the treatment of aphthous ulceration, Br. Med. J. **2:**147, 1968.

Mani, N. J., and Singh, B.: Studies on oral submucous fibrosis. III. Epithelial changes, Oral Surg. **41:**203, 1976.

Marefat, M. P., Albright, J. T., and Shklar, G.: Ultrastructural alterations in experimental lingual leukoplakia and carcinoma, Oral Surg. **47:**334, 1979.

Marlette, R. H.: Generalized melanoses and nonmelanotic pigmentations of the head and neck, J. Am. Dent. Assoc. **90:**141, 1975.

Martin, J. L., Buenahora, A. M., and Bolden, T. E.: Leukoedema of the buccal mucosa, Meharri-Dent. **29:**7, 1970.

Martin, J. L.: Epidemiology of leukoedema in the Negro, J. Oral Med. **28:**41, 1973.

Martin, J. L., Buenahorn, A. M., and Bolden, T. E.: Cyto-histology of leukoedema of the buccal mucosa, J. D. C. Dent. Soc. **44:**47, 1969.

Martin, J. L., and Crump, E. P.: Leukoedema of the buccal mucosa in Negro children and youth, Oral Surg. **34:**49, 1972.

Mashberg, A.: Erythroplasia: the earliest sign of asymptomatic oral cancer, J. Am. Dent. Assoc. **96:**615, 1978.

Mason, R. M., and Barnes, C. G.: Behçet's syndrome with arthritis, Ann. Rheum. Dis. **28:**95, 1969.

McCarthy, P. L.: Benign mucous membrane pemphigoid, Oral Surg. **33:**75, 1972.

McClatchey, K. D., Silverman, S., Jr., and Hansen, L. S.: Studies on oral lichen planus. III. Clincial and histologic correlations in 213 patients, Oral Surg. **39:**122, 1975.

McGinnis, J. P., and Turner, J. E.: Ultrastructure of the white sponge nevus, Oral Surg. **40:**644, 1975.

McKinney, R. V.: Hand, foot, and mouth disease: a viral disease of importance to dentists, J. Am. Dent. Assoc. **91:**122, 1975.

McKinney, R. V., Jr., and Singh, B. B.: Basement membrane changes under neoplastic oral mucous membrane, Oral Surg. **44:**875, 1977.

Melish, M. E., Hicks, R. M., and Larson, E. J.: Mucocutaneous lymph node syndrome in the United States, Am. J. Dis. Child. **130**:599, 1976.

Merchant, H. W.: Oral pigmentation associated with bronchogenic carcinoma, Oral Surg. **36**:675, 1973.

Merchant, H. W., Hayes, L. E., and Ellison, L. T.: Soft-palate pigmentation in lung disease, including cancer, Oral Surg. **41**:726, 1976.

Miller, M. F., Garfunkel, A. A., Ram, C., and Ship, I. I.: Inheritance patterns in recurrent aphthous ulcers: twin and pedigree data, Oral Surg. **43**:886, 1977.

Miller, M. F., Garfunkel, A. A., Ram, C. A., and Ship, I.: The inheritance of recurrent aphthous stomatitis, Oral Surg. **49**:409, 1980.

Miller, M. F., Ship, I. I., and Ram, C.: A retrospective study of the prevalence and incidence of recurrent aphthous ulcers in a professional population, 1958-1971, Oral Surg. **43**:532, 1977.

Mincer, H. H., Turner, J. E., and Sebelius, C. L.: Juvenile pemphigus vulgaris, Oral Surg. **40**:257, 1975.

Monteleone, L.: Periadenitis mucosa necrotica recurrens, Oral Surg. **23**:586, 1967.

Mosadomi, A., Shklar, G., Loftus, E. R., and Chauncey, H. H.: Effects of tobacco smoking and age on the keratinization of palatal mucosa: a cytologic study, Oral Surg. **46**:413, 1978.

Murti, P. R., Bhonsle, R. B., Daftary, D. K., and Mehta, F. S.: Oral lichen planus associated with pigmentation, J. Oral Med. **34**:23, 1979.

Naib, Z. M., Nahmias, A. J., Josey, W. E., and Kramer, J. H.: Genital herpetic infection: association with cervical dysplasia and carcinoma, CA **23**:940, 1969.

Nairn, R. I.: Nystatin and amphotericin B in the treatment of denture-related candidiasis, Oral Surg. **40**:68, 1975.

Nally, F. F.: Behçet's syndrome with autoimmune findings, Oral Surg. **25**:357, 1968.

Nally, F. F., and James, L. D.: Primary herpes simplex: report of an unusual case, Oral Surg. **29**:680, 1970.

Nally, F. F., and James, L. D.: Primary herpes simplex; report of an unusual case, Oral Surg. **29**:680, 1970.

Nisengard, R. J., Jablonska, S., Beutner, E. H., Shu, S., Chorzelski, T. P., Jarzabek, M., Blaszczyk, M., and Rzesa, G.: Diagnostic importance of immunofluorescence in oral bullous diseases and lupus erythematosus, Oral Surg. **40**:365, 1975.

Nitzan, D. W., Pisanti, S., and Dishon, T.: Comparison and evaluation of fluorescent antibody techniques in the detection of herpes simplex virus in oral infection, Oral Surg. **45**:207, 1978.

O'Brien, T. K., Saunders, D. R., and Templeton, F. E.: Chronic gastric erosions and oral aphthae, Am. J. Dig. Dis. **19**:447, 1972.

Olsson, K. A.: A comparison of two prosthetic methods for the treatment of denture stomatitis, Acta Odontol. Scand. **29:**745, 1971.

Page, L. R., Corio, R. L., Crawford, B. E., Giansanti, J. S., and Weathers, D. R.: The oral melanotic macule, Oral Surg. **44:**219, 1977.

Pearson, R. W., Potter, B., and Strauss, F.: Epidermolysis bullosa hereditaria letalis, Arch. Dermatol. **109:**349, 1974.

Pisanty, S.: Oral psoriasis, Oral Surg. **30:**351, 1970.

Puga, A., Rosenthal, J. D., Openshaw, H., and Notkins, A. L.: Herpes simplex virus DNA and RNA sequences in acutely and chronically infected trigeminal ganglia of mice, Virology **89:**102, 1978.

Ramanathan, K., Canaganayagam, A., Keat, T. C., and Retnanesan, A.: Frequency of oral precancerous conditions in 407 Malaysians—with correlation to oral habits, Med. J. Malaya **27:**173, 1973.

Ramulu, C., Raju, M. V. S., Ratnam, G. V., and Reddy, C. R. R. M.: Stomatitis nicotina and its relation to carcinoma of hard palate in reverse smokers of Chuttas, J. Dent. Res. **52:**711, 1973.

Rapidis, A. D., Langdon, J. D., and Patel, M. F.: Recurrent oral and oculogenital ulcerations (Behçet's syndrome), Oral Surg. **41:**457, 1976.

Reddy, C. R. R. M., Kameswari, V. R., Raju, M. V. S., and Ramulu, C.: Palatal epithelial changes in reverse smokers having carcinoma of hard palate, Indian J. Med. Res. **62:**195, 1974.

Reddy, C. R. R. M., Kameswari, V. R., Ramulu, C., and Reddy, P. G.: Histopathological study of stomatitis nicotina, Br. J. Cancer **25:**403, 1971.

Reddy, C. R. R. M., Rajakumari, K., and Ramulu, C.: Regression of stomatitis nicotina in persons with a long-standing habit of reverse smoking, Oral Surg. **38:**571, 1974.

Reddy, C. R. R. M., Ramulu, C., Raju, M. V. S, and Reddy, P. G.: Changes in the ducts of the glands of the hard palate in reverse smokers, CA **30:**231, 1972.

Reddy, C. R. R. M., Ramulu, C., Raju, M. V. S., and Reddy, P. G.: Relation of reverse smoking and other habits to the development of stomatitis nicotina, Indian J. Cancer **9:**223, 1972.

Regezi, J. A., Deegan, M. J., and Hayward, J. R.: Lichen planus: immunologic and morphologic identification of the submucosal infiltrate, Oral Surg. **46:**44, 1978.

Reisman, R. J., Schwartz, A. E., Friedman, E. W., and Gerry, R. G.: The malignant potential of oral lichen planus—diagnostic pitfalls, Oral Surg. **38:**227, 1974.

Renner, R. P., Lee, M., Anders, L., and McNamara, T. F.; The role of C. *albicans* in denture stomatitis, Oral Surg. **47:**323, 1979.

Rickles, N. H.: Allergy in surface lesions of the oral mucosa, Oral Surg. **33:**744, 1972.

Roed-Peterson, B., and Pindborg, J. J.: Prevalence of oral leukoedema in Uganda, Arch. Oral Biol. **18:**1191, 1973.

Roenigk, H. H., Jr., Ryan, J. G., and Bergfeld, W. F.: Epidermolysis bullosa acquisita; report of three cases and review of all published cases, Arch. Dermatol. **103**:1, 1971.

Rowell, N. R.: Systemic lupus erythematosus, Br. Med. J. **2**:427, 1969.

Royston, I., and Aurelian, L.: The association of genital herpesvirus with cervical atypia and carcinoma in situ, Am. J. Epidemiol. **91**:531, 1970.

Rubright, W. C., Walker, J. A., Karlsson, V. L., and Diehl, D. L.: Oral slough caused by dentifrice detergents and aggravated by drugs with antisialic activity, J. Am. Dent. Assoc. **97**:215, 1978.

Russell, A. S., Brisson, E., and Grace, M.: A double-blind, controlled trial of levamisole in the treatment of recurrent herpes labialis, J. Infect. Dis. **137**:597, 1978.

Sadeghi, E. K., and Witkop, C. J.: Ultrastructural study of hereditary benign intraepithelial dyskeratosis, Oral Surg. **44**:567, 1977.

Sadeghi, E. M., and Witkop, C. J.: The presence of Candida albicans in hereditary benign intraepithelial dyskeratosis, Oral Sug. **48**:342, 1979.

Salmon, T. N., Robertson, G. R., Jr., Tracy, N. H., and Hiatt, W. R.: Oral psoriasis, Oral Surg. **38**:48, 1974.

Samit, A. M., and Greene, G. W., Jr.: Atypical benign migratory glossitis, Oral Surg. **42**:780, 1976.

Sapp, J. P., and Brooke, R. I.: Intranuclear inclusion bodies in recurrent aphthous ulcers with a herpetiform pattern, Oral Surg. **43**:416, 1977.

Schlesinger, S. L., Borbotsina, J., and O'Neill, L.: Petechial hemorrhages of the soft palate secondary to fellatio, Oral Surg. **40**:376, 1975.

Schwartz, A. W.: Median rhomboid glossitis, Plast. Reconstr. Surg. **52**:91, 1973.

Schwartz, D. L.: Stomatitis nicotina of the palate, Oral Surg. **20**:306, 1965.

Shapiro, L., and Zegerelli, D. J.: The solitary labial lentigo; a clinicopathologic study of twenty cases, Oral Surg. **31**:87, 1971.

Shapiro, S., Olson, D. L., and Chellemi, S. J.: The association between smoking and aphthous ulcers, Oral Surg. **30**:624, 1970.

Shear, M.: Erythroplakia of the mouth, Int. Dent. J. **22**:460, 1972.

Shedd, D. P.: Clinical characteristics of early oral cancer, J.A.M.A. **215**:955, 1971.

Sheridan, P. J., and Herrman, E. C.: Intraoral lesions of adults associated with herpes simplex virus, Oral Surg. **32**:390, 1971.

Shiau, Y. Y., and Kwan, H. W.: Submucous fibrosis in Taiwan, Oral Surg. **47**:453, 1979.

Shillitoe, E. J., Wilton, J. M. A., and Lehner, T.: Sequential changes in cell-mediated immune responses to herpes simplex virus after recurrent herpetic infection in humans, Infect. Immun. **18**:130, 1977.

Ship, I. I.: Epidemiologic aspects of recurrent aphthous ulcerations, Oral Surg. **33**:400, 1972.

Ship, I. I., Brightman, V. F., and Lastep, L. L.: The patient with recurrent aphthosis ulcers and the patient with recurrent herpes labialis: a study of two population samples, J. Am. Dent. Assoc. **75:**645, 1967.

Ship, I. I., and Ram, C.: A retrospective study of recurrent herpes labialis (RHL) in a professional population, 1958–1971, Oral Surg. **44:**723, 1977.

Shklar, G.: Recent research on oral mucous membrane diseases, Oral Surg. **30:**242, 1970.

Shklar, G.: Lichen planus as an oral ulcerative disease, Oral Surg. **33:**376, 1972.

Shklar, G., Flynn, E., and Szabo, G.: Basement membrane alteration in oral lichen planus, J. Invest. Dermatol. **70:**45, 1978.

Shklar, G., and Sapiro, S. M.: Stomatitis areata migrans, Oral Surg. **36:**28, 1973.

Silverman, N. A., Alexander, J. C., Jr., Hollinshead, A. C., and Chretien, P. B.: Correlation of tumor burden with in vitro lymphocyte reactivity and antibodies to herpesvirus tumor-associated antigens in head and neck squamous carcinoma, CA **37:**135, 1976.

Silverman, S., Jr., and Beumer, III: Primary herpetic gingivostomatitis of adult onset, Oral Surg. **36:**496, 1973.

Silverman, S., Jr., and Griffith, M.: Studies on oral ichen planus. II. Follow-up on 200 patients, clinical characteristics, and associated malignancy, Oral Surg. **37:**705, 1974.

Sklar, S. H., and Buimovici-Klein, E.: Adenosine in the treatment of recurrent herpes labialis, Oral Surg. **48:**416, 1979.

Snyder, M. L, Church, D. H., and Rickles, N. H.: Primary herpes infection of right second finger: report of a case, Oral Surg. **27:**598, 1969.

Southam, J. C., Colley, I. T., and Clarke, N. G.: Oral herpetic infection in adults: clinical, histological and cytological features, Br. J. Dermatol. **80:**248, 1968.

Southam, J. C., and Ettinger, R. L.: A histological study of sublingual varices, Oral Surg. **38:**879, 1974.

Stanley, H. R.: Aphthous lesions, Oral Surg. **33:**407, 1972.

Stanley, H. R.: Management of patients with persistent recurrent aphthous stomatitis and Sutton's disease, Oral Surg. **35:**174, 1973.

Ström, J.: Ectodermosis erosiva pluriorificalis, Stevens-Johnson's syndrome and other febrile mucocutaneous reactions, and Behçet's syndrome in cold-agglutination-positive infections, Lancet **1:**457, 1965.

Tagami, H., and Imamura, S.: Benign mucous membrane pemphigoid, Arch. Dermatol. **109:**711, 1974.

Tenser, R. B. Miller, R. L., and Rapp, F.: Trigeminal ganglion infection by Thymidine Kinase–negative mutants of herpes simplex virus, Science **205:**915, 1979.

Terezhalmy, G. T.: Mucocutaneous lymph node syndrome, Oral Surg. **47:**26, 1979.

Terezhalmy, G. T., Tyler, M. T., and Ross, G. R.: Eczema herpeticum: atopic dermatitis complicated by primary herpetic gingivostomatitis, Oral Surg. **48:**513, 1979.

Thoma, G. W., and Robbins, G. B.: Blue nevus of the oral mucosa, Texas Dent. J. **86:**4, 1968.

Verhaegen, H., De Cree, J., and Brugmans, J.: Treatment of aphthous stomatitis, Lancet **2:**842, 1973.

Waldron, C. A., and Shafer, W. G.: Leukoplakia revisited: a clinicopathologic study of 3,256 oral leukoplakias, Cancer **36:**1386, 1975.

Walker, D. M.: Identification of subpopulations of lymphocytes and macrophages in the infiltrate of lichen planus lesions of skin and oral mucosa, Br. J. Dermatol. **94:**529, 1976.

Walker, D. M.: The inflammatory infiltrate in lichen planus lesions; an autoradiographic and ultrastructural study, J. Oral Pathol. **5:**277, 1976.

Weathers, D. R., Baker, G., Archard, H. O., and Burkes, E. J.: Psoriasiform lesions of the oral mucosa (with emphasis on "ectopic geographic tongue"), Oral Surg. **37:**872, 1974.

Weathers, D. R., Corio, R. L., Crawford, B. E., Giansanti, J. S., and Page, L. R.: The labial melanotic macule, Oral Surg. **42:**196, 1976.

Weathers, D. R., and Griffin, J. W.: Intraoral ulcerations of recurrent herpes simplex and recurrent aphthae: two distinct clinical entities, J. Am. Dent. Assoc. **81:**81, 1970.

Weathers, D. R., and Waldron, C. A.: Intraoral cellular nevi, Oral Surg. **20:**467, 1965.

Weedon, D., and Little, J. H.: Spindle and epithelioid cell nevi in children and adults: a review of 211 cases of the Spitz nevus, CA **40:**217, 1977.

White, D. K., Leis, H. J., and Miller, A. S.: Intraoral psoriasis associated with widespread dermal psoriasis, Oral Surg. **41:**174, 1976.

WHO Collaboration Centre for Oral Precancerous Lesions: Definition of leukoplakia and related lesions: an aid to studies on oral precancer, Oral Surg. **46:**518, 1978.

Wilgram, G. F.: A possible role of the Merkel cell in aphthous stomatitis, Oral Surg. **34:**231, 1972.

Williamson, J. J.: Erythroplasia of Queyrat of the buccal mucous membrane, Oral Surg. **17:**308, 1964.

Witkop, C. J., Jr., and Gorlin, R. J.: Four hereditary mucosal syndromes, Arch. Dermatol. **84:**762, 1961.

Witkop, C. J., Jr., White, J. G., Sauk, J. J., and King, R. A.: Clinical, histologic, cytologic, and ultrastructural characteristics of the oral lesions from hereditary mucoepithelial dysplasia, Oral Surg. **46:**645, 1978.

Young, S. K., Rowe, N. H., and Buchanan, R. A.: A clinical study for the control of facial mucocutaneous herpes virus infections. I. Characterization of natural history in a professional school population, Oral Surg. **41:**498, 1976.

Zakay-Rones, Z., Ehrlich, J., Hochman, N., and Levy, R.: The sulcular epithelium as a reservoir for herpes simplex virus in man, J. Periodontol. **44:**779, 1973.

Zegarelli, E. V., Everett, F. G., and Kutscher, A. H.: Familial white folded dysplasia of the mucous membranes. Oral Surg. **14:**1436, 1961.

Zegarelli, E. V., Kutscher, A. H., Mercadante, J. L., Kupferberg, N., and Piro, J. D.: An atlas of oral lesions observed in the syndrome of oral melanosis with associated intestinal polyposis (Peutz-Jeghers syndrome), Oral Surg. **15:**411, 1962.

Zegarelli, D. J., and Zegarelli, E. V.: Intraoral pemphigus vulgaris, Oral Surg. **44:**384, 1977.

CHAPTER 14

Cysts of soft tissues

The majority of cysts in oral regions occur within the jaws. However, the following are limited to the soft tissues:

1. Mucocele (mucous retention cyst; retention phenomenon)
2. Mucous cyst
3. Ranula
4. Gingival cyst
5. Epidermoid cyst
6. Nasoalveolar cyst
7. Branchial cyst
8. Lymphoepithelial cyst
9. Thyroglossal cyst

Mucocele (mucous retention cyst; retention phenomenon). The mucocele is a mucus-containing cyst that occurs in the salivary gland–bearing areas of the oral mucosa and consitutes 2.8% of all cysts found at oral biopsies.

The cyst presents as a small, circumscribed, usually elevated, translucent bluish lesion of the mucosa. If deep seated, it can be palpated as a circumscribed, freely movable lesion (Fig. 14-1). Except in the anterior half of the hard palate (which is devoid of salivary glands), the lesion can occur anywhere in the oral cavity. The lip and tongue are the preferred sites. Superficial lesions frequently rupture, discharge a sticky mucoid material, and collapse. As soon as they appear to have healed, they recur. This cycle of rupture, discharge, and recurrence may go on for months.

Microscopically the fully developed lesion consists of a cystic cavity filled with a lightly basophilic homogeneous material that is mucus (Fig. 14-2). Round, swollen, apparently degenerating cells are dispersed throughout this material. The lining of the cyst is usually formed only by granulation tissue and, under extremely rare circumstances, by epithelium (Fig. 14-2). The sal-

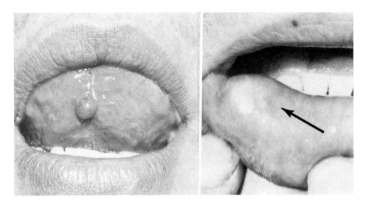

Fig. 14-1. A mucocele can present as an elevated (left) or partially sub-merged (right) lesion.

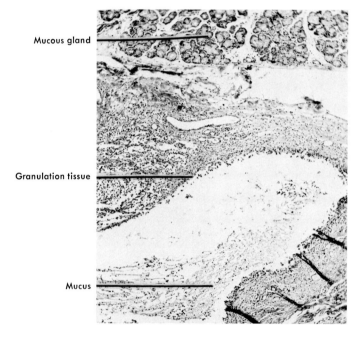

Mucous gland

Granulation tissue

Mucus

Fig. 14-2. Microscopically a mucocele appears as a mucus-containing cyst lined by granulation tissue.

ivary gland, as well as the connective tissue in the vicinity of the mucocele, is infiltrated by neutrophils, plasma cells, and lymphocytes. In an early mucocele or in one that has ruptured, a clear-cut cystic cavity cannot be identified; the lesion consists of a diffuse permeation of the affected area by mucus.

Mucoceles are formed because of a traumatic rupture of the excretory duct of a salivary gland and the subsequent accumulation of saliva in the tissues. Treatment therefore consists of removal of the cyst as well as the associated gland. Since the minor salivary glands lie close to the surface, they usually are removed with the mucoceles and a cure is accomplished.

Mucous cyst. A rare cystic lesion of the oral cavity, the mucous cyst usually occurs in the lip, cheek, or tongue.

This lesion is a small compressible growth that seldom reaches a size larger than a few millimeters. Microscopically it is characterized by a mucus-containing cystic cavity lined by epithelium that is either cuboidal or columnar or consists of mucous cells.

The lesion differs from a mucocele insofar as it is not caused by severance of the duct, is lined by epithelium, and usually is not associated with mucous glands. Surgical excision is curative.

Ranula. The ranula is a large soft, mucus-containing swelling in the floor of the mouth (Fig. 14-3).

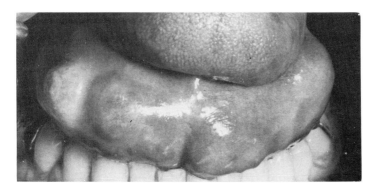

Fig. 14-3. The ranula is a large compressible lesion of the floor of the mouth.

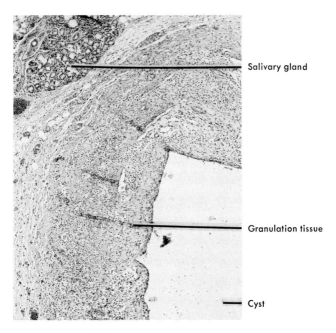

Salivary gland

Granulation tissue

Cyst

Fig. 14-4. Microscopically a ranula is lined by granulation tissue and, except for its size, is identical to a mucocele.

Microscopically and in its formation, a ranula is identical to a mucocele except that it is associated with larger glands and is therefore of greater size (Fig. 14-4). It is produced by a defect in Wharton's duct (submaxillary gland) or Bartholin's duct (major sublingual gland).

Sometimes the treatment consists of excision of the cyst and gland. It is better, however, to do a so-called Partsch procedure and establish a surface connection for the severed duct (marsupialization).

Gingival cyst. The gingival cyst presents as a circumscribed, elevated, somtimes movable, nonulcerated lesion of the attached gingiva and alveolar mucosa (Fig. 14-5).

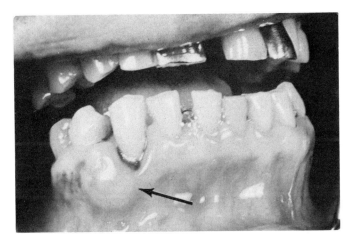

Fig. 14-5. Gingival cyst. Note the raised circumscribed lesion of the gingiva (arrow).

These cysts appear twice as frequently in the mandible as in the maxilla, and about 90% occur in the buccal gingiva. The area from the lateral incisor to the premolar is involved in almost 80% of cases. The most common site, therefore, is the buccal aspect of the region from the mandibular lateral incisor to the second premolar. The lesion occurs with about equal frequency in both sexes, and the greatest incidence is in the sixth decade.

Although the cysts occur in the soft tissues, about 50% erode the cortical plate from the periosteal side and there is a circumscribed radiolucency (Fig. 14-6). The radiolucency may be mistaken for a mental foramen, a lateral periodontal cyst, or a lateral radicular cyst. However, the teeth in the area are vital, and this establishes the correct diagnosis.

Microscopically a cyst lined by cuboidal, squamous, or stratified squamous epithelium or by a double layer of cuboidal epithelium (Fig. 14-7) is seen. The connective tissue is either free of inflammatory cells or shows minimal infiltrate. Treatment consists of excision.

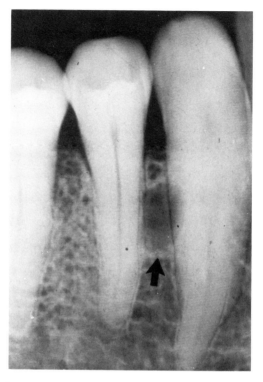

Fig. 14-6. Gingival cyst. Note the circumscribed radiolucency between the canine and premolar (arrow).

Epidermoid cyst. This lesion is sometimes referred to as a *dermoid cyst, epidermal cyst,* or *dermal cyst.*

The epidermoid cyst is a freely movable well-circumscribed mass that is usually seen in the floor of the mouth or in the cheek (Fig. 14-8). In the former location it may elevate the tongue and interfere with speech and mastication. It has a doughlike feel but may be fluctuant. The cut sections reveal cheesy or liquid material.

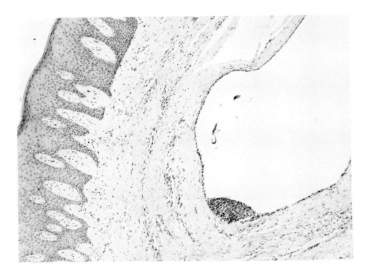

Fig. 14-7. Gingival cyst. The cystic cavity (right) is lined by epithelial cells that in one area are piled up in the form of a plaque.

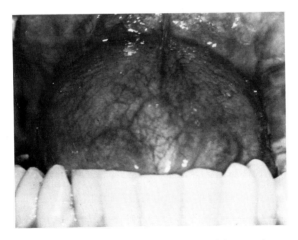

Fig. 14-8. Epidermoid cyst of the floor of the mouth.

Microscopically the cyst shows a lining of keratinized stratified squamous epithelium, and the cyst cavity usually contains keratin. The connective tissue wall of the cyst may contain sebaceous glands, sweat glands, and hair follicles.

The term *dermoid*, sometimes employed for this lesion, should be reserved for neoplastic teratomatous lesions that are occasionally seen in the midline of the oral cavity (p. 640).

Nasoalveolar cyst. The nasoalveolar cyst is a fissural cyst and is the only member of the group of fissural cysts that occurs in

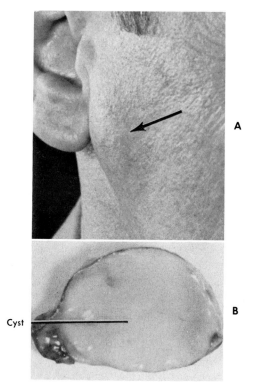

A

Cyst

B

Fig. 14-9. A, Branchial cyst at the angle of the mandible (arrow). **B,** Bisected gross specimen.

the soft tissues. It is a soft tissue cyst and is described earlier in the book (p. 237).

Branchial cyst. The circumscribed movable swelling usually occurs on the lateral side of the neck. However, 10% to 15% are seen at the angle of the mandible (Fig. 14-9). Rarely one may be seen on the floor of the mouth. The lesion occurs between the ages of 20 and 40 years.

Although at one time this cyst was believed to be derived from the branchial arch remnants, it has been shown to arise

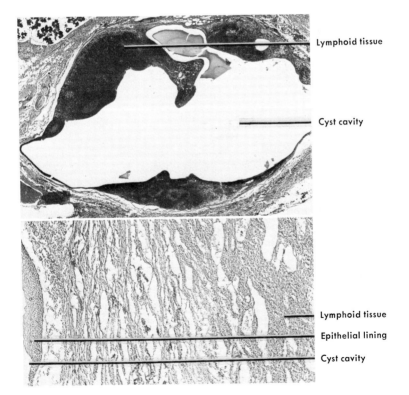

Fig. 14-10. The branchial cyst is an epithelium-lined cyst that lies in a dense aggregate of lymphocytes.

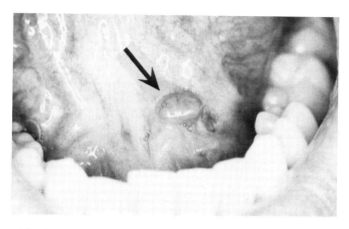

Fig. 14-11. Lymphoepithelial cyst (arrow) of the floor of the mouth.

from the epithelial inclusions within the cervical lymph nodes. Its great frequency after sexual maturity is due to the fact that the glandular epithelium entrapped in the lymph nodes probably begins to proliferate after puberty.

Microscopic sections show that branchial cysts are usually lined by stratified squamous epithelium and are surrounded by lymphoid tissue. The lymphoid tissue has all the characteristics of a lymph node. However, if the cyst is large, it may compress the lymph node architecture—in which case the lymphoid tissue is seen only as a zone of densely packed cells (Fig. 14-10). If aspirated or drained, branchial cysts recur. Excision therefore is the treatment of choice.

Lymphoepithelial cyst. An lymphoepithelial cyst of the oral cavity is usually 3 × 3 mm to 1.5 × 1.5 cm in size, is nonulcerated, and is freely movable with a duration of a few months to many years (Fig. 14-11).

This lesion is seen more often in males than in females and occurs between the ages of 15 and 65 years (mean, 36 years). About 60% occur on the floor of the mouth, and 40% on the

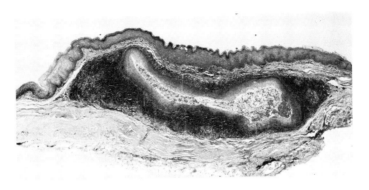

Fig. 14-12. Lymphoepithelial cyst of the floor of the mouth. It is lined by stratified squamous epithelium and has dense lymphoid aggregates in its wall.

lateral and ventral surfaces of the tongue. Rarely the cyst may occur in the soft palate or palatoglossal area.

Microscopically it is well circumscribed, lined by stratified squamous epithelium, and surrounded by a dense zone of lymphocytes. The entire lesion is covered by oral mucosa (Fig. 14-12).

Treatment of a lymphoepithelial cyst consists of simple enucleation. This lesion is believed to arise in a recently described structure in the mucosa of the oral cavity called the *oral tonsil*. In about 20% of the population, these 1- to 3-mm circumscribed nodular structures are observed on the mucosa of the soft palate, ventral surface of the tongue, and floor of the mouth. They consist of an epithelium-lined crypt surrounded by dense lymphoid tissue.

Thyroglossal cyst. This cyst of the embryonic thyroglossal duct remnants is discussed later in the book (p. 635).

REFERENCES

Baker, B. R., and Mitchell, D. F.: The pathogenesis of epidermoid implantation cysts, Oral Surg. **19:**494, 1965.

Bahaskar, S. N.: Histogenesis of branchial cysts, Am. J. Pathol. **35:**407, 1959.

Bhaskar, S. N.: Gingival cyst and the keratinizing ameloblastoma, Oral Surg. **19:**796, 1965.

Bhaskar, S. N.: Lymphoepithelial cysts of the oral cavity, Oral Surg. **21**:120, 1966.

Bhaskar, S. N., Bolden, T. E., and Weinmann, J. P.: Pathogenesis of mucoceles, J. Dent. Res. **35**:863, 1956.

Bhaskar, S. N., and Laskin, D. M.: Gingival cysts, Oral Surg. **8**:803, 1955.

Buchner, A., and Hansen, L. S.: The histomorphologic spectrum of the gingival cyst in the adult, Oral Surg. **48**:532, 1979.

Cohen, L.: Mucoceles of the oral cavity, Oral Surg. **19**:365, 1965.

Giunta, J., and Cataldo, E.: Lymphoepithelial cysts of the oral mucosa, Oral Surg. **35**:77, 1973.

Grand, N. G., and Marwah, A. S.: Pigmented gingival cyst, Oral Surg. **17**:635, 1964.

Harrison, J. D.: Salivary mucoceles, Oral Surg. **39**:268, 1975.

Jaques, D. A., Chambers, R. G., and Oertel, J. E.: Thyroglossal tract carcinoma, a review of the literature and addition of 18 cases, Am. J. Surg. **120**:439, 1970.

Kelln, E. E.: Oral epidermal cysts and probably histogenesis, Oral Surg. **19**:359, 1965.

Knapp, M. J.: Oral tonsils: location, distribution, and histology, Oral Surg. **29**:155, 1970.

Knapp, M. J.: Pathology of oral tonsils, Oral Surg. **29**:295, 1970.

Korchin, L.: Dermoid cyst with lingual sinus tract, Oral Surg. **37**:175, 1974.

Main, D. M. G.: Tooth identity in ovarian teratomas, Br. Dent. J. **129**:328, 1970.

Melhado, R. M., Rulli, M. A., and Martinelli, C.: The etiopathogenesis of gingival cysts, Oral Surg. **35**:510, 1973.

Meyer, I.: Dermoid cysts (dermoids) of the floor of the mouth, Oral Surg. **8**:1149, 1955.

Mirsky, I., and Doyle, J. L.: Sublingual teratoid cyst with unusual giant-cell reaction, Oral Surg. **23**:428, 1967.

Portales, C., and Loscalzo, L. J.: Unusual epidermal cyst, Oral Surg. **24**:581, 1967.

CHAPTER 15

Benign tumors and tumorlike proliferations of soft tissues

The benign tumors and tumorlike proliferations of the oral soft tissue constitute about 20% of all oral lesions biopsied by the dentist. Statistically, seven of the fifteen most frequently observed lesions of the oral cavity (except caries and periodontal disease) are benign tumors or tumorlike soft tissue growths (Table 17).

Benign tumors or tumorlike growths that arise in the soft tissues of the oral cavity may be classified as follows:

Epithelial tumors

1. Verruca vulgaris
2. Condyloma acuminatum
3. Papilloma
4. Focal epithelial hyperplasia (Heck's disease)

5. Pseudoepitheliomatous hyperplasia (keratoacanthoma)
6. Inflammatory papillary hyperplasia

Mesenchymal tumors

1. Irritation fibroma
2. Peripheral fibroma and peripheral fibroma with calcification
   a. Giant cell fibroma
   b. Oral focal mucinosis
3. Myxoma (of soft tissues)
4. Epulis fissuratum
5. Pseudoepitheliomatous hyperplasia (keratoacanthoma)
6. Inflammatory papillary hyperplasia
7. Pyogenic granuloma

8. Pregnancy tumor (granuloma gravidarum)
9. Hemangiomas
   a. Capillary and cavernous hemangiomas
   b. Juvenile hemangioma
10. Lymphangioma
11. Cystic hygroma (cystic lymphangioma; hygroma cysticum colli)
12. Neuroma (traumatic neuroma)
13. Schwannoma (neurilemoma)

473

Table 17. Fifteen most common oral lesions* biopsied in dental offices

Lesion	Number†	Percent
Dental granuloma	2,231	12.24
Radicular cyst	2,046	11.23
Irritation fibroma	1,378	7.56
Benign hyperkeratosis	1,337	7.34
Dentigerous cyst	1,194	6.55
Gingivitis, chronic	1,111	6.09
Mucocele	522	2.86
Peripheral fibroma	515	2.82
Epulis fissuratum	515	2.82
Papilloma	349	1.91
Pyogenic granuloma	323	1.77
Inflammatory papillary hyperplasia	295	1.50
Ulcer (benign)	197	1.08
Leukoplakia (premalignant)	187	1.02
Squamous cell carcinoma	132	0.72
TOTAL	12,332	67.51

*Exclusive of caries and periodontal disease.
†Out of a total of 18,214 cases.

Mesenchymal tumors—cont'd

14. Neurofibroma
15. Generalized neurofibromatosis (multiple neurofibromatosis; von Recklinghausen's disease); tuberous sclerosis
16. Lipoma
17. Granular cell myoblastoma
18. Congenital epulis
19. Nevoxanthoendothelioma (juvenile xanthogranuloma; xanthogranuloma)
20. Verruciform xanthoma
21. Soft tissue plasmacytoma (extramedullary plasmacytoma)
22. Plasma cell granuloma
23. Leiomyoma
24. Rhabdomyoma
25. Juvenile nasopharyngeal angiofibroma
26. Hamartoma and choristoma

EPITHELIAL TUMORS

Of the epithelial tumors, only the papilloma and inflammatory papillary hyperplasia occur with any frequency. The rest are rare and are discussed only for completeness.

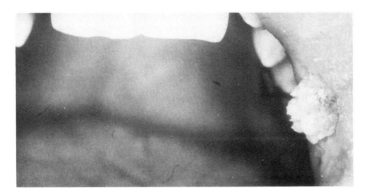

Fig. 15-1. Verruca vulgaris. Note the raised, broad-based growth at the corner of the mouth.

Verruca vulgaris. Verruca vulgaris is caused by a virus, and the incubation period is from about 6 weeks to a year. Although primarily a lesion of the skin, it does occur in the oral cavity, particularly on the lips and palate.

Clinically the verruca vulgaris is a sessile, soft, cauliflower-like lesion only a few millimeters in size (Fig. 15-1). Microscopically it is a papillomatous lesion in which the epithelium is thrown into folds, and it shows alternating hyperkeratosis and parakeratosis and long epithelial ridges. The ridges at the margin of the verruca are bent inward toward the center (Fig. 15-2). Under the electron microscope characteristic viral inclusions can be demonstrated within the epithelium.

The lesion may disappear spontaneously, or it may be excised or treated with liquid nitrogen. Whereas recurrence of a spontaneously involuted verruca vulgaris is rare, recurrence following therapy is common.

Condyloma acuminatum. This virus-produced verrucous broad-based epithelial lesion usually occurs in the anogenital area (venereal condyloma, verruca acuminata, moist wart, venereal wart); but its occurrence in the oral cavity is now established (Fig. 15-3).

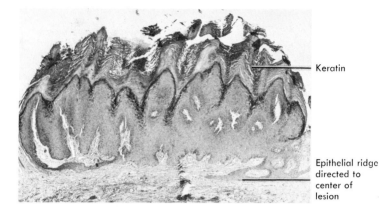

Keratin

Epithelial ridge
directed to
center of
lesion

Fig. 15-2. Verruca vulgaris. The lesion is papillary and covered by keratin.

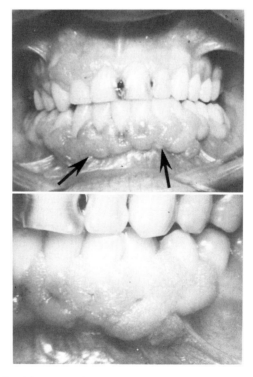

Fig. 15-3. Condyloma acuminatum. Note the multiple papillary growths (arrows). (Courtesy Milton J. Knapp, D.D.S., Portland, Ore.)

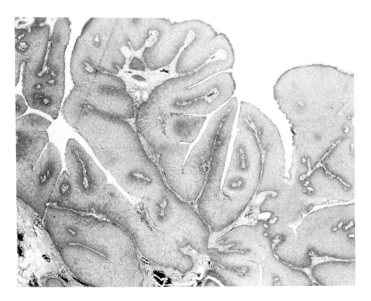

Fig. 15-4. Condyloma acuminatum. The lesion consists of a papillary growth of epithelium. There is no dyskeratosis.

The lesion may be multiple and may spread by autoinoculation. Microscopically it is papillary and covered by parakeratotic stratified squamous epithelium (Fig. 15-4). The subepithelial tissue had lymphocytic infiltrate. Surgical excision is the treatment of choice, but recurrence is likely.

Papilloma. This benign epithelial neoplasm constitutes about 2% of all oral biopsy specimens (Table 17). The mean age of oral papilloma is about 35 years, and it is slightly more common in the male and in the white race. The hard and soft palate and uvula are the most common site (35%), but the lesion can occur anywhere in the oral mucosa (tongue 23%, lips 13%, other sites 29%).

Clinically the oral papilloma is a white, pedunculated, cauliflower-like growth (Fig. 15-5). Lesions within the oral cavity

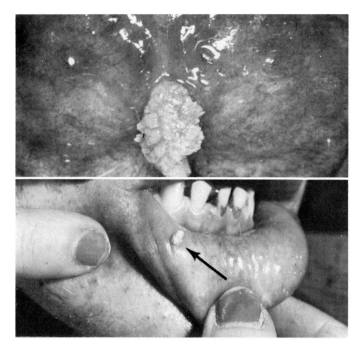

Fig. 15-5. Papilloma of the floor of the mouth and lip (arrow).

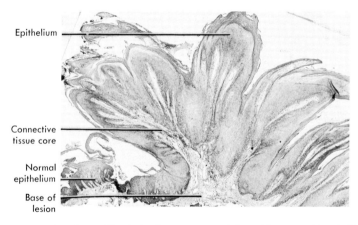

Epithelium

Connective
tissue core

Normal
epithelium

Base of
lesion

Fig. 15-6. Papilloma. The lesion has a narrow stalk and is covered by stratified squamous epithelium.

are soft, whereas those on the exposed areas of the lips are usually rough and scaly.

Microscopic sections show a cauliflower-like lesion that has a narrow stalk and that is formed by many fingerlike projections. The latter are covered by stratified squamous epithelium and have a core of loose connective tissue (Fig. 15-6). The epithelium may show hyperkeratosis or parakeratosis but is otherwise normal. The connective tissue shows evenly distributed chronic inflammatory infiltrate.

If the lesion is excised from its base, it does not recur. Unlike papillomas in other areas (e.g., urinary bladder, gastrointestinal tract), the oral lesions do not undergo malignant changes.

On rare occasion, multiple papillomas may occur in the oral cavity. These have a tendency to recur and are probably of viral origin.

Focal epithelial hyperplasia (Heck's disease). Primarily in American and South American Indian children (but also in other races such as the Eskimo), multiple bumpy soft lesions of the oral mucosa have been described (Fig. 15-7).

The lesions are quite prominent after 25 years of age and occur most often on the lower lip; but they can involve any area of the mouth (especially the buccal mucosa, upper lip, tongue, gingiva, and anterior pillar of the fauces). They range in size from a pinhead to about 0.5 cm and cause no symptoms. Microscopic sections show local piling up of normal epithelium (Fig. 15-8).

The cause of the disease is not known. Electron microscopy studies, however, have shown intranuclear virus particles that were classified as belonging to the papova (*pa*pilloma, *po*lyoma, *va*cuolating agent) group. For this reason, a viral etiology is most likely. The lesion may regress spontaneously, and no treatment is necessary.

A condition similar to focal epithelial hyperplasia called *multiple fibroepithelial hyperplasia* has been described. It is different from focal epithelial hyperplasia in that the raised nodular

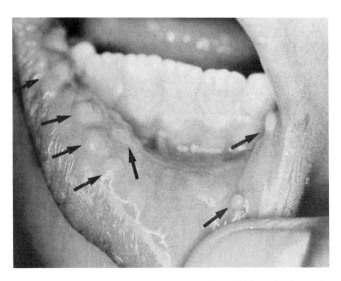

Fig. 15-7. Focal epithelial hyperplasia. Note the multiple raised growths on the mucous membrane (arrows).

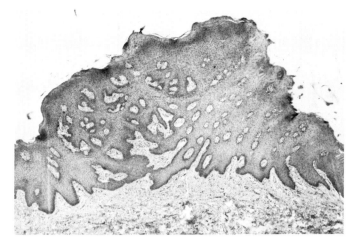

Fig. 15-8. Focal epithelial hyperplasia. The raised lesion is covered by hyperplastic epithelium.

lesions of the oral mucosa are composed of connective tissue that is covered by stratified squamous epithelium.

Pseudoepitheliomatous hyperplasia (keratocanthoma). In the presence of a variety of conditions (e.g., chronic ulcers, fungous infections, bony sequestra), the oral epithelium can undergo prominent though benign tumorlike proliferation. Furthermore, epithelial hyperplasia and tumorlike growths may occur without any apparent cause. Such proliferations are called pseudoepitheliomatous hyperplasia; and from the description just given, it should be apparent that the hyperplasia may be *primary* (idiopathic) or *secondary* (as a result of a known cause).

Clinically the lesion can be an ulcer, a nodule, or a plaque. Usual locations are the lip, tongue, and alveolar ridges. Microscopic features are most important and are the only means of diagnosis. These consist of marked proliferation of epithelium and apparent invasion of underlying tissues.

An epithelial proliferation superficially resembles a squamous cell carcinoma, but all epithelial cells are normal and do not show dyskeratosis. The absence of dyskeratosis is the only criterion for differential diagnosis between the two.

The lesion has no capacity for metastasis. Since it may be locally infiltrating, excision is the best treatment. Some lesions regress spontaneously.

The term *keratoacanthoma* (also called *molluscum sebaceum*, *self-healing carcinoma*, and *verrucoma*) is applied to an exuberant pseudoepitheliomatous hyperplasia. Although primarily of the skin, this condition does occur on the lip, tongue (Fig. 15-9), and alveolar ridge. It usually develops in whites in or after the third decade. It is five times more common in males than in females, and of the lip lesions the lower lip is the preferred site (6:1).

Keratoacanthoma presents as a craterlike lesion containing a mass of keratin and ranges in size from 0.5 to 2 cm. Microscopic sections show a central trough of keratin surrounded by marked epithelial proliferation (pseudoepitheliomatous hyperplasia). However, dyskeratosis is absent—which is the most important

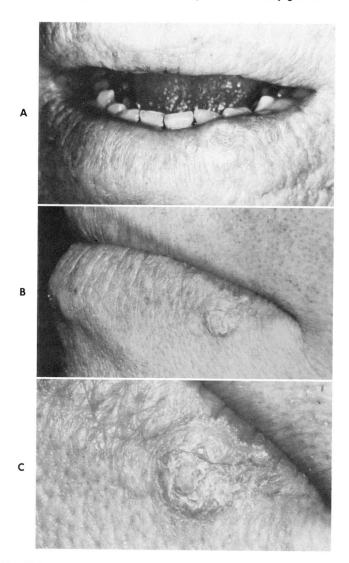

Fig. 15-9. Keratoacanthoma of the lip **(A)** and of the mucocutaneous junction **(B** and **C).** (Courtesy A. Acevedo, D.D.S., Iowa City, and J. Ward, D.D.S., Washington, D.C.)

distinction between a keratoacanthoma and a squamous cell carcinoma.

Treatment of keratoacanthoma consists of surgical excision of the lesion.

Squamous acanthoma is the term applied to a very rare, white, flat or raised, sometimes granular, verrucous, sessile or pedunculated lesion of the oral cavity. It is probably of traumatic origin and histologically shows a localized area of pseudoepitheliomatous hyperplasia of oral epithelium.

Inflammatory papillary hyperplasia. Although on rare occasion, inflammatory papillary hyperplasia does occur on the mandibular and maxillary alveolar ridges, the palate is by far the most common site.

This overgrowth constitutes 1.5% of all oral lesions (Table 17) and usually is associated with an ill-fitting complete or partial denture; poor oral hygiene is a contributing factor. How-

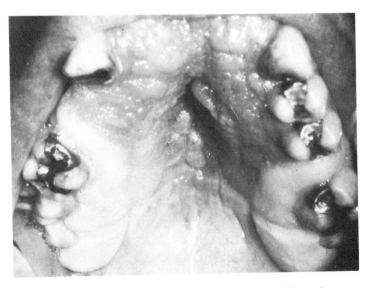

Fig. 15-10. Inflammatory papillary hyperplasia of the palate. The patient wore an ill-fitting partial denture.

ever, the lesion may occur without apparent cause. The majority of patients are in the fourth or fifth decade of life, and males are afflicted more frequently than females.

Inflammatory papillary hyperplasia consists of numerous small wartlike or papillary growths on the palate (Fig. 15-10). Food debris may collect between them and give rise to secondary inflammation. Ulceration is absent, and the lesion is usually asymptomatic.

Microscopic sections show numerous papillary growths covered by hyperplastic, usually nonkeratinized, stratified squamous epithelium. The epithelium is not dyskeratotic but may extend deep into the underlying connective tissue. The connective tissue is densely infiltrated by plasma cells and lymphocytes (Fig. 15-11). On extremely rare occasion, the lesion has been described as undergoing malignant change. However, this is equivocal.

Treatment of inflammatory papillary hyperplasia consists of

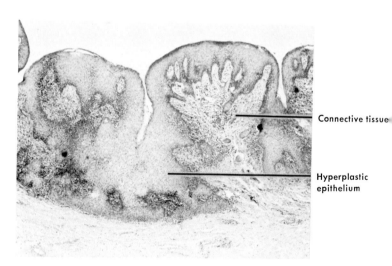

Connective tissue

Hyperplastic epithelium

Fig. 15-11. Inflammatory papillary hyperplasia. Note the multiple papillary growths, which are covered by stratified squamous epithelium.

removal of dentures at night, preparation of a well-fitting denture if necessary, and excision of the lesion. Although electrocautery, liquid nitrogen, cryotherapy, and surgical excision all have been used, removal of the lesion with a large curette (e.g., uterine curette) followed by the use of a tissue conditioner or a periodontal pack dressing is the best treatment.

MESENCHYMAL TUMORS

Irritation fibroma. This benign lesion constitutes 7.5% of all biopsy specimens (Table 17) and is the most common tumorlike growth of the oral cavity.

Occurring as a response to some local irritation, the irritation fibroma is an elevated pedunculated or sessile lesion that is typically of normal color but may appear paler than the normal mucosa (Fig. 15-12). It ranges in size from a few millimeters to a few centimeters. It may occur anywhere in the oral cavity, but the tongue, buccal mucosa, and lip are the sites most commonly affected. It usually is associated with a local irritation such as sucking in of the cheek through an interdental or edentulous space, lip biting, or thrusting of the tongue against a diastema.

An irritation fibroma consists predominantly of dense collagen with areas of hyalinization and a paucity of blood vessels (Fig. 15-13). Inflammatory cells, if present, are minimal; and the entire lesion is covered by stratified squamous epithelium that may show parakeratosis or hyperkeratosis.

Treatment of an irritation fibroma consists of excision. However, if the contributory cause persists, the lesion will recur.

Peripheral fibroma and peripheral fibroma with calcification. These are variants of each other. They appear as pale to red, firm, sessile or pedunculated lesions that arise from the interdental papilla (Fig. 15-14). They constitute 2.8% of all oral lesions (Table 17).

The majority (64%) occur in females, with the average age being 34 years. The average duration of the lesions is 18 months; and the maxilla is involved slightly more frequently

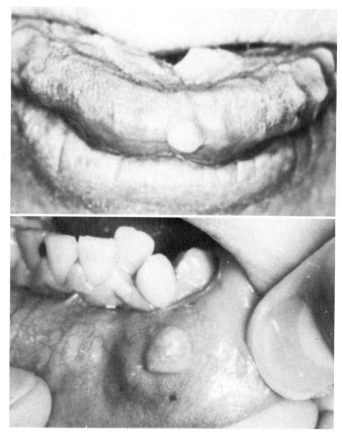

Fig. 15-12. Irritation fibroma of the oral mucous membrane (two cases). These are raised, pale, firm lesions.

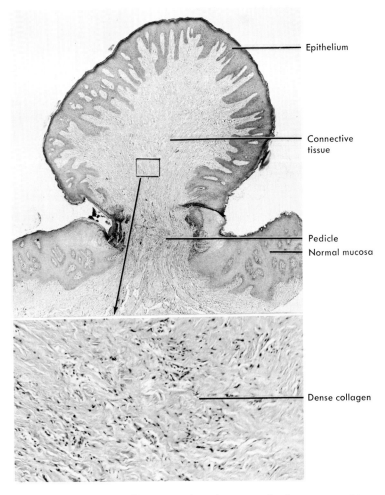

Epithelium

Connective
tissue

Pedicle
Normal mucosa

Dense collagen

Fig. 15-13. An irritation fibroma consists of a mass of collagen covered by epithelium.

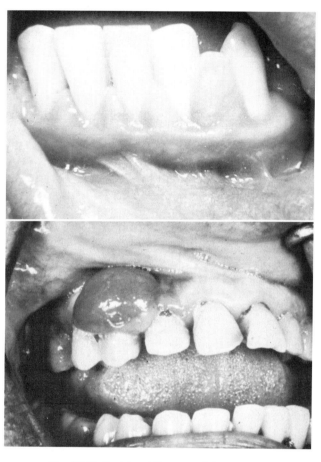

Fig. 15-14. Peripheral fibromas of the gingiva.

than the mandible, with the anterior part of the mouth the preferred site. Lesions vary in size from 0.5 to 8 cm and may cause migration of teeth. About 22% are ulcerated.

Microscopic sections reveal a tumor consisting of fibroblasts and collagen fibers in varying proportions. The lesion is more cellular than the irritation fibroma, and some show myxomatous degeneration. The tumor is covered by thin stratified squamous epithelium, but in certain areas ulceration can be seen. Such areas show infiltration by neutrophils, plasma cells, and lymphocytes.

About 50% of the lesions contain calcified material and therefore are called peripheral fibroma with calcification (Fig. 15-15). Excision is the treatment of choice.

Giant cell fibroma. This term is sometimes applied to fibromas of the gingiva and other parts of the oral mucosa. These lesions show, in addition to other microscopic features of the peripheral fibroma, giant fibroblasts with single or multiple nuclei (Fig. 15-15, *C*). The cells are usually stellate or spindle shaped and lie close to the epithelium. The giant cell fibroma is not unique but represents only a minor variation of the peripheral and irritation fibromas.

Oral focal mucinosis. This term applies to solitary lesions of the oral mucosa that consist primarily of myxomatous tissue. These are the oral counterpart of a cutaneous entity of the same name (cutaneous focal mucinosis), and they are clinically indistinguishable from small peripheral fibromas or irritation fibromas (Figs. 15-12 and 15-14). Whether separate entity or merely small fibromas with complete myxomatous degeneration, these lesions are benign and local removal is curative.

Myxoma (of soft tissues). This is a very rare, slow growing, insidious, infiltrative tumor that occurs in all age groups, with the average age being 40 years. The most frequent location is the cheek, floor of the mouth, and palate. Lesions are from a few weeks' to a few years' duration. Histologic sections show a circumscribed mass that is composed of stellate cells in abundant myxomatous stroma. Local excision is curative.

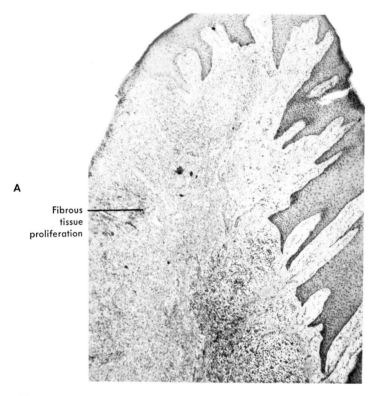

A

Fibrous
tissue
proliferation

Fig. 15-15. Histologic features of a peripheral fibroma of the gingiva **(A)**, a peripheral fibroma with calcification **(B)**, and a giant cell fibroma **(C)**. (In **C**, the dark areas represent giant cells.)

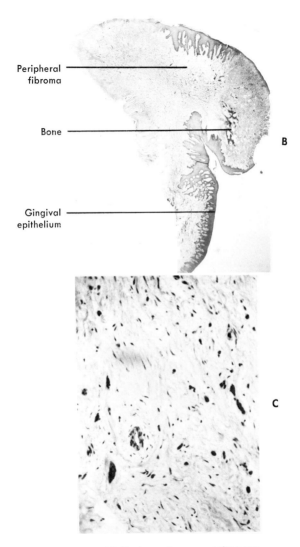

Fig. 15-15, cont'd. For legend see opposite page.

Epulis fissuratum. This tumorlike growth constitutes 2.8% of all material found at oral biopsy (Table 17).

The epulis fissuratum is associated with the flanges of ill-fitting dentures and is therefore seen in the upper and lower buccal and labial vestibule (Fig. 15-16). It is a soft, painful, redundant growth of tissue that bleeds easily and extends from under the offending denture flange. When the denture is removed, a gutter is seen in the lesion. Patients are usually elderly.

Microscopic sections show large amounts of fibrous connective tissue infiltrated by plasma cells and lymphocytes. There may be areas of ulceration, but most of the lesion's surface is covered by stratified squamous epithelium (Fig. 15-17).

Treatment consists of correcting the denture and excising the excessive tissue.

Epulis granulomatosa. This benign tumorlike growth is seen in association with extraction wounds or small exfoliating sequestra. Clinically the extraction socket is filled by exuberant red, easily bleeding granular tissue (Fig. 15-18).

Microscopic sections show young edematous connective tis-

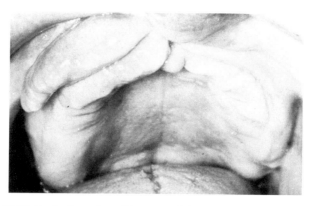

Fig. 15-16. Epulis fissuratum. The mass of tissue in the maxillary vestibule was a response to an ill-fitting denture.

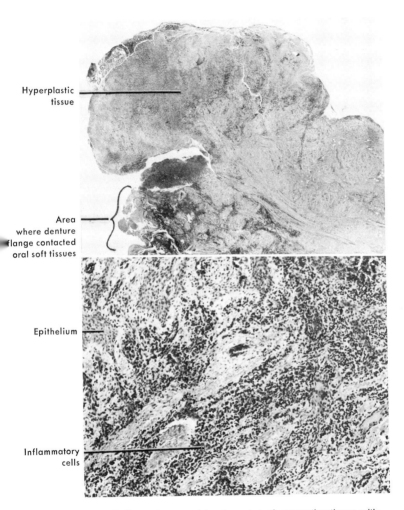

Hyperplastic
tissue

Area
where denture
flange contacted
oral soft tissues

Epithelium

Inflammatory
cells

Fig. 15-17. An epulis fissuratum consists of a mass of connective tissue with dense infiltration by plasma cells and lymphocytes.

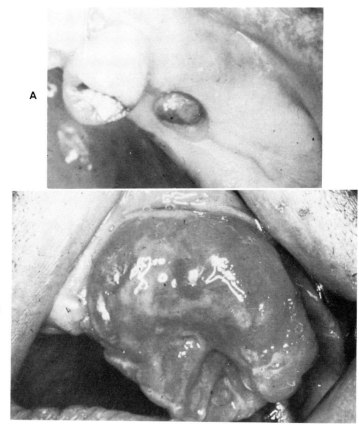

Fig. 15-18. A, Epulis granulomatosa in an extraction socket. **B,** Extensive epulis granulomatosa arising from an extraction socket.

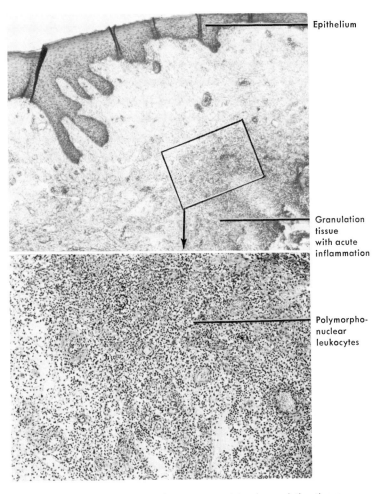

Epithelium

Granulation
tissue
with acute
inflammation

Polymorpho-
nuclear
leukocytes

Fig. 15-19. An epulis granulomatosa consists of granulation tissue.

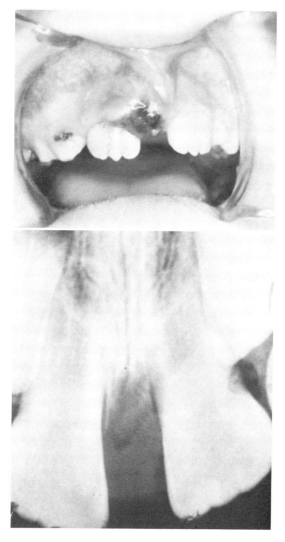

Fig. 15-20. Clinical and radiographic appearances of a peripheral giant cell granuloma in a child. Note the migration of the permanent incisors.

sue with infiltration by neutrophils, plasma cells, and lymphocytes; there are many capillaries and a thin covering of stratified
squamous epithelium (Fig. 15-19). If the tissue is too exuberant,
currettage may be necessary.

   ***Peripheral giant cell granuloma (myeloid epulis; giant cell
epulis).*** The peripheral giant cell granuloma is a pedunculated
or broad-based growth that has a smooth surface, is reddish
blue and sometimes lobulated, and bleeds easily (Figs. 15-20
and 15-21).

   The peripheral giant cell granuloma is limited to the gingiva
or to the soft tissues of edentulous ridges, and the mandible is
involved more frequently than the maxilla. The vast majority of
lesions occur after the age of 20 years, 40% in the fourth and
fifth decades, with the average age at occurrence being 44
years. This is in contrast to the central giant cell granuloma,
which occurs before the age of 20 years. Sex distribution is
about equal. Duration is usually a few weeks to a few months,

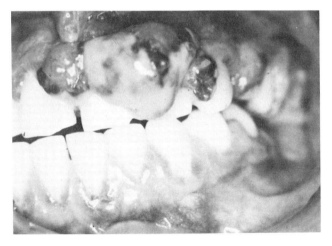

Fig. 15-21. Peripheral giant cell granuloma arising from the interdental papilla.
The lesion bleeds easily and has a hemorrhagic appearance.

and the lesion is limited to the gingiva and soft tissue covering of the alveolar ridges. Often there is a history of trauma, such as tooth extraction.

Radiographs are negative; but on rare occasion, the underlying bone includes a radiolucency. Microscopic sections are diagnostic and are identical to those of central giant cell granuloma. The tumor is made up of fibroblasts, mast cells, blood vessels, and multinucleated giant cells (Fig. 15-22). Electron microscopic studies have shown that the giant cells have abundant cell organelles, especially mitochondria. Fibroblasts are seen to be of two types. One type has a small number of cytoplasmic organelles, while the other has a large number of mitochondria. Fibroblasts of the latter type often form aggregates and may be the precursors of the giant cells. All lesions contain mild to marked amounts of hemosiderin (Fig. 15-22). The tumor is completely covered by stratified squamous epithelium or may be partly ulcerated.

A peripheral giant cell granuloma does not recur following its local removal.

Pyogenic granuloma. A tumorlike growth that occurs at all ages, the pyogenic granuloma constitutes 1.8% of all material found at oral biopsy (Table 17).

The pyogenic granuloma occurs slightly more frequently in females than in males, and about 75% of the lesions involve the gingiva. The remainder occur in the cheek, lip, tongue, palate, mucobuccal fold, and frenum (in descending order of frequency). Gingival lesions involve the maxilla (56%) more often than the mandible (44%), the buccal aspect more often than the lingual aspect, and the anterior part of the jaws more often than the posterior regions. Except for the lingual area of the mandibular molars, lesions occur in all regions of the gingiva.

The pyogenic granuloma usually presents as an elevated, soft, pedunculated or broad-based growth, has a smooth red surface, is often ulcerated, bleeds easily, and may have a raspberry-like appearance (Fig. 15-23). It has a duration of weeks or months. The lesion is partly or completely covered by stratified

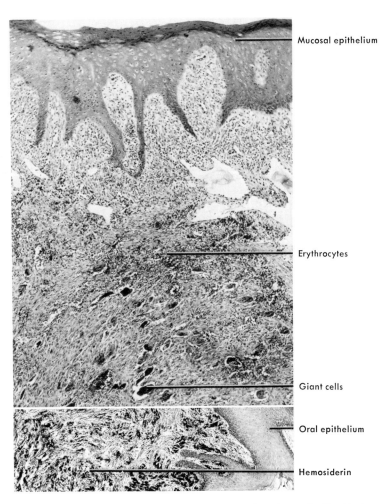

Fig. 15-22. A peripheral giant cell granuloma contains giant cells, fibroblasts, fibrous tissue, blood vessels, and hemosiderin.

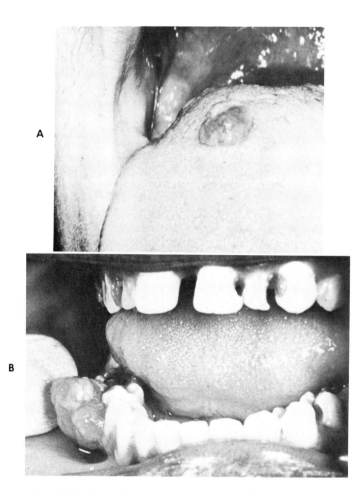

Fig. 15-23. Pyogenic granuloma of the tongue **(A)** and gingiva **(B).**

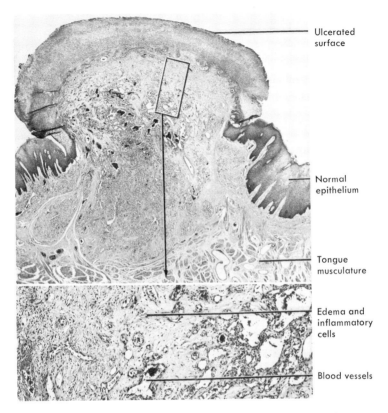

Ulcerated
surface

Normal
epithelium

Tongue
musculature

Edema and
inflammatory
cells

Blood vessels

Fig. 15-24. A pyogenic granuloma appears as a raised lesion with many
blood vessels and a partial or complete covering of stratified squamous epithelium.

squamous epithelium (Fig. 15-24). About 65% are partly or almost completely ulcerated, and the ulcerated regions are covered by a fibrinous exudate. The major mass of the tumor is
composed of small capillaries arranged in islands and lobules
and interspersed with edematous connective tissue (Fig. 15-24).
The lesion shows mild to dense infiltration by polymorphonuclear leukocytes, plasma cells, and lymphocytes.

The cause of pyogenic granuloma is unknown. However, since the lesion consists essentially of granulation tissue, it is believed to represent an overzealous response of tissues to some local trauma.

Treatment consists of excision. Although these lesions are benign, 16% recur following removal.

Pregnancy tumor (granuloma gravidarum). A very small percentage (1%) of women with pregnancy gingivitis develop tumorlike growths on the gingiva that both clinically and microscopically are identical to the pyogenic granuloma. These lesions are called pregnancy tumors (Fig. 15-25).

Pregnancy tumors appear about the third month of pregnancy and in some instances regress spontaneously after parturition. There may be a recurrence at the same site in a subsequent pregnancy.

The lesions are benign, and excision after parturition is the treatment of choice. Their microscopic features are the same as for a pyogenic granuloma (Fig. 15-24).

Hemangiomas. Tumors or tumorlike malformations that consist of blood vessels have been subdivided into numerous types; the most important as far as the oral tissues are concerned are the *capillary*, *cavernous*, and *juvenile* types.

Capillary and cavernous hemangiomas. These lesions in the oral cavity may be seen at any age and in either sex. However, most are congenital and become clinically apparent at an early age. They present as elevated, partly elevated, or submerged, circumscribed or diffuse, reddish or bluish, smooth-surfaced lesions of varying size. They are usually soft and compressible to palpation and may blanch on pressure.

The most common sites are the tongue (Fig. 15-26) and cheek, but the lesions may occur elsewhere (Fig. 15-27). They can produce considerable enlargement of the involved site and therefore interfere with speech and mastication. Hemangiomas are benign and seldom if ever become malignant. Either they do not grow at all or they grow very slowly. Due to internal bleeding, thrombosis, and organization, they may undergo fibrosis and regress spontaneously.

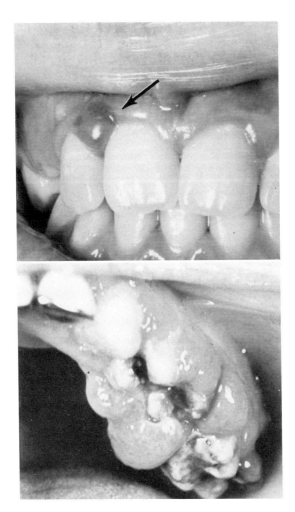

Fig. 15-25. Pregnancy tumors (two cases). The lesion (arrow) usually presents as a red, easily bleeding growth of the gingiva.

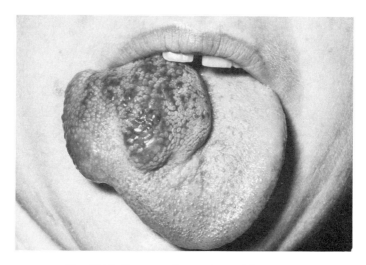

Fig. 15-26. Cavernous hemangioma of the tongue.

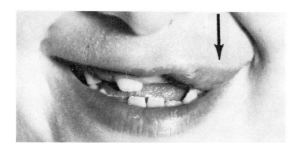

Fig. 15-27. Capillary hemangioma of the lip.

A capillary hemangioma consists of numerous blood-containing, endothelium-lined capillaries that may diffusely infiltrate the mucosa or may be present in clusters (Fig. 15-28). By contrast, a cavernous hemangioma consists of a few or numerous large, thin-walled, blood-containing spaces lined by flattened endothelial cells (Fig. 15-29). The epithelium covering the lesions is usually intact.

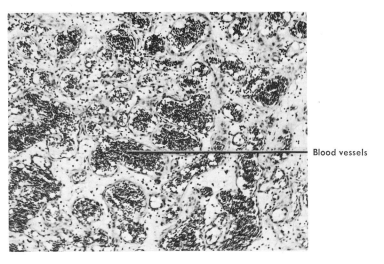

Blood vessels

Fig. 15-28. A capillary hemangioma consists of numerous small blood vessels.

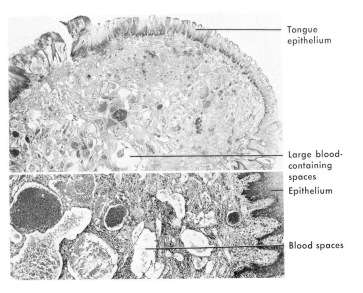

Tongue epithelium

Large blood-containing spaces

Epithelium

Blood spaces

Fig. 15-29. Cavernous hemangioma involving almost the entire tongue.

Superficial lesions can be removed surgically; or fibrosis may be induced by sclerosing solutions (sodium psylliate, sodium morrhuate, sodium tetradecyl sulfate), carbon dioxide snow, injections of boiling water, cryotherapy, or electrocautery. Spontaneous regression following accidental injury is also possible. Radiation of the lesions is contraindicated.

Juvenile hemangioma. This tumor of infancy occur most frequently in the parotid and submaxillary glands or on the lip (Fig. 15-30).

Patients are usually under 2 or 3 years of age, and many are only a few months old. The involved site is diffusely enlarged, and the tumor is not red or bluish but presents as a firm mass of normal mucosal color. It grows slowly.

Microscopic features consist of numerous small blood ves-

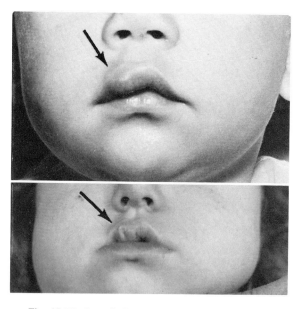

Fig. 15-30. Juvenile hemangioma of the lip (arrows).

sels, many of which are not yet canalized and which diffusely infiltrate the involved site (Fig. 15-31). The salivary gland lobules may be completely replaced by these blood vessels, and only the presence of a few ducts identify the tissue as a salivary gland. Similarly the lip musculature is replaced and infiltrated by some blood vessels and endothelial buds.

Juvenile hemangioma is treated in the same manner as the cavernous and capillary types, but it has a better chance of spontaneous regression.

Lymphangioma. This tumor or tumorlike growth may occur anywhere on the skin or mucous membrane, but the oral cavity is one of the most common sites (Fig. 15-32).

In the mouth lymphangiomas are seen most frequently on the tongue. When superficial, they present as a cluster of colorless, thin-walled, soft excrescences on the mucosa; when deep

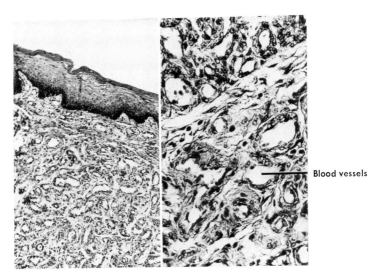

Blood vessels

Fig. 15-31. Juvenile hemangioma of the lip. The entire area is replaced by blood vessels.

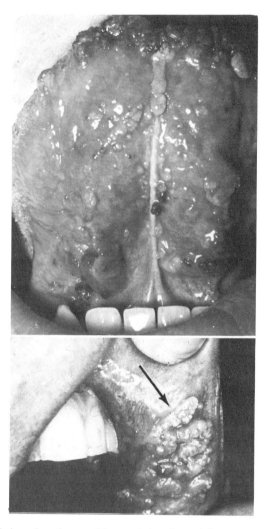

Fig. 15-32. Lymphangiomas of the ventral surface of the tongue and of the cheek. Arrow shows the pebbly surface caused by dilated lymph channels (which can extend into the basement membrane).

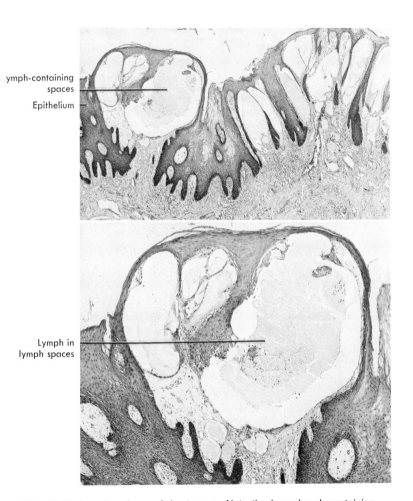

Lymph-containing
spaces

Epithelium

Lymph in
lymph spaces

Fig. 15-33. Lymphangioma of the tongue. Note the large lymph-containing spaces underneath the epithelium.

seated, they produce a diffuse enlargement of the tongue and obliterate its surface characteristics so that it appears smooth and devoid of papillae. The tongue may be markedly enlarged (macroglossia lymphomatosa).

Microscopically most oral lymphangiomas consist of large, thin-walled, lymph-containing spaces. In superficial lesions these cavernous spaces lie immediately beneath the epithelium (Fig. 15-33).

Lymphangiomas do not undergo malignant change. They do not respond to radiation or sclerosing solutions. Surgical excision, whenever possible, is the treatment of choice.

Cystic hygroma (cystic lymphangioma; hygroma cysticum colli). This congential malformation is composed of large lymph-containing cystic spaces that develop in the neck.

The lesion occurs in infancy and childhood and may be unilateral or bilateral. Although it primarily involves the neck, it may extend upward and replace and enlarge the parotid gland, floor of the mouth, cheek, and tongue (Fig. 15-34).

Microscopic sections show one or numerous lymph-containing cysts lined by thin, flat endothelium and containing varying amounts of collagen in their walls (Fig. 15-35).

A cystic hygroma is nonencapsulated and its removal is almost impossible, but surgical excision is the only course of treatment.

Neuroma (traumatic neuroma). When a nerve is cut, its proximal end regenerates in an attempt to close the gap. This regeneration conisits of proliferation by Schwann cells and fibroblasts as well as the growth of axis cylinders. If the axis cylinders contact the distal end of the nerve, repair is complete. However, if they do not, proliferation continues and a mass of fibroblasts, Schwann cells, and axis cylinders is formed. This mass constitutes a neuroma.

In the oral cavity, neuromas are seen most frequently in the region of the mental foramen. Other common sites are the lips and tongue, or they may occur within the jaw.

The lesions usually present as movable nodules in the oral

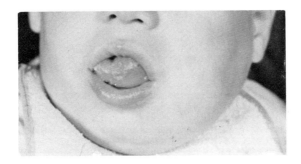

Fig. 15-34. Cystic hygroma involving the cheek and the tongue.

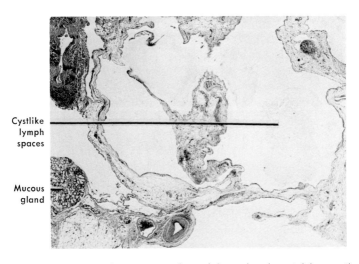

Cystlike
lymph
spaces

Mucous
gland

Fig. 15-35. A cystic hygroma consists of large lymph-containing cystic spaces.

Nerve fibers, fibroblasts, and Schwann cells

Nerve trunk

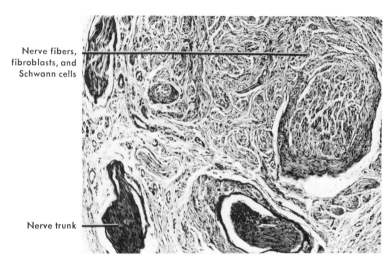

Fig. 15-36. Traumatic neuroma. Note the dense mass of nerve fibers.

mucosa that may be painful. Microscopic sections show a variable amount of scar tissue (collagenous tissue) in which numerous transversely and longitudinally cut nerve trunks can be seen (Fig. 15-36).

Treatment of neuroma consists of excision.

The *Sipple syndrome*, also called *neuropolyendocrine syndrome* or *multiple endocrine adenomatosis type II*, is a hereditary disease that is transmitted as an autosomal dominant trait and consists of multiple neuromas of the lips, tongue, eyelids, and larynx. The lesions are often present at birth and histologically are indistinguishable for traumatic neuromas. Between 20 and 35 years of age, patients develop medullary carcinomas of the thyroid and/or pheochromocytomas of the adrenal glands.

Schwannoma (neurilemoma) and neurofibroma. The schwannoma and the neurofibroma are two distinct entities. Because of their many similarities, however, they will be considered together.

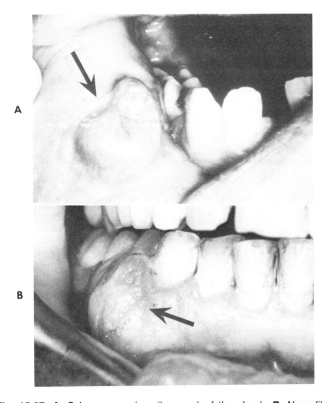

Fig. 15-37. A, Schwannoma (neurilemoma) of the cheek. **B,** Neurofibroma of the gingiva.

Continued.

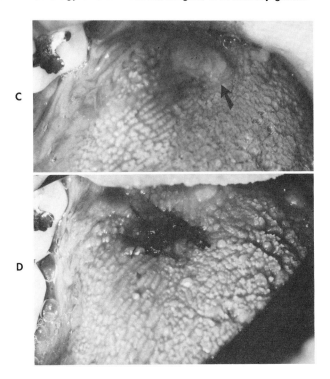

Fig. 15-37, cont'd. C and **D,** Neurofibroma of the posterior dorsal surface of the tongue before **(C)** and after **(D)** excision.

Schwannomas and neurofibromas are benign tumors of nerve sheath origin. In the oral cavity, the neurofibroma is far more common than the schwannoma (8:1); patients are usually white; the lesions are usually asymptomatic; and although they can occur at any age, patients are usually in the third or fourth decade of life. The usual sites in the oral cavity in order of frequency are the cheek, palate, tongue, lips, and alveolar ridge. Schwannoma and neurofibroma usually present as small sessile, smooth-surfaced growths on the oral mucosa (Fig. 15-37). Deep-seated lesions can be felt as circumscribed nodules. Both tumors grow extremely slowly and are asymptomatic.

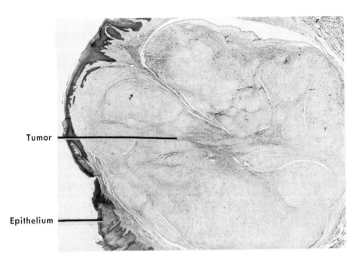

Tumor

Epithelium

Fig. 15-38. Schwannoma (neurilemoma). The tumor is covered by epithelium and is encapsulated.

Microscopically the schwannoma is an encapsulated tumor consisting of Schwann cells and fibroblastic proliferation (Fig. 15-38). The cells form twisted bundles or line up in such a way that their nuclei lie shoulder to shoulder (palisading or regimentation). Rows of nuclei and nucleus-free bands of cytoplasm are therefore seen. A number of Schwann cells lie together in groups, forming what is called Verocay bodies (Fig. 15-39). The part of a tumor composed of Verocay bodies is called *Antoni type A* tissue. Schwannomas also consist of a varying amount of *Antoni type B* tissue (Fig. 15-40), which is merely a loose, haphazard, sometimes cystic mixture of Schwann cells, fibroblasts, and fibers.

The neurofibroma is not encapsulated. It consists only of Antoni type B tissue (Fig. 15-40). Verocay bodies and Antoni type A tissue are absent. The tumor also contains neurites (axons).

Electron microscopic studies show the neurofibroma to be

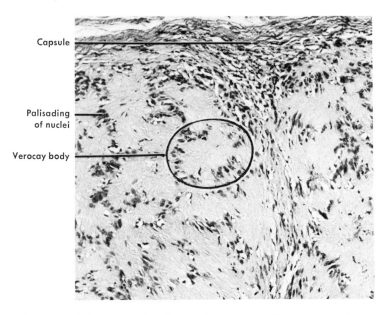

Capsule

Palisading
of nuclei

Verocay body

Fig. 15-39. Schwannoma (neurilemoma). Verocay bodies are a prominent feature.

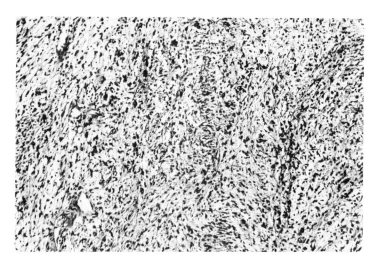

Fig. 15-40. Antoni type B tissue from a neurofibroma.

composed of elongated, spindle-shaped cells with bundles of collagen fibrils scattered between them. Cytoplasm contains microfilaments, rough endoplasmic reticulum, ribosomes, mitochondria, and a well-developed Golgi complex. Junctional complexes are seen between adjacent cells. These features indicate that the neurofibroma arises from the perineural cells. Ultrastructure of the schwannoma shows that the cells are surrounded by a basal lamina, have many cytoplasmic processes, and in areas surround collagen and axonlike structures. These findings confirm the view that schwannomas arise from the Schwann cells.

Generalized neurofibromatosis (multiple neurofibromatosis; von Recklinghausen's disease); tuberous sclerosis. Multiple neurofibromatosis is a hereditary disease with numerous malformations.

Abnormalities of the peripheral nerves are the most spectacular. There are neurofibromas in the skin, oral cavity, gastrointestinal tract, and bones as well as brown (melanin) pigmented spots on the skin (café au lait spots) (Fig. 15-41). Because of neurogenic tumors within the marrow, the bones may be markedly deformed. Besides neurogenic tumors, lipomas, sebaceous adenomas, fibromas, and excessive hair may be seen in this disease.

In the oral cavity, lesions occur in the soft tissues and/or the jaws. The tongue is the most commonly affected site. If the neurofibromas are deep, the tongue appears enlarged (macroglossia); if they are superficial, it appears fissured (scrotal). Tumors also occur on the gingiva, palate, and buccal mucous membrane (Fig. 15-41, *B*). Neurofibromas may occur within the periodontal membrane and lead to the migration of teeth. Lesions within the jaw appear as radiolucencies and may present a diagnostic problem.

The microscopic features of the lesions in von Recklinghausen's disease are the same as those described for solitary neurofibromas. Lesions of multiple neurofibromatosis appear in childhood and may stop growing at any time. However, neurofibromas seen in this disease may undergo malignant change

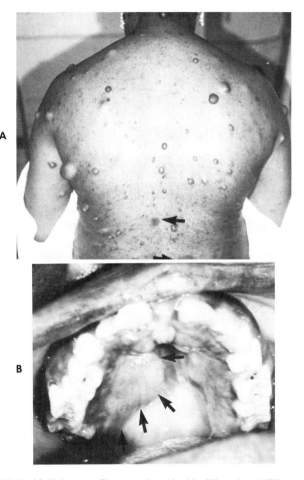

Fig. 15-41. Multiple neurofibromatosis with skin **(A)** and oral **(B)** lesions. In **A,** note the brown areas of pigmentation (arrows). **B** shows a large neurofibroma of the palate (arrows).

into neurofibrosarcomas. About 50% of malignant nerve sheath tumors arise in patients with von Recklinghausen's disease.

Tuberous sclerosis is a syndrome related to generalized neurofibromatosis and is characterized by dominant inheritance, mental retardation, epilepsy, skin tumors (adenoma sebaceum), and café au lait spots (pigmented patches) on the skin. Oral lesions consist of fibromas of the anterior gingiva, lips, tongue, or palate. These nodules vary in color from bluish to normal and are seen in 11% of cases. Enamel hypoplasia, cysts of the mandible, hypercalcified areas of the jaws, and cleft lip and palate may also be seen. Seventy-five percent of patients usually die before 25 years of age.

Lipoma. Although one of the commonest of all neoplasms, a lipoma is rare in the oral cavity. When present, it is usually seen in the cheek, where it forms a soft, fairly well-defined mass (Fig. 15-42).

Lipomas may be pedunculated or submerged. Microscopi-

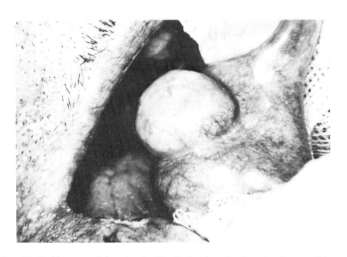

Fig. 15-42. Lipoma of the cheek. The lesion is raised and yellow and has a broad base.

cally they consist of normal fat cells often arranged in lobules (Fig. 15-43). Oral lipomas grow very slowly, and recurrence following excision is rare.

Granular cell myoblastoma. The exact nature of this benign soft tissue tumor is unknown.

Although an origin from muscle cells, fibroblasts, and histiocytes has been reported, recent histochemical and electron microscopic studies indicate that the granular cell myoblastoma arises from the Schwann cells of the nerve sheath. It may occur anywhere on the skin, mucous membrane, or gastrointestinal tract; but the oral cavity is one of the most commonly affected

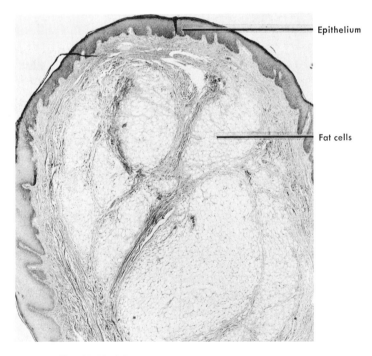

Epithelium

Fat cells

Fig. 15-43. A lipoma consists predominantly of fat cells.

sites. Multiple lesions have been reported, as well as spontaneous regression in some instances.

In the oral cavity, by far the largest number of lesions occur on the lateral and dorsal surfaces of the tongue. The tumor presents as a small, slightly elevated, smooth-surfaced, nonulcerated growth of the mucous membrane (Fig. 15-44).

The epithelium overlying the granular cell myoblastoma usually shows pseudoepitheliomatous hyperplasia (Fig. 15-45, A). The epithelial hyperplasia is often marked, and an erroneous diagnosis of squamous cell carcinoma may be made. The tumor lies under the epithelium. Although nonencapsulated, it is sometimes circumscribed and consists of large granular cells that have small round nuclei (Fig. 15-45, B) These cells lie in sheets and are associated with muscle fibers and nerve sheaths. Electron microscopic studies show the granules seen in these cells to be compatible with liposomes.

Treatment of a granular cell myoblastoma consists of excision, which is curative.

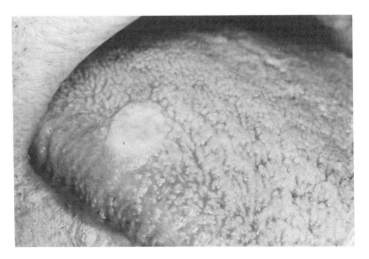

Fig. 15-44. Granular cell myoblastoma of the tongue.

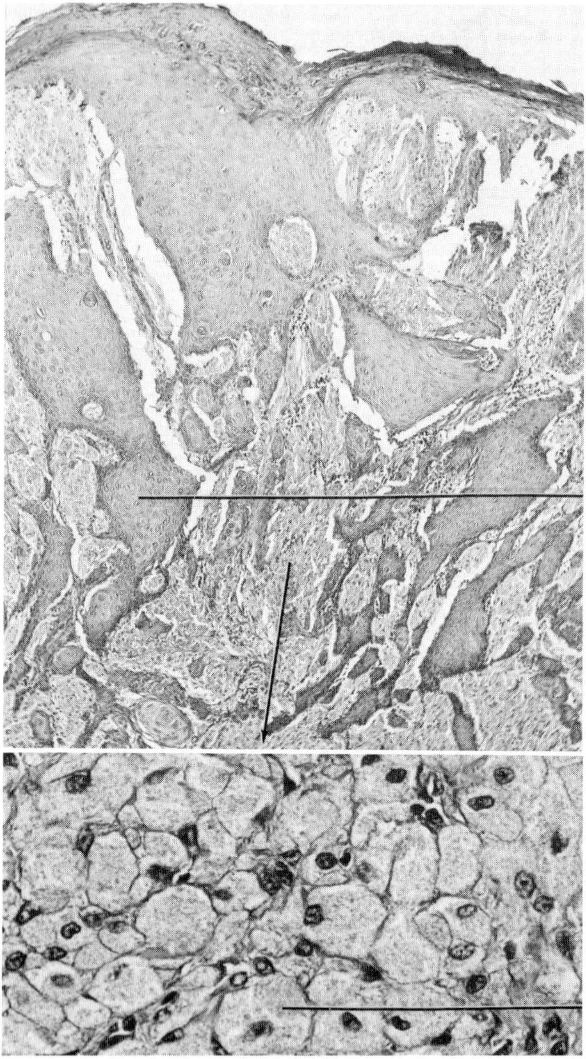

Fig. 15-45. Granular cell myoblastoma. **A,** Note the marked pseudoepithe-liomatous hyperplasia. **B,** Enlargement of an area in **A.** Note the granular cells with small round nuclei.

Congenital epulis. This benign tumor is seen only in new-born infants.

Although considered by some authors to be a granular cell myoblastoma, the congenital epulis is a separate entity, a pedunculated, smooth-surfaced, soft tissue growth (Fig. 15-46). It arises from the maxillary or mandibular alveolar mucosa, but maxillary lesions are about four times as common as those of the mandible. There is a marked sexual predilection for females (10:1).

A congenital epulis consists mainly of large granular cells that lie in sheets and resemble those seen in a granular cell myoblastoma. Some fusiform cells resembling fibroblasts inter-weave between the sheets of granular cells. Unlike the granular cell myoblastoma, however, pseudoepitheliomatous hyperplasia is not present and the epithelium covering the epulis is atrophic and usually devoid of ridges. Islands of odontogenic epithelium may be seen in the lesion (Fig. 15-47).

Treatment consists of excision. Since the lesion is often pedunculated, this is usually a simple procedure. There is no recurrence following excision.

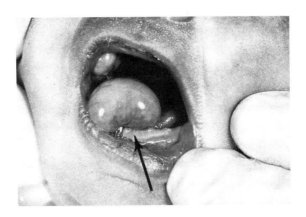

Fig. 15-46. Congenital epulis arising from the alveolar mucosa of the mandible.

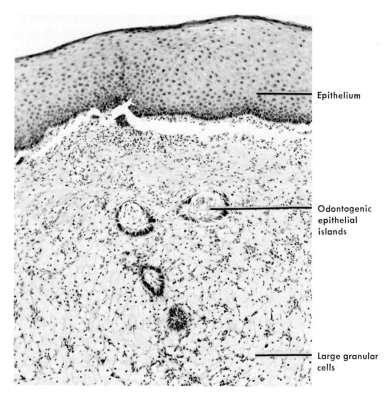

Epithelium

Odontogenic
epithelial
islands

Large granular
cells

Fig. 15-47. A congenital epulis consists of granular cells and fibroblasts and often contains odontogenic epithelium.

Nevoxanthoendothelioma (juvenile xanthogranuloma; xanthogranuloma). In contrast to various well-known forms of xanthoma that are associated with metabolic disturbances, a nevoxanthoendothelioma appears spontaneously.

This lesion of infancy or childhood is usually solitary, occurs predominantly on the head and face, and regresses without treatment. It rarely occurs in the oral cavity; but when it does, the tongue is affected more often than any other site.

Microscopically a nevoxanthoendothelioma shows a predom-

inance of polygonal and fusiform histiocytes, varying numbers
of Touton giant cells, fat-laden histiocytes, and infiltration by
lymphocytes and eosinophils. The histiocytic elements often reveal mitoses, and the eosinophils are very prominent. Because
of its microscopic features, the lesion may be mistaken for an
eosinophilic granuloma or some form of malignant mesenchymal neoplasm. The presence of inflammatory cells, Touton
giant cells, and fat-laden histiocytes, however, aids in arriving
at the correct diagnosis.

The lesion is benign and may regress spontaneously. If excised, it does not recur.

Verruciform xanthoma. This verrucous or papillary lesion of
the oral mucosa ranges in size from less than 1 mm to 2 cm and
occurs usually after 40 years of age. It is more common in
whites than in blacks and in females than in males. Almost 65%
of the lesions occur on the gingiva and the alveolar ridge, but
they can occur in any other site in the oral mucosa.

Microscopic features consist of a papillary lesion covered by
parakeratotic stratified squamous epithelium. The unique feature is the presence of foam cells or xanthoma cells in the connective tissue between the epithelial ridges. The connective tissue around the cells may be hyalinized. The lesion is treated by
conservative excision.

Soft tissue plasmacytoma (extramedullary plasmacytoma).
Two of the lesions composed of plasma cells—the multiple myeloma and the solitary intraosseous myeloma—are described
elsewhere (p. 322). The remaining two, the soft tissue plasmacytoma and the plasma cell granuloma, occur in soft tissues.
(Plasma cell gingivitis [p. 191] is probably related to the plasma
cell granuloma.)

The soft tissue plasmacytoma occurs after the age of 40 years
and is more common in males than in females. The upper respiratory tract and oral cavity are the sites usually affected. In
the oral region the soft palate, maxillary mucosa, maxillary
sinus, and tonsillar area are involved; and the lesion presents as
a tumor mass or granulomatous lesion (Fig. 15-48).

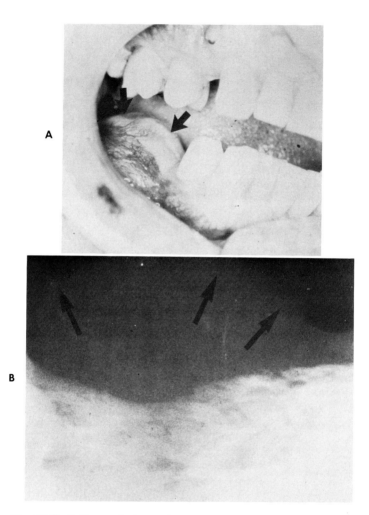

Fig. 15-48. Solitary soft tissue plasmacytoma of the mandibular ridge (arrows). This growth produced minimal bone destruction **(B).** Arrows in **B** show the faint outline of the soft tissue lesion.

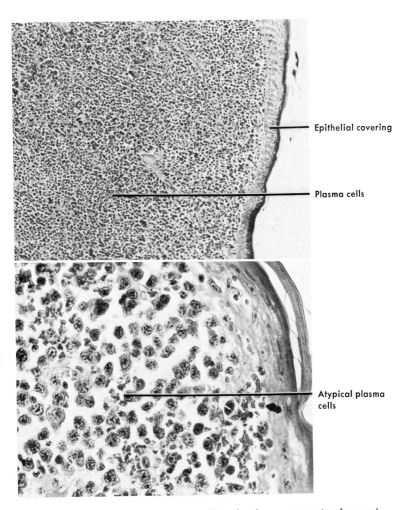

Epithelial covering

Plasma cells

Atypical plasma cells

Fig. 15-49. Soft tissue plasmacytoma. Note the dense aggregate of normal and abnormal plasma cells.

Microscopically a soft tissue plasmacytoma consists exclusively of a dense aggregation of typical and atypical plasma cells (Fig. 15-49). Laboratory tests that are positive in the multiple myeloma are negative in soft tissue lesions; but in certain patients, electrophoretic studies on the serum show a sharp gamma peak.

Some of these lesions are benign, and surgical excision is curative. However, others represent early stages of multiple myeloma. For this reason patients with a soft tissue plasmacytoma should be observed at frequent intervals.

Plasma cell granuloma. This lesion is a rare benign growth of the gingival and other oral soft tissues (Fig. 15-50).

Microscopically a plasma cell granuloma is covered by stratified squamous epithelium and is composed of a dense mass of normal plasma cells and occasional lymphocytes (Fig. 15-51). It is probably related to plasma cell gingivitis (p. 191) and is treated conservatively.

Leiomyoma. An extremely rare tumor of the oral cavity, leiomyoma is composed of smooth muscle (Fig. 15-52).

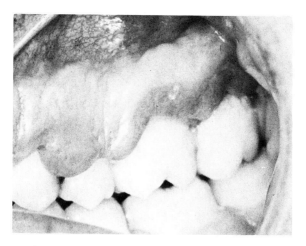

Fig. 15-50. Plasma cell granuloma of the gingiva.

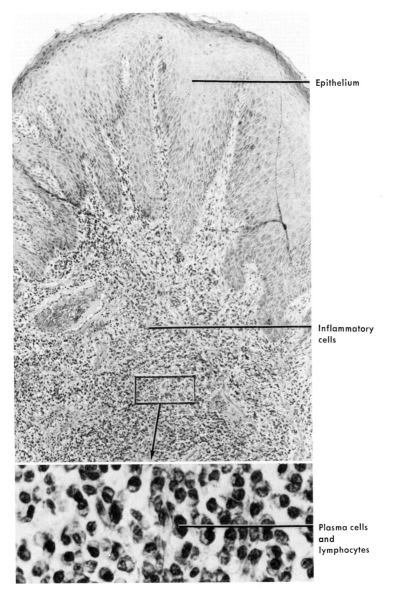

Epithelium

Inflammatory cells

Plasma cells and lymphocytes

Fig. 15-51. A plasma cell granuloma consists of a dense mass of many plasma cells and some lymphocytes.

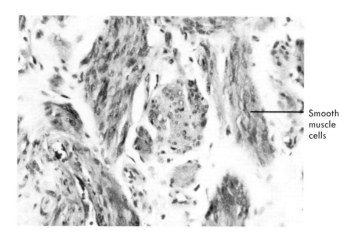

Smooth
muscle
cells

Fig. 15-52. Photomicrograph of a leiomyoma showing bundles of smooth muscle cells. (Courtesy J. Adrian, D.D.S., Washington, D.C.)

Most recorded cases have occurred in patients between 40 and 60 years of age, and in females twice as frequently as in males. The lesions are usually in the tongue; they are small and grow slowly. Excision is curative.

Rhabdomyoma. Rhabdomyoma is a rare soft tissue tumor of muscle that is very rare in the oral cavity. About 30 cases have been reported. It occurs primarily in adults (mean age 56 years) and in males more often than in females (2:1). The majority of cases have occurred in the floor of mouth. Other sites are the soft palate, tongue, and buccal mucosa. Histologic sections show circumscribed, very vascular lesions that are composed of ovoid, polygonal, or elongated cells with granular eosinophilic cytoplasm in which cross striations can be identified. Local excision is the treatment of choice, but about 30% of the lesions have recurred.

Juvenile nasopharyngeal angiofibroma. This vascular tumor occurs primarily in males, and most patients are from 15 to 18 years of age. More than 75% of cases occur in whites.

A juvenile nasopharyngeal angiofibroma may extend from

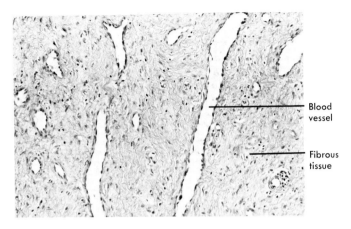

Fig. 15-53. Photomicrograph of an angiofibroma. Note the dense fibrous tissue surrounding many blood vessels.

the nasopharynx to the oral cavity. It is noncapsulated and expansile, produces nasal obstruction, and may appear as a mass in the palate.

Microscopic features consist of numerous blood vessels surrounded by and lying within a dense stroma of fibrous connective tissue (Fig. 15-53). Surgical excision and/or radiation are methods of therapy. Recurrences are common, but malignant degeneration does not occur.

Hamartoma and choristoma. When an excessive amount of normal tissue is seen in its usual location, the resulting tumorlike mass is called a hamartoma. When it occurs in an abnormal location, it is called a choristoma. These lesions constitute 7% of all oral tumors in children and usually are located on the dorsum of the tongue or on the lip.

Hamartomas and choristomas are circumscribed, slowgrowing masses that microscopically consist of one or more of the following tissues: salivary gland, cartilage, bone, striated muscle, nerves, and fat. In the oral cavity the tongue is the most common site. Such lesions often contain bone or cartilage and

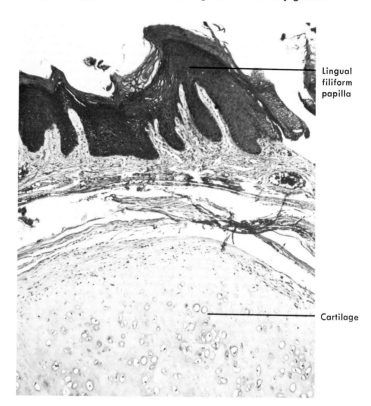

Lingual
filiform
papilla

Cartilage

Fig. 15-54. Lingual chondromatous choristoma. Note the presence of carti-lage under the lingual epithelium.

are referred to as *lingual osseous choristoma* or *lingual chon-dromatous choristoma* (Fig. 15-54). Excision is curative.

REFERENCES

Abbey, L. M., Page, D. G., and Sawyer, D. R.: The clinical and histopathologic features of a series of 464 oral squamous cell papillomas, Oral Surg. **49**:419, 1980.

Abbey, L. M., Sawyer, D. R., and Syrop, H. M.: Oral squamous acanthoma, Oral Surg. **45**:255, 1978.

Adkins, K. F., Martinez, M. G., and Hartley, M. W.: Ultrastructure of giant-cell lesions: a peripheral giant-cell reparative granuloma, Oral Surg. **28**:713, 1969.

Andersen, L., Arwill, T., Fejerskov, O., Heyden, G., and Philipsen, H. P.: Oral giant-cell granulomas: an enzyme histochemical and ultrastructural study, Acta Pathol. Microbiol. Scand. (A) **81**:617, 1973.

Anderson, D. R.: Focal epithelial hyperplasia; report of a case in a South African caucasoid, J. Dent. Assoc. S. Afr. **26**:32, 1971.

Archard, H. O., Heck, J. W., and Stanley, H. H.: Focal epithelial hyperplasia: an unusual oral mucosal lesion found in Indian children, Oral Surg. **20**:201, 1965.

Arwill, T., Heyden, G., and Ramstedt, A.: Follicular choristoma of the gingiva, Oral Surg. **35**:89, 1973.

Baden, E., and Fischer, R. J.: Multiple neurofibromatosis and neurofibroma of the palate, Oral Surg. **16**:1356, 1963.

Badger, G. R.: Solitary neurofibromatosis in the maxilla: report of oral findings, J. Am. Dent. Assoc. **100**:213, 1980.

Bartel, H., and Piatowska, D.: Electron microscopic study of peripheral giant-cell reparative granuloma, Oral Surg. **43**:82, 1977.

Baughman, R. A.: Pedunculated lesions. I. Papillary type, Florida Dent. J. **44**:10, 1973.

Bhaskar, S. N.: Oral tumors of infancy and childhood, J. Pediatr. **63**:195, 1963.

Bhaskar, S. N.: Oral pathology in the dental office; survey of 20,575 biopsy specimens, J. Am. Dent. Assoc. **76**:761, 1968.

Bhaskar, S. N., and Akamine, R.: Congenital epulis (congenital granular cell fibroblastoma), Oral Surg. **8**:517, 1955.

Bhaskar, S. N., and Dubit, J.: Central and peripheral hemangioma, Oral Surg. **23**:385, 1967.

Bhaskar, S. N., and Frisch, J.: Neurofibroma of oral tissues, Oral Surg. **22**:662, 1966.

Bhaskar, S. N., and Jacoway, J. R.: Pyogenic granuloma, clinical features, incidence histology and results of treatment: report of 242 cases, J. Oral Surg. **24**:391, 1966.

Bhaskar, S. N., and Jacoway, J. R.: Peripheral fibroma and peripheral fibroma with calcification: report of 376 cases, J. Am. Dent. Assoc. **4**:1312, 1967.

Bhaskar, S. N., Levin, M. P., and Frisch, J.: Plasma cell granuloma of periodontal tissues: report of 45 cases, Periodontics **6**:272, 1968.

Blair, A. E., and Edwards, D. M.: Congenital epulis of the newborn, Oral Surg. **43**:687, 1977.

Bloem, J. J., and van der Waal, I.: Paraffinoma of the face, Oral Surg. **38**:675, 1974.

Borghelli, R. F., Stirparo, M. A., Paroni, H. C., Barros, R. E., and Dominquez, F. V.: Focal epithelial hyperplasia, Oral Surg. **40**:107, 1975.

Buchner, A.: Focal epithelial hyperplasia in Israeli families of Libyan origin, Oral Surg. **46:**64, 1978.

Buchner, A., and Mass, E.: Focal epithelial hyperplasia in an Israeli family, Oral Surg. **36:**507, 1973.

Buchner, A., and Ramon, Y.: Focal epithelial hyperplasia: report of two new cases from Israel and review of the literature, Arch. Dermatol. **107:**97, 1973.

Buchner, A., and Sandbank, M.: Multiple fibroepithelial hyperplasias of the oral mucosa, Oral Surg. **46:**34, 1978.

Burkes, E. J., Jr., Patterson, J. E., and Bowman, T. O.: Lingual sebaceous glands: report of case, J. Am. Dent. Assoc. **94:**1166, 1977.

Caputo, R., Bellone, A. G., and Tagliavini, R.: Ultrastructure of the granular cell myoblastoma, Arch. Dermatol. Forsch. **242:**127, 1972.

Chen, S. Y., and Miller, A. S.: Neurofibroma and schwannoma of the oral cavity, Oral Surg. **47:**522, 1979.

Cherrick, H. M., Dunlap, C. L., and King, O. H.: Leiomyomas of the oral cavity, Oral Surg. **35:**54, 1973.

Christensen, R. E., Jr., Hertz, R. S., and Cherrick, H. M.: Intraoral juvenile xanthogranuloma, Oral Surg. **45:**586, 1978.

Corio, R. L., and Lewis, D. M.: Introral rhabdomyomas, Oral Surg. **48:**525, 1979.

Custer, R. P., and Fust, J. A.: Congenital epulis, Am. J. Clin. Pathol. **22:**1044, 1952.

Damm, D. D., and Neville, B. W.: Oral leiomyomas, Oral Surg. **47:**343, 1979.

del Rio, C. E.: Chondroma of the tongue: review of the literature and a case report, J. Oral Med. **33:**54, 1978.

Dutescu, N., Georgescu, L., and Mihai, H.: Lipoma of submandibular space with osseous metaplasia, Oral Surg. **35:**611, 1973.

Edwards, M. B., and Hamza, A. E.: Focal epithelial hyperplasia in Abu Dhabi, Oral Surg. **45:**902, 1978.

El-Khashab, M. M., and Abdelaziz, A. M.: Focal epithelial hyperplasia (Heck's disease), Oral Surg. **31:**637, 1971.

Ellis, G. L., Abrams, A. M., and Melrose, R. J.: Intraosseous benign neural sheath neoplasms of the jaws, Oral Surg. **44:**731, 1977.

Elzay, R. P., and Dutz, W.: Myxomas of the paraoral-oral soft tissues, Oral Surg. **45:**246, 1978.

Eversole, L. R., and Sorenson, H. W.: Oral florid papillomatosis in Down's syndrome, Oral Surg. **73:**202, 1974.

Eveson, J. W., and Merchant, N. E.: Sublingual rhabdomyoma, Int. J. Oral Surg. **7:**27, 1978.

Fisher, E. R., and Wechsler, H.: Granular cell myoblastomanomer, CA **15:**936, 1962.

Freedman, P. D., Kerpel, S. M., Begel, H., and Lumerman, H.: Solitary intraoral keratoacanthoma, Oral Surg. **47:**74, 1979.

Freeman, M. J., and Standish, S. M.: Facial and oral manifestations of familial disseminated neurofibromatosis, Oral Surg. **19**:52, 1965.

Frithiof, L., and Wersall, J.: Virus-like particles in human oral papilloma, Acta Otolaryngol. **64**:263, 1967.

Goldblatt, L. I., and Edesess, R. B.: Central leiomyoma of the mandible, Oral Surg. **43**:591, 1977.

Greer, R. O.: Inverted oral papilloma, Oral Surg. **36**:400, 1973.

Greer, R. O., and Goldman, H. M.: Oral papillomas, Oral Surg. **38**:435, 1974.

Greer, R. O., and Richardson, J. F.: The nature of lipomas and their significance in the oral cavity, Oral Surg. **36**:551, 1973.

Gutman, J., Cifuentes, C., Balzarini, M. A., Sobarzo, V., and Vicuna, R.: Chondroma of the tongue, Oral Surg. **37**:75, 1974.

Hanks, C. T., Fischman, S. L., and Genzman, N. D.: Focal epithelial hyperplasia, Oral Surg. **33**:934, 1972.

Hatziotis, J. C., and Mylona-Hatziotou, A. J.: Blue nevi of the oral cavity: review of the literature and report of two cases, J. Oral Surg. **31**:772, 1973.

Helsham, R. W., and Buchanan, G.: Keratoacanthoma of the oral cavity, Oral Surg. **13**:844, 1960.

Henefer, E. P., Abaza, N. A., and Anderson, S. P.: Congenital granular-cell epulis: report of a case, Oral Surg. **47**:515, 1979.

Hicks, J. L., and Nelson, J. F.: Juvenile nasopharyngeal angiofibroma, Oral Surg. **35**:807, 1973.

Hollander, C. F., van Noord, M. J., and Rijswijk, Z. H.: Focal epithelial hyperplasia: a virus-induced oral mucosal lesion in the champanzee, Oral Surg. **33**:220, 1972.

Jarvis, A., and Gorlin, R. J.: Focal epithelial hyperplasia in an Eskimo population, Oral Surg. **33**:227, 1972.

Kist, J., and Bhaskar, S. N.: Leiomyoma of the palate, J. Oral Surg. **22**:346, 1964.

Kjaerheim, A., and Stokke, T.: Juvenile xanthogranuloma of the oral cavity, Oral Surg. **38**:414, 1974.

Knapp, M. J., and Uohara, G. I.: Oral condyloma acuminatum, Oral Surg. **23**:538, 1967.

Krolls, S. O., Jacoway, J. R., and Alexander, W. N.: Osseous choristomas (osteomas) of intraoral soft tissues, Oral Surg. **32**:588, 1971.

Mark, H. I., and Kaplan, S. L.: Blue nevus of the oral cavity, Oral Surg. **24**:151, 1967.

Martinelli, C., and Rulli, M. A.: Primary plasmacytoma of soft tissue (gingiva), Oral Surg. **25**:607, 1968.

McClendon, E. H.: Lingual osseous choristoma, Oral Surg. **39**:39, 1975.

McGavran, M. H., Sessions, D. G., Dorfman, R. F., Davis, D. O., and Ogura, J. H.: Nasopharyngeal angiofibroma, Arch. Otolaryngol. **90**:68, 1969.

Merrill, R. G., and Downs, J. R.: Oral leiomyomas, Oral Surg. **23**:438, 1967.

Miller, A. S., and Elzay, R. P.: Verruciform xanthoma of the gingiva: report of six cases, J. Periodontol. **44**:103, 1973.

Miller, A. S., Leifer, C., Chen, S. Y., and Harwick, R. D.: Oral granular-cell tumors, Oral Surg. **44**:227, 1977.

Milobsky, S. A., and Thompson, C. W.: Neurilemmoma of the cheek, Oral Surg. **24**:124, 1967.

Mincer, H. H., and Spears, K. D.: Nerve sheath myxoma in the tongue, Oral Surg. **37**:428, 1974.

Morgan, G. A., and Morgan, P. R.: Neurilemmoma—neurofibroma, Oral Surg. **25**:182, 1968.

Moscovic, A. M., and Azar, H. A.: Multiple granular cell tumors (myoblastomas), CA **20**:2032, 1967.

Neville, B. W., and Weathers, D. R.: Verruciform xantnoma, Oral Surg. **49**:429, 1980.

Perriman, A., and Uthman, A.: Focal epithelial hyperplasia; report of seven cases from Iraq, Oral Surg. **31**:221, 1971.

Pisanti, S., Sharav, Y., Kaufman, E., and Posner, L. N.: Pemphigus vulgaris: incidence in Jews of different ethnic groups, according to age, sex, and initial lesion, Oral Surg. **38**:382, 1974.

Pisanty, S.: Keratoacanthoma of the face, Oral Surg. **21**:506, 1966.

Pisanty, S.: Bilateral lipomas of the tongue, Oral Surg. **42**:451, 1976.

Praetorius-Clausen, F.: Histopathology of focal epithelial hyperplasia, Tandlaegebladet **73**:1013, 1969.

Praetorius-Clausen, F.: Rare oral viral disorders (molluscum contagiosum, localized keratoacanthoma, verrucae, condyloma acuminatum, and focal epithelial hyperplasia), Oral Surg. **34**:604, 1972.

Praetorius-Clausen, F., and Willis, J. M.: Papova virus-like particles in focal epithelial hyperplasia, Scand. J. Dent. Res. **50**:722, 1971.

Quinn, J. H.: Calcified bodies in the buccal soft tissues, Oral Surg. **19**:292, 1965.

Rasmussen, O. C.: Painful traumatic neuromas in the oral cavity, Oral Surg. **49**:191, 1980.

Regezi, J. A., Courtney, R. M., and Kerr, D. A.: Fibrous lesions of the skin and mucous membranes which contain stellate and multinucleated cells, Oral Surg. **39**:605, 1975.

Rittersma, J., Kate, L. P., and Westerink, P.: Neurofibromatosis with mandibular deformities, Oral Surg. **33**:718, 1972.

Rosenberg Gertzman, G. B., Clark, M., and Gaston, G.: Multiple hamartoma and neoplasia syndrome (Cowden's syndrome), Oral Surg. **49**:314, 1980.

Rossi, E. P., and Hirsch, S. A.: A survey of 4,793 oral lesions with emphasis on neoplasia and premalignancy, J. Am. Dent. Assoc. **94**:883, 1977.

Scofield, H. H., Werning, J. T., and Shukes, R. C.: Solitary intraoral keratoacanthoma, Oral Surg. **37**:889, 1974.

Scully, C.: Orofacial manifestations in tuberous sclerosis, Oral Surg. **44:**706, 1977.

Seibert, J. S., Shannon, C. J., Jr., and Jacoway, J. R.: Treatment of recurrent condyloma acuminatum, Oral Surg. **27:**398, 1969.

Silverman, S., Jr., Greenspan, J. S., and Christie, T. M.: Junctional nevus of the oral mucosa, Oral Surg. **39:**259, 1975.

Sist, T. C., Jr., and Greene, G. W., Jr.: Benign nerve sheath myxoma: light and electron microscopic features of two cases, Oral Surg. **47:**441, 1979.

Snyder, S. R., and Merkow, L. P.: Traumatic granuloma of the tongue, Oral Surg. **36:**397, 1973.

Sobel, H. J., Arvin, E., Marquet, E., and Schwarz, R.: Reactive granular cells in sites of trauma, Am. J. Clin. Pathol. **61:**223, 1974.

Sobel, H. J., Schwarz, R., and Marquet, E.: Light- and electron-microscopic studies of the origion of granular-cell myoblastoma, J. Pathol. **109:**101, 1973.

Soga, J., Saito, K., Suzuki, N., and Sakai, T.: Plasma cell granuloma of the stomach, Cancer **25:**618, 1970.

Southam, J. C., and Venkataraman, B. K.: Calcification and ossification in epulides in man (excluding giant-cell epulides), Arch. Oral Biol. **18:**1243, 1973.

Summers, L., and Booth, D. R.: Intraoral condyloma acuminatum, Oral Surg. **38:**273, 1974.

Svirsky, J. A., Freedman, P. O., and Lumerman, H.: Solitary intraoral keratoacanthoma, Oral Surg. **43:**116, 1977.

Teles, J. C. B., Cardoso, A. S., and Goncalves, A. R.: Blue nevus of the oral mucosa, Oral Surg. **38:**905, 1974.

Thawley, S. E., and Ogura, J. H.: Granular cell myoblastoma of the head and neck, South Med. J. **67:**1020, 1974.

Tomich, C. E.: Oral focal mucinosis, Oral Surg. **38:**714, 1974.

Tornes, K., and Bang, G.: Traumatic eosinophilic granuloma of the gingiva, Oral Surg. **38:**99, 1974.

Tucker, K. M., and Heget, H. R.: The incidence of inflammatory papillary hyperplasia, J. Am. Dent. Assoc. **93:**610, 1976.

Urbach, F., Wine, S. S., Johnson, W. C., and Davies, R. E.: Generalized paraffinoma (sclerosing lipogranuloma), Arch, Dermatol. **103:**277, 1971.

van Gemert, R. J., Yamashita, D. D. R., and Goodsell, J. F.: Multiple neurofibromatosis (von Recklinghausen's disease) with concurrent micrognathia, Oral Surg. **43:**165, 1977.

Wallace, J. R.: Focal epithelial hyperplasia (Heck's disease): report of case, J. Am. Dent. Assoc. **93:**118, 1976.

Weathers, D. R., and Callihan, M. D.: Giant cell fibroma, Oral Surg. **37:**374, 1974.

Weathers, D. R., and Campbell, W. G.: Ultrastructure of the giant-cell fibroma of the oral mucosa, Oral Surg. **38:**550, 1974.

Weathers, D. R., and Waldron, C. A.: Intraoral cellular nevi, Oral Surg. **20**:467, 1965.

Westwood, R. M., Alexander, R. W., and Bennett, D. E.: Giant odontogenic myxofibroma, Oral Surg. **37**:83, 1974.

Winther, L. K.: Rhabdomyoma of the hypopharynx and larynx: report of two cases and a review of the literature, J. Laryngol. Otol. **90**:1041, 1976.

Wysocki, G. P., and Hardie, J.: Ultrastructural studies of intraoral verruca vulgaris, Oral Surg. **47**:58, 1979.

Yrastorza, J. A.: Inflammatory papillary hyperplasia of the palate, J. Oral Surg. **21**:330, 1963.

Zegarelli, D. J.: Solitary intraoral keratoacanthoma, Oral Surg. **40**:785, 1975.

Zegarelli, D. J., Zegarelli-Schmidt, E. C., and Zegarelli, E. V.: Verruciform xanthoma: a clinical, light microscopic, and electron microscopic study of two cases, Oral Surg. **38**:725, 1974.

Zegarelli, D. J., Zegarelli-Schmidt, E. C., and Zegarelli, E. V.: Verruciform xanthoma: further light and electron microscopic studies, with the addition of a third case, Oral Surg. **40**:246, 1975.

CHAPTER 16

Malignant tumors of soft tissues

The following malignant tumors may arise on the soft tissues of the oral cavity:

Epithelial tumors

1. Squamous cell carcinoma (epidermoid carcinoma)
2. Spindle cell carcinoma
3. Adenoid squamous cell carcinoma
4. Verrucous carcinoma
5. Transitional cell carcinoma
6. Lymphoepithelioma
7. Melanoma
8. Malignant tumors of salivary glands

Mesenchymal tumors

1. Fibrosarcoma
2. Fasciitis
3. Rhabdomyosarcoma
4. Embryonal rhabdomyosarcoma
5. Soft tissue plasmacytoma
6. Malignant lymphoma
   a. Lymphosarcoma
   b. Reticulum cell sarcoma
7. Leukemia
8. Midline lethal granuloma and Wegener's granulomatosis
9. Kaposi's sarcoma

Metastatic tumors

EPITHELIAL TUMORS

Squamous cell carcinoma (epidermoid carcinoma). Although only 0.5% of lesions biopsied by dentists are squamous cell carcinoma, this lesion is the most common malignant tumor of the oral cavity, representing slightly more than 90% of all oral malignancies (Fig. 16-1). It is about four times as common in males as in females, and its highest incidence is after the fourth decade. It occurs more frequently on the lips than intraorally.

Whereas in the United States oral cancer is the eighth most

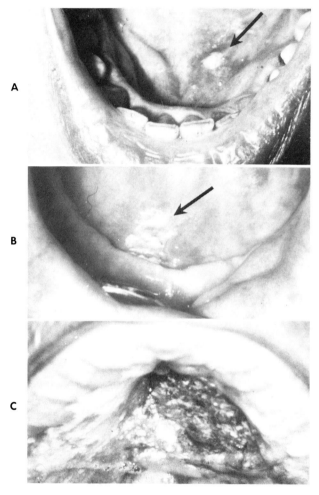

Fig. 16-1. Early and late squamous cell carcinomas of the mouth. **A** and **B,** Early lesions (arrows) of the floor of the mouth, **C,** Late lesion of the palate.

common form of cancer in males and the twelfth most common in females, in some areas of the world (e.g., Hong Kong) it is the most common form of human cancer. In the United States oral cancer (lip, tongue, salivary gland, floor of the mouth and other oral mucosa, and pharynx) constitutes about 3.5% of all malignant tumors in the male and 2% in the female. However, in some areas of the Far East it accounts for almost 70% of malignant disease in man.

In the United States more than 24,000 new cases of oral cancer occur every year, and more than 9,000 patients die of this disease annually. Three percent of all cancer deaths in males and 1% of cancer deaths in females is due to oral cancer. Five-year cures are obtained in about 75% of patients in whom oral cancer is localized at the site of origin, but these cures are obtained in only 25% if there is regional node involvement. The importance of early diagnosis, therefore, is extremely important.

Of the *lip carcinomas*, 95% occur on the lower lip. The lesions usually are on the lateral areas rather than in the midline. Lip carcinoma appears as an ulcer, wart, sore, or scale and occurs more frequently in members of fair-skinned races than in those of dark-skinned races. Carcinomas of the lip are discovered early, and at the time of treatment only a small percentage show lymph node metastases. However, cancer of the upper lip metastasizes six times as often as cancer of the lower lip. The ten-year cure rate for the upper and lower lip carcinomas is 80% and 92% respectively.

Of the *intraoral carcinomas*, 50% occur on the tongue, 16% in the floor of the mouth, and the remaining 34% (with about equal incidence) on the alveolar mucosa, palate, and cheek. Sixty percent of intraoral carcinomas present as ulcers, and 30% as "growths." The remaining 10% are seen as white lesions or as other abnormalities in the mucosa. The lesions are usually indurated. Tumors of the palate, gingiva, and tongue are largest in size.

Carcinomas of the tongue occur in the posterior two thirds

and on the lateral borders; only rarely is the anterior third of the dorsal surface affected. Since carcinomas of the tongue metastasize earlier than those of the lip, at the time of treatment more than 40% of patients show regional lymph node metastases; and in about 25% distant organs are affected. Of the cervical lymph node metastases, 75% occur on the side of the tumor, 20% occur bilaterally, and 3% involve only the contralateral side. The relative malignancy of tongue cancer can be correlated roughly with its location—the further back the location of the tumor, the greater its malignancy. About one third of the patients with tongue cancer survive for two years, and one fifth live longer than five years. Alcoholism and syphilitic glossitis are believed to predispose to lingual cancer.

Carcinoma of the floor of the mouth, like that of the tongue, metastasizes early and carries a poor prognosis. Carcinoma of the cheek is not common (about 9% of all intraoral carcinomas), but 40% of these tumors metastasize to distant organs.

The cause of oral squamous cell carcinoma is unknown. However, ill-fitting oral prostheses, actinic radiation, smoking, jagged teeth, syphilitic glossitis, and alcoholism are believed to play a role in its production. Smoking may be an important factor not only in the production of oral cancer but also in the development of a second tumor after the first one has been cured.

In squamous cell carcinoma the epithelial cells show all the evidences of dyskeratosis (p. 379)—pleomorphism, normal and abnormal mitoses, loss of polarity, and hyperchromatism. Also, there is invasion of the underlying tissues (Fig. 16-2). Islands, cords, strands, and clusters of tumor cells can be seen between muscle bundles and minor salivary glands, in connective tissue, and in other tissues that may be present in the area.

The degree to which a squamous cell carcinoma infiltrates or invades the underlying tissues depends on many factors—the most important being the duration and the degree of differentiation of the tumor. The epithelium forms whorllike structures called *epithelial pearls* (Fig. 16-2). When these undergo

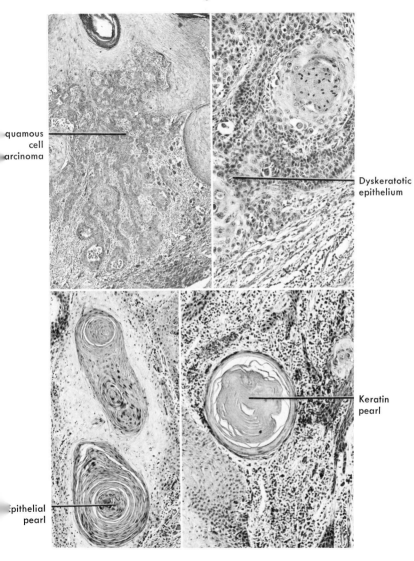

Squamous
cell
carcinoma

Dyskeratotic
epithelium

Keratin
pearl

Epithelial
pearl

Fig. 16-2. A squamous cell carcinoma is characterized by dyskeratotic epithelium, keratin pearl formation, and invasion of the underlying connective tissue.

partial or complete keratinization, they are called *keratin pearls*. The degree of malignancy of a tumor depends on the degree of its differentiation. In other words, the closer a malignant tumor resembles the tissues from which it is derived, the less malignant it is. On this premise is based the *Broders classification* of tumors.

According to the Broders concept, a squamous cell carcinoma (or any other cancer) may be classified as grade I to grade IV, in an ascending order of malignancy. In grade I tumors, 75% or more of the cells are normally differentiated; in grade II, from 50% to 75%; in grade III, from 25% to 50%; and in grade IV, from 0% to 25%. As a rule, carcinomas of the lip are better differentiated than those within the mouth; and, of the latter, carcinomas of the tongue and floor of the mouth are least differentiated. Squamous cell carcinoma of the oral regions metastasizes to the regional lymph nodes and only later to the distant organs.

The treatment for oral cancer is surgery, radiation, and chemotherapy. Excision of the lip tumors produces a high percentage of cures. This is partly because of the high degree of differentiation of these lesions and partly because of their location and early diagnosis. Chemotherapy and radiation of lesions that are not completely manageable by surgery offers the best prognosis.

Spindle cell carcinoma. The variant of the squamous cell carcinoma usually occurs on the lip. Although clinically it has the same appearance as squamous cell carcinoma, microscopically it is characterized by spindle-shaped cells and can be mistaken for a fibrosarcoma. If this type of a tumor follows radiation or physical injury, its prognosis is grave.

Adenoid squamous cell carcinoma. This rare variant of the squamous cell carcinoma usually occurs in elderly white males and involves the lips (lower lip more often than the upper). Clinically it is an ulcer, a wart, or a keratotic lesion about 1 cm in diameter (Fig. 16-3).

Microscopic features are those of a squamous cell carcinoma

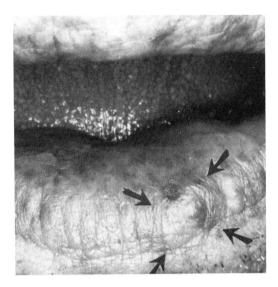

Fig. 16-3. An adenoid squamous cell carcinoma (arrows) is a rare variation of the squamous cell carcinoma. (Courtesy J. R. Jacoway, D.D.S., Washington, D.C.)

whose deep aspects reveal ductlike or glandular arrangement (Fig. 16-4). The tumor can metastasize and should be widely excised.

Verrucous carcinoma. This cauliflower-like tumor is usually seen after the age of 50 years (Fig. 16-5). It is almost always intraoral in location, with the alveolar ridge the favored site, and it usually occurs in tobacco chewers.

The verrucous carcinoma is exophytic; that is, it grows away from the mucosal surface, in contradistinction to the usual squamous cell carcinoma (which grows into the tissues) (Fig. 16-6). The tumor has a papillary appearance and a wide or a narrow stalk. The epithelial cells show all characteristics of malignancy.

The verrucous carcinoma has a much better prognosis than the usual infiltrating type of carcinoma. Surgical excision is the treatment of choice.

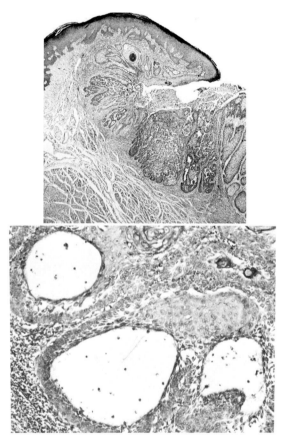

Fig. 16-4. An adenoid squamous cell carcinoma is composed of glandlike structures and also has the features of the usual squamous cell carcinoma.

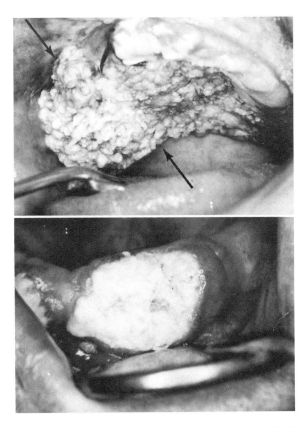

Fig. 16-5. Verrucous carcinoma of the palate (arrows) and mandibular alveolar ridge.

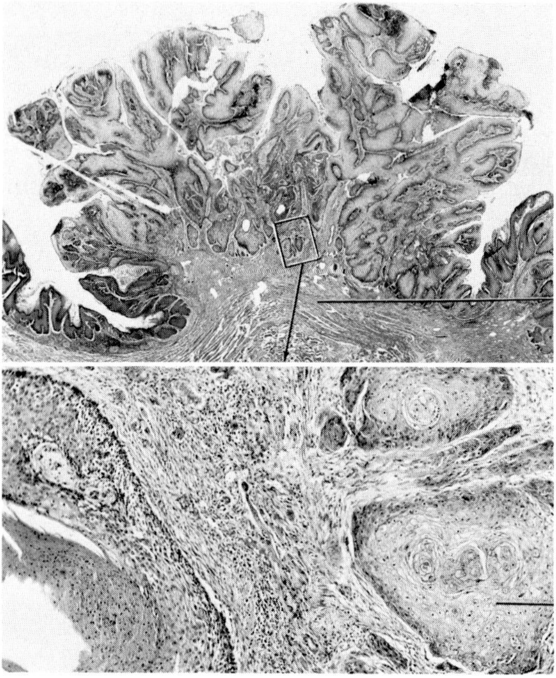

Base of tumor

Tumor cells invading lamina propria

Fig. 16-6. A verrucous carcinoma is characterized by an exophytic growth. Usually the tumor does not infiltrate too far into the deep tissues.

Transitional cell carcinoma. The transitional cell carcinoma has certain clinical, histologic, and behavioristic features that distinguish it from other intraoral carcinomas.

The tumor frequently occurs at the base of the tongue and in the oropharynx and usually afflicts males. It presents as a small red raspberry–like or velvety lesion that may show erosion but in which the deep ulceration of squamous cell carcinoma is absent. Most patients (65% to 70%) have a primary lesion that is insignificant; a palpable cervical node is the earliest sign of the disease.

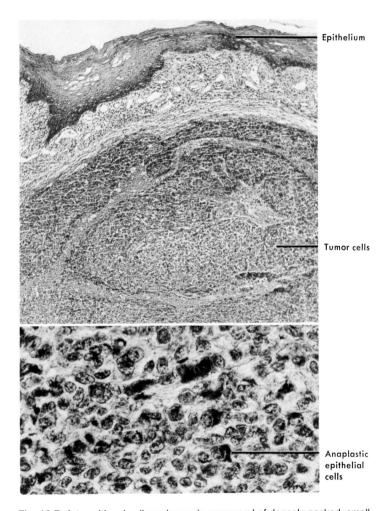

Epithelium

Tumor cells

Anaplastic
epithelial
cells

Fig. 16-7. A transitional cell carcinoma is composed of densely packed, small dark-staining epithelial cells.

The tumor is composed of sheets, folded ribbons, and islands of densely packed epithelial cells with hyperchromatic nuclei and scanty cytoplasm (Fig. 16-7). Sections stained by hematoxylin and eosin and viewed under the low-power microscope show marked basophilia. Some epithelial islands have central areas of necrosis. Mitoses are numerous. The cells of a transitional cell carcinoma lack the spinous processes, keratinization, and pearl formation characteristically seen in squamous cell carcinomas.

A transitional cell carcinoma metastasizes early. It is radiosensitive, so both surgical excision and radiation are used in its treatment. However, the prognosis is poor.

Lymphoepithelioma. The clinical features of a lymphoepithelioma resemble those of a transitional cell carcinoma; that is, it presents as a small insignificant ulcer or growth that may go unnoticed and is observed only when the patient develops a metastatic enlargement of one of the cervical lymph nodes. Patients are much younger (usually in their third decade) than those who have transitional cell or squamous cell carcinoma.

A lymphoepithelioma usually occurs in the nasopharynx or in the tonsillar area. It consists of islands of large polyhedral cells with indistinct boundaries. These cells may show mitoses and hyperchromatic nuclei. The epithelial islands lie in a sea of lymphocytes (Fig. 16-8).

A lymphoepithelioma is radiosensitive but not radiocurable. The prognosis is poor.

Melanoma. This highly malignant melanin-containing tumor of the skin, mucous membranes, and eyes may develop from a junctional or compound nevus; or it may originate without a precursor. It rarely occurs before puberty.

A malignant melanoma of the oral cavity is rare; only 1.5% occur in this region. Patients are usually past 50 years of age, and males are afflicted more frequently than females. The most common sites in the oral cavity are the hard palate and maxillary alveolar ridge (Fig. 16-9); but the lesion also occurs on the upper lip, buccal mucosa, and inferior alveolar ridge. It gener-

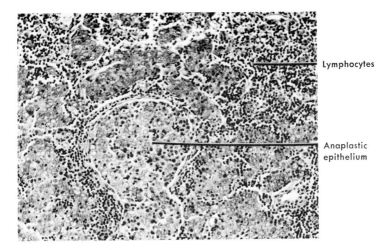

Lymphocytes

Anaplastic
epithelium

Fig. 16-8. A lymphoepithelioma is composed of islands and sheets of epithelium in a "sea" of lymphocytes.

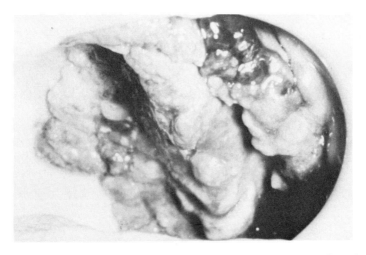

Fig. 16-9. Melanoma of the maxillary ridge in an edentulous patient. Part of the tumor is pigmented (dark areas).

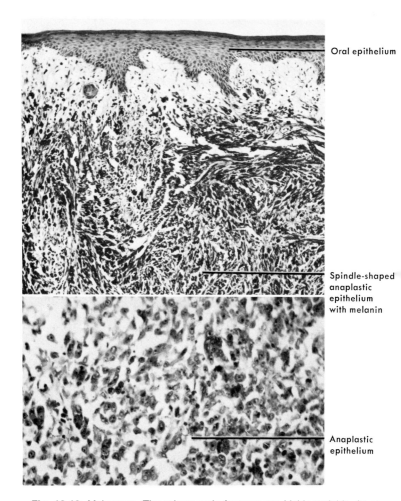

Oral epithelium

Spindle-shaped
anaplastic
epithelium
with melanin

Anaplastic
epithelium

Fig. 16-10. Melanoma. The microscopic features are highly variable. In essence, the tumor consists of noncohesive epithelial cells that may contain varying amounts of melanin.

ally starts as a painless pigmented or nonpigmented area of variable duration (weeks to years), which later become ulcerated, bleeds, has a red border, and rapidly increases in pigmentation. Induration is rare.

The microscopic appearance of a melanoma is quite varied. Some tumors resemble squamous cell carcinomas with large noncohesive cells; others are composed of spindle cells resembling those seen in sarcomas (Fig. 16-10); still others are made up of cells lying in alveolar formations and resembling nevus cells. When the tumor cells contain pigment, the diagnosis is relatively easy. However, the nonpigmented tumors, called *amelanotic melanomas,* may pose a problem in microscopic diagnosis. Certain special stains (e.g., dihydroxyphenylalanine, or dopa) will reveal the melanin-forming cells.

With regard to behavior, two forms of oral melanomas have been observed—those that spread superficially in the mucosa and those that extend vertically into the deeper tissues. While the prognosis of a malignant melanoma of the oral cavity is extremely poor and death within five years is highly likely, the superficially spreading lesions have a somewhat better outcome.

Malignant tumors of salivary glands. Malignant tumors arising in the salivary glands are discussed in Chapter 17 (p. 599).

MESENCHYMAL TUMORS

Malignant mesenchymal tumors of the soft tissues are rare, and in the oral cavity they are even rarer. For this reason detailed information concerning their behavior is lacking.

Fibrosarcoma. The oral fibrosarcoma is an uncommon tumor that afflicts males more often than females, usually between the third and fifth decades of life. It is found in the cheek, lip, and periosteum of the maxilla and mandible (Fig. 16-11).

Fibrosarcomas may grow slowly or rapidly with intervening periods of inactivity. The five-year survival rate for patients who have a peripheral lesion is better than for patients with a lesion in the jaws.

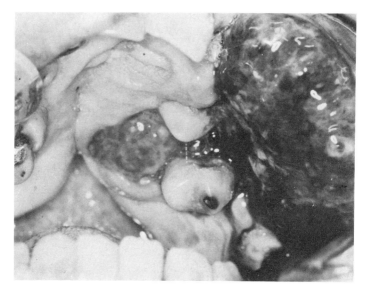

Fig. 16-11. Advanced case of fibrosarcoma of the maxillary soft tissues.

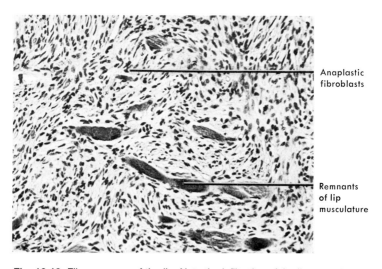

Anaplastic
fibroblasts

Remnants
of lip
musculature

Fig. 16-12. Fibrosarcoma of the lip. Note the infiltration of the lip musculature by abnormal fibroblasts.

A fibrosarcoma consists of fibroblasts and collagen fibers, and both the cells and the fibers appear to run in streams (Fig. 16-12). In the well-differentiated fibrosarcoma the fibroblasts are spindle shaped, have fusiform nuclei, show very few mitoses, and resemble normal cells. Collagen fibers may be fine and obscure, or dense and pronounced. The less-differentiated (more malignant) fibrosarcomas are more cellular and show many mitoses in hyperchromatic and bizarre fibroblasts.

Most fibrosarcomas are locally infiltrative and persistent, but they do not metastasize; these tumors have a favorable prognosis. The less common poorly differentiated fibrosarcomas metastasize widely and are fatal. Treatment consists of wide excision.

Fasciitis. Also called nodular fasciitis, this tumorlike growth is often mistaken for a fibrosarcoma and therefore is included in the present chapter.

It occurs in subcutaneous tissues; in the oral region it may be seen in the cheek. The lesion has a short history and rapid

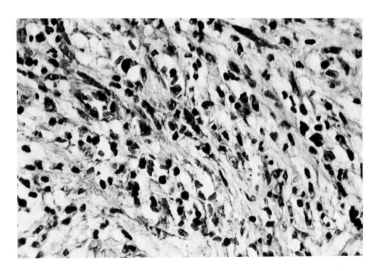

Fig. 16-13. Fasciitis. Note the edematous appearance and the fibroblastic proliferation.

growth, is tender, and afflicts patients in their second, third, and fourth decades of life.

The microscopic picture of fasciitis superficially resembles that of a fibrosarcoma. The lesion consists of young fibroblasts, numerous capillaries, interstitial hemorrhage, edematous or mucoedematous stroma, and a few lymphocytes (Fig. 16-13). Many fibroblasts and plump endothelial cells of the capillaries show mitoses. The lesion is benign and may regress spontaneously.

Rhabdomyosarcoma. On rare occasion, a rhabdomyosarcoma may arise in the mouth, with the tongue the favored site. Congenital rhabdomyosarcomas of the tongue also may occur.

Clinically the mass grows very rapidly and is associated with induration and hemorrhage and frequently with cervical lymphadenopathy.

Microscopic features include the presence of highly bizarre cells (e.g., tadpole cells, racquet cells), strap-shaped cells whose nuclei are arranged in tandem, and giant cells with wide variations in the number of nuclei and amount of cytoplasm (Fig. 16-14). The cytoplasm of some cells shows cross striations, as exist in voluntary muscle.

The tumor is highly malignant. Its prognosis is poor, and it requires extensive surgical excision.

Embryonal rhabdomyosarcoma. This rare tumor is seen most frequently in the head and neck area and in the genitourinary tract.

About 73% of these tumors occur in the first decade of life. Intraoral lesions arise around Stensen's duct, the soft palate, and the oropharynx—where they present as soft polypoid, grapelike masses or as a single submucosal mass.

Microscopic sections show a highly undifferentiated mesenchymal tumor in which small cells resembling lymphocytes with slightly eosinophilic cytoplasm, fusiform cells, and striated cells may be seen.

The embryonal rhabdomyosarcoma is highly malignant and invariably fatal.

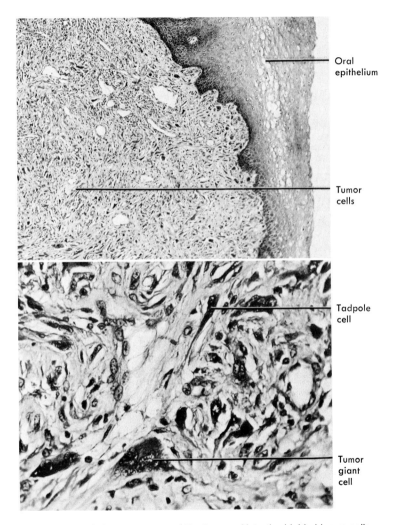

Oral
epithelium

Tumor
cells

Tadpole
cell

Tumor
giant
cell

Fig. 16-14. Rhabdomyosarcoma of the tongue. Note the highly bizarre cells, which are derived from striated muscle.

Soft tissue plasmacytoma. Some soft tissue plasmacytomas are benign, while others represent an early manifestation of multiple myeloma (p. 322 and 528).

Malignant lymphoma. This tumor of lymphoid tissue has been subject to numerous and varied classifications. It usually arises in lymphoid organs (e.g., lymph nodes; spleen; diffuse lymphoid tissue of the body, such as the lingual and pharyngeal tonsils; lymphoid tissue of the gastrointestinal tract). However, some tumors also arise in apparently nonlymphoid areas (e.g., palate, gingiva).

Malignant lymphomas are essentially of four types: lymphosarcoma, reticulum cell sarcoma, Hodgkin's disease, and giant follicular lymphoma. Since only lymphosarcoma and reticulum cell sarcoma occur as primary lesions in the oral cavity, they are discussed here.

Lymphosarcoma. The primary oral lesion of lymphosarcoma may arise in the hard palate, gingiva, or tonsils. It usually oc-

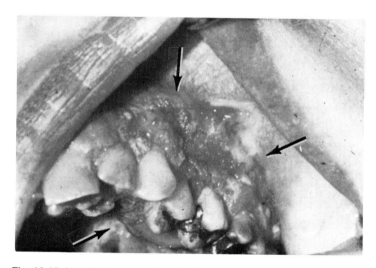

Fig. 16-15. Lymphosarcoma of the gingiva. Note the enlargement, ulceration, and necrosis of the tissue (arrows).

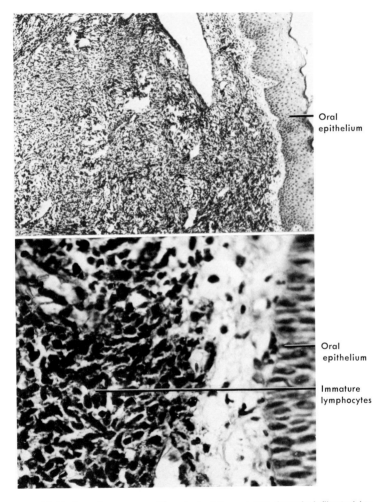

Oral
epithelium

Oral
epithelium

Immature
lymphocytes

Fig. 16-16. Lymphosarcoma. The gingival tissues are densely infiltrated by
immature lymphocytes.

curs in adults but may appear at any age. Males are afflicted more often than females.

Clinically the lesion is a palatal or gingival hyperplasia or a tumor mass. Ulceration, necrosis, and foul breath are common (Fig. 16-15).

Microscopic sections show that the tumor mass consists of sheets and masses of round cells resembling mature and immature lymphocytes (Fig. 16-16). Mitoses are variable. The tumor cells extend into every available space. Viewed under low-power magnification, the boundary between the involved and the uninvolved tissues appears irregular but sharp. In lesions that are not ulcerated, a tumor-free connective tissue zone separates the tumor from the covering epithelium.

Lymphosarcomas are occasionally mistaken for inflammatory lesions; but the latter have no subepithelial cell-free zone, present more than one type of cellular infiltrate (e.g., lymphocytes, plasma cells, neutrophils), and show graded intensities of cellular infiltrate in the periphery of the lesion.

Lymphosarcomas are radiosensitive. Remissions are temporary, however, and sooner or later the oral disease becomes generalized.

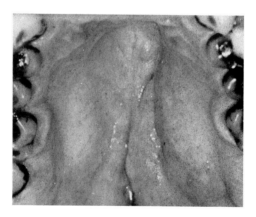

Fig. 16-17. Lymphoproliferative disease of the hard palate.

Reticulum cell sarcoma. The primary lesion of reticulum cell sarcoma may arise in the soft tissues or within the jaws. In the soft tissues its clinical features are the same as have been described for lymphosarcoma.

The term *lymphoproliferative disease of the hard palate* is sometimes applied to the *primary* lesion of malignant lymphoma of the palate. This lesion occurs in elderly patients (average age, 70 years), usually in the hard palate, and presents as a soft unilateral or bilateral swelling that may be ulcerated (Fig. 16-17).

Leukemia. The term leukemia is applied to those malignant tumors of white blood cells (lymphoid and myelogenous) that extend into the bloodstream. Thus leukemias may be acute and chronic lymphocytic, acute and chronic myelogenous, or acute and chronic monocytic.

The acute leukemias begin as generalized infections (i.e., with fever, chills, and malaise) and later may present enlargement of the spleen and lymph nodes. They usually occur in children and young adults and within a few weeks or months run a rapidly fatal course. Due to the replacement of all blood cells by the leukemic component, patients have anemia, hemorrhages of the mucosa, and petechiae.

Oral lesions are a most common and constant finding in acute leukemia: enlargement, bleeding, and necrosis of the gingiva and bleeding and oozing of blood around the teeth (Fig. 16-18). There may be ecchymoses with necrosis of the oral mucosa. Tooth extraction is followed by profuse bleeding. The peripheral blood in acute forms of leukemia shows a marked increase (15 to 50,000 per milliliter) in the number of the respective cells.

Chronic leukemias occur in adults or older patients and have a protracted course extending up to many years. However, acute exacerbation and death may occur at any time. These leukemias have an insidious beginning; enlarged spleen and lymph nodes may be the first symptoms, and the patient may complain of weakness. Oral symptoms are usually present and consist of

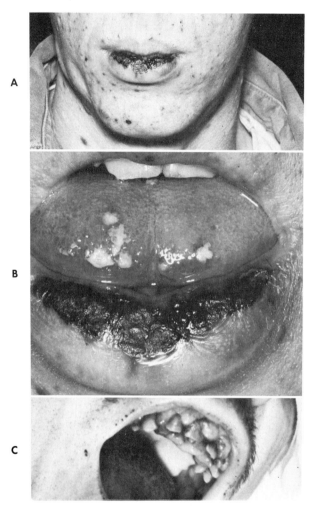

Fig. 16-18. A and **B,** Acute myelogenous leukemia. **C,** Acute lymphocytic leukemia.

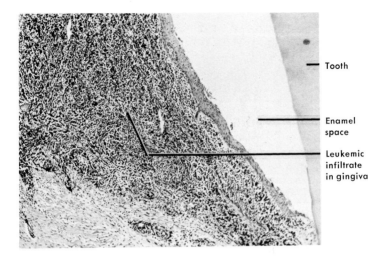

Tooth

Enamel
space

Leukemic
infiltrate
in gingiva

Fig. 16-19. Leukemic infiltrate in the interdental gingival papilla.

gingival hyperplasia. Although seen in all types of leukemias, they are early and constant in the monocytic form. The peripheral blood contains a much greater number of leukemic cells than is seen in the acute form (50,000 to 500,000 per milliliter).

Microscopic sections prepared from the oral lesions show a dense infiltration of the connective tissue by immature cells of the lymphoid, myelogenous, or monocytic series (Fig. 16-19). In lymphocytic leukemia the infiltrate consists of cells resembling lymphocytes or with slightly larger round hyperchromatic nuclei. In myelogenous leukemia the infiltrating cells have lobed nuclei and varying amounts of cytoplasmic granules and thus resemble myeloblasts and myelocytes. In monocytic leukemia the infiltrating cells resemble either atypical monocytes or histiocytes.

Midline lethal granuloma and Wegener's granulomatosis. Midline lethal granuloma is a malignant lesion of obscure cause that involves the nasal cavity and maxilla. Lesions may begin in

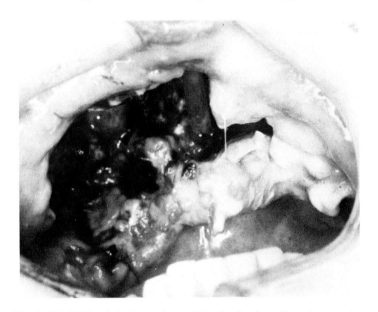

Fig. 16-20. Midline lethal granuloma of the hard palate. Note the complete destruction and necrosis of a large area of the palate. The dark area partly represents necrosis and destruction in the nasal cavity.

the palate as a nonspecific ulcer that does not respond to any treatment but progressively destroys the soft and hard tissues of the palate and nose and ultimately kills the patient by exhaustion, bleeding, malnutrition, and cachexia (Fig. 16-20).

During the course of the disease, the patient may complain of weakness; but there are no systemic symptoms. The disease may last from a few months to five years.

Microscopic features include nonspecific inflammation composed of immature and atypical lymphocytes, histiocytes, and plasma cells with necrosis of tissue. The prognosis is grave.

Wegener's granulomatosis is a lesion that is sometimes considered identical to the midline lethal granuloma. However, oral lesions are not so common, and the sites usually involved are the larynx, trachea, kidneys, and lungs. Death is usually due to renal failure.

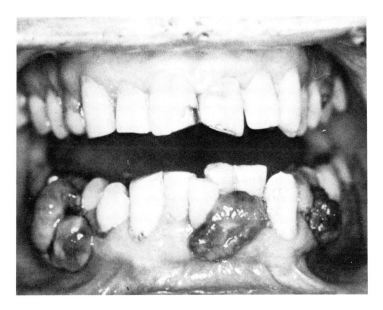

Fig. 16-21. Oral lesions of Kaposi's sarcoma. Note the multiple dark, hemorrhagic growths. (Courtesy Milton J. Knapp, D.D.S., Portland, Ore.)

When oral lesions occur, they involve the gingiva and consist of painful, bleeding growths of the interdental papillae. In some cases the gingival lesions are the earliest sign of the disease.

The histologic picture consists of necrosis, inflammation of vessels, and inflammatory cells.

Kaposi's sarcoma. Also called *multiple idiopathic hemorrhagic sarcoma of Kaposi*, this rare tumor of blood vessels appears as multiple lesions in the skin and internal organs (Fig. 16-21).

Patients develop malignant lymphomas or other types of cancer in addition to this disease. It occurs most often in the fifth to seventh decades of life, and almost 90% of patients are male. Oral lesions can occur anywhere and are reddish nodules or masses.

Microscopic features are varied but consist primarily of

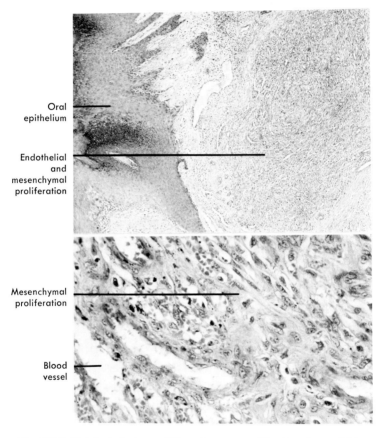

Oral
epithelium

Endothelial
and
mesenchymal
proliferation

Mesenchymal
proliferation

Blood
vessel

Fig. 16-22. Histologic features of Kaposi's sarcoma. (Courtesy James Adrian, D.D.S., Washington, D.C.)

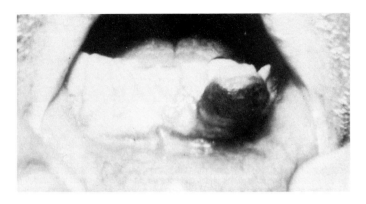

Fig. 16-23. Adenocarcinoma of the kidney, metastatic to the gingiva.

blood vessel proliferation with numerous foci of mesenchymal tissue (Fig. 16-22).

METASTATIC TUMORS

About 1% of the malignant tumors of the body metastasize to the oral cavity, and only 1% of oral malignancies are metastatic foci. The majority (90%) of oral metastases occur in the jaws, and only about 10% occur in the soft tissues. Of the latter, 5% are in the tongue, 4% in the gingiva and cheek, and 1% elsewhere (Fig. 16-23). Patients range in age from 40 to 60 years, and the primary site is usually the breast, thyroid, kidney, lung, genitourinary system, or gastrointestinal tract.

Clinically these lesions are characterized by rapid onset and growth, but diagnosis is confirmed only at biopsy.

REFERENCES

Ah Moo, E. W.: Lethal midline granuloma of the face, Oral Surg. **23:**578, 1967.

Allen, A. C., and Spitz, S.: Malignant melanoma: a clinicopathological analysis of the criteria for diagnosis and prognosis, CA **6:**1, 1953.

American Cancer Society: CA **29:**6, 1979.

Azaz, B., and Lustmann, J.: Keratoacanthoma of the lower lip, Oral Surg. **38:**918, 1974.

Baden, E., and Newman, R.: Liposarcoma of the oropharygeal region, Oral Surg. **44:**889, 1977.

Ballard, B. R., Suess, G. R., Pickren, J. W., Greene, G. W., and Shedd, D. P.: Squamous-cell carcinoma of the floor of the mouth, Oral Surg. **45:**568, 1978.

Berg, J. W., Schottenfeld, D., and Ritter, F.: Incidence of multiple primary cancers, J. Natl. Cancer Inst. **44:**263, 1970.

Bhaskar, S. N.: Oral pathology in the dental office: survey of 20,575 biopsy specimens, J. Am. Dent. Assoc. **76:**761, 1968.

Bhaskar, S. N.: Oral manifestations of metastatic tumors, Postgrad. Med. **49:**155, 1971.

Bhaskar, S. N., and Frisch, J.: Reticulum cell sarcoma of the gingiva, Oral Surg. **21:**236, 1966.

Birkholz, H., and Reed, J. H.: Bronchogenic carcinoma metastatic to the lip and the mandible, J. Am. Dent. Assoc. **98:**414, 1979.

Blok, P., van Delden, L., and van der Waal, I.: Non-Hodgkin's lymphoma of the hard palate, Oral Surg. **47:**445, 1979.

Bollinger, T. E., and Hiatt, W. R.: Basal-cell adenoma of the upper lip, Oral Surg. **35:**600, 1973.

Borello, E. D., Sedano, H. O., Rossi- Maino, O., and Martinez-Ramseyer, R.: Primary malignant melanoma of the oral cavity, Oral Surg. **21:**67, 1966.

Broders, A. C.: The grading of carcinoma, Minn. Med. **8:**726, 1925.

Brooke, R. I.: Wegener's granulomatosis involving the gingivae, Br. Dent. J. **127:**34, 1969.

Brown, C. H.: Malignant granuloma, Br. Med. J. **3:**471, 1969.

Brown, R. L., Suh, J. M., Scarborough, J. E., Wilkins, S. A., and Smith, R. R.: Snuff dipper's intraoral cancer, clinical characteristics and response to therapy, CA **18:**2, 1965.

Calderwood, R. G.: Primary reticulum-cell sarcoma of gingiva, Oral Surg. **24:**71, 1967.

Catlin, D.: Mucosal melanomas of the head and neck, Am. J. Roentgenol **99:**809, 1967.

Catlin, D., Das, G. T., and McNeer, G.: Noncutaneous melanoma: primary mucosal melanoma of the head and neck region, CA **15:**75, 1966.

Charkondian, G. K.: Primary malignant melanoma of the oral cavity, Oral Surg. **28:**464, 1969.

Chaudhry, A. P., Hampel, A., and Gorlin, R. J.: Primary malignant melanoma of the oral cavity: a review of 105 cases, CA **11:**923, 1958.

Chen, S.-Y., and Harwick, R. D.: Ultrastructure of oral squamous-cell carcinoma, Oral Surg. **44:**744, 1977.

Cline, R. E, and Stenger, T. G.: Histiocytic lymphoma (reticulum-cell sarcoma), Oral Surg. **43:**422, 1977.

Cochran, A. J.: Histology and prognosis in malignant melanoma, J. Pathol. **97:**459, 1969.

Cook, H. P.: Oral lymphomas, Oral Surg. **14:**690, 1961.

Curran, J. B., and Whittaker, J. S.: Primary malignant melanoma of the oral cavity, Oral Surg. **36:**701, 1973.

Danforth, R. A., and Baughman, R. A.: Chievitz's organ: a potential pitfall in oral cancer diagnosis, Oral Surg. **48:**231, 1979.

Del Carmen, B. V., and Korbitz, B. C.: Oral metastasis from hypernephroma, J. Am. Geriatr. Soc. **18:**743, 1970.

Edwards, M. B., and Buckerfield, J. P.: Wegener's granulomatosis: a case with primary mucocutaneous lesions, Oral Surg. **46:**53, 1978.

Einhoen, J., and Wersal, J.: Incidence of oral carcinoma in patients with leukoplakia of the oral mucosa, CA **20:**2189, 1967.

Ellis, G. L., Jensen, J. L., Reingold, I. M., and Barr, R. J.: Malignant neoplasms metastatic to gingivae, Oral Surg. **44:**238, 1977.

Eversole, L. R., Schwartz, W. D., and Sabes, W. R.: Central and peripheral fibrinogenic and neurogenic sarcoma of the oral regions, Oral Surg. **36:**49, 1973.

Falsom, T. C., White, C. P., Bromer, L., Canby, H. F., and Garrington, G. E.: Oral exfoliative study, Oral Surg. **33:**61, 1972.

Fantasia, J. E., and Chen, L. C.: A testicular tumor with gingival metastasis, Oral Surg. **48:**64, 1979.

Farman, A. G., and Kay, S.: Oral leiomyosarcoma, Oral Surg. **43:**402, 1977.

Fisher, E. R., McCoy, M. M., and Wechsler, H. L.: Analysis of histopathologic and electron-microscopic determinants of keratoacanthoma and squamous cell carcinoma, CA **29:**1387, 1972.

Frazell, E. L., and Lucas, J. C.: Cancer of the tongue, CA **15:**1085, 1962.

Friedlander, A. H., and Singer, R.: Renal adenocarcinoma of the kidney with metastasis to the tongue, J. Am. Dent. Assoc. **97:**989, 1978.

Gelfman, W. E., and Williams, A.: Spindle-cell carcinoma of the tongue, Oral Surg. **27:**659, 1969.

Gerughty, R. M., Henninger, G. R., and Brown, F. M.: Adenosquamous carcinoma of the nasal, oral, and laryngeal cavities: a clinicopathological survey of ten cases, CA **22:**1140, 1968.

Giraldo, G., Beth, E., Henle, W., Henle, G., Mike, V., Safai, B. Huraux, J. M., McHardy, J., and de-The, G.: Antibody patterns to herpesviruses in Kaposi's sarcoma. II. Serological association of American Kaposi's sarcoma with cytomegalovirus, Int. J. Cancer **22:**126, 1978.

Giunta, J. L., Gomez, L. S. A., and Greer, R. O.: Oral focal acantholytic dyskeratosis (warty dyskeratoma), Oral Surg. **39:**474, 1975.

Godby, A. F., Sonntag, R. W., and Cosentino, B. J.: Hypernephroma with metastasis to the mandibular gingiva, Oral Surg. **23:**696, 1967.

Grinspan, D., Abulafia, J., Diaz, J., and Berdichesky, R.: Melanoma of the oral mucosa: a case of infiltrating melanoma originating in Hutchinson's malignant lentigo or precancerous melanosis of Dubreuilh, Oral Surg. **28:**1, 1969.

Gulmen, S., and Pullon, P. A.: Sweat gland carcinoma of the lips, Oral Surg. **41:**643, 1976.

Hatziotis, J. C, Constaninidou, H., and Papanayotou, P. H.: Metastatic tumors of the oral soft tissue, Oral Surg. **36**:544, 1973.

Hormia, M., and Vuori Esa, E. J.: Mucosal melanomas of the head and neck, J. Laryngol. **83**:349, 1969.

Jackson, D., and Simpson, H. E.: Primary malignant melanoma of the oral cavity, Oral Surg. **39**:553, 1975.

Jacoway, J. R., Nelson, J. F., and Boyers, R. C.: Adenoid squamous cell carcinoma (adenoacanthoma) of the oral labial mucosa, Oral Surg. **32**:444, 1971.

Johnson, H. A.: Query: Keratoacanthoma of mucous membrane? Plast. Reconstr. Surg. **41**:373, 1968.

Johnson, W. C., and Helwig, E. B.: Adenoid squamous cell carcinoma (adenoacanthoma): a clinicopathologic study of 155 patients, CA **19**:1639, 1966.

Jones, H. J., and Coyle, J. I.: Squamous carcinoma of the lip: a study of the interface between neoplastic epithelium and the underlying mesenchyma, J. Dent. Res. (suppl.) **48**:702, 1969.

Jones, S. E.: Non-Hodgkin's lymphomas, J.A.M.A. **234**:635, 1975.

Kakehaski, S., Hamner, J. E, Baer, P. N., and McIntire, J. A.: Wegener's granulomatosis Oral Surg. **19**:120, 1965.

Kempson, R. L., and Kyriakos, M.: Fibroxanthosarcoma of the soft tissues, CA **29**:961, 1972.

Kohn, M. W., and Eversole, L. R.: Keratoacanthoma of the lower lip, J. Oral Surg. **30**:522, 1972.

Koop, C. E., and Tewarson, I. P.: Rhabdomyosarcoma of the head and neck in children, Ann. Surg. **160**:95, 1964.

Krause, C. J: Carcinoma of oral cavity, Arch. Otolaryngol. **97**:354, 1973.

Krolls, S. O., and Hoffman, S.: Squamous cell carcinoma of the oral soft tissues: a statistical analysis of 14,253 cases by age, sex, and race of patients, J. Am. Dent. Assoc. **92**:571, 1976.

Lehrer, S., Roswit, B., and Federman, Q.: The presentation of malignant lymphoma in the oral cavity and pharynx, Oral Surg. **41**:441, 1976.

Lukes, R. J., and Collins, R. D.: Immunologic characterization of human malignant lymphomas, CA **34**:1488, 1974.

Lumerman, H., Bodner, B., and Zambito, R.: Intraoral (submucosal) pseudosarcomatous nodular fasciitis: report of a case, Oral Surg. **34**:239, 1972.

Lynch, M. A., and Ship, I. I.: Oral manifestations of leukemia: a postdiagnostic study, J. Am. Dent. Assoc. **75**:1139, 1967.

McGovern, V. J.: Edidemiological aspects of melanoma: a review, Pathology **9**:233, 1977.

Michaud, M., Baerhner, R. L., Bixler, D., and Kafrawy, A. H.: Oral manifestations of acute leukemia in children, J. Am. Dent. Assoc. **95**:1145, 1977.

Miller, A. S., and Pullon, P. A.: Metastatic malignant melanoma of the tongue, Arch. Dermatol. **103**:201, 1971.

Miller, R., Cheris, L., and Stratigos, G. T.: Nodular fasciitis, Oral Surg. **40**:399, 1975.

Milton, G. W., and Lane-Grown, M. M.: Malignant melanoma of the nose and mouth, Br. J. Surg. **52**:484, 1965.

Mittelman, G. J., Pickle, D. E., Scopp, I. W., and Greene, G. W., Jr.: Spindle-cell carcinoma of the floor of the mouth, Oral Surg. **20**:399, 1965.

Mittelman, D., and Kaban, L. B.: Recurrent "non-Hodgkin's lymphoma" presenting with gingival enlargement, Oral Surg. **42**:792, 1976.

Moffat, D. A.: Metastatic adenocarcinoma of the rectum presenting as an epulis: a case report, Br. J. Oral Surg. **14**:90, 1976.

Moore, C.: Smoking and cancer of the mouth, pharynx, and larynx, J.A.M.A. **191**:283, 1965.

Moran, E. M., Ultmann, J. E., Ferguson, D. J., Hoffer, P. B., Ranninger, K., and Rappaport, H.: Staging laparotomy in non-Hodgkin's lymphoma, Br. J. Cancer, **31**(Suppl. 2):228, 1975.

Mosby, E. L., Sugg, W. E., and Hiatt, W. R.: Gingival and pharyngeal metastasis for a malignant melanoma, Oral Surg. **36**:6, 1973.

O'Day, R. A., Soule, E. H., and Gores, R. J.: Embryonal rhabdomyosarcoma of the oral soft tissues, Oral Surg. **20**:85, 1965.

Omar-Ahmad, V., and Ramanathan, K.: Oral carcinoma, Med. J. Malaya **22**:172, 1968.

Parkes, C. R., and Bottomley, W. F.: Lymphoblastic lymphosarcoma, Oral Surg. **33**:297, 1972.

Paymaster, J. C.: Some observations on oral and pharyngeal carcinomas in the State of Bombay, CA **15**:578, 1962.

Perlmutter, S., Buchner, A., and Smukler, H.: Metastasis to the gingiva, Oral Surg. **38**:749, 1974.

Pliskin, M. E., Mastrangelo, M. J., Brown, A. M., and Custer, R. P.: Metastatic melanoma of the maxilla presenting as a gingival swelling, Oral Surg. **41**:101, 1976.

Price, E. B., Silliphant, W. M., and Shuman, R.: Nodular fasciitis: a clinicopathologic analysis of 65 cases, Am. J. Clin. Pathol. **35**:122, 1961.

Quick, D., and Cutler, M.: Transitional cell epidermoid carcinoma; a radiosensitive type of intraoral tumor, Surg. Gynceol. Obstet. **45**:320, 1927.

Raitt, J. W.: Wegener's granulomatosis: treatment with cytotoxic agents and adrenocorticoids, Ann. Intern. Med. **74**:344, 1971.

Rakower, W.: Fasciitis, an unusual diagnosis, and the clinician's dilemma: report of a case, J. Oral Surg. **29**:503, 1971.

Rosenberg, C. J., Salcedo, M., and Rojas, R.: Melanocarcinoma of the buccal mucosa, Oral Surg. **22**:498, 1966.

Schuler, S., McDonald, J. S., Strull, N. J., and Alpert, B.: Soft-tissue reticulum-cell sarcoma of the oral cavity, Oral Surg. **45**:894, 1978.

Scott, J., and Finch, L. D.: Wegener's granulomatosis presenting as gingivitis, Oral Surg. **34**:920, 1972.

Shafer, W. G.: Initial mismanagement and delay in diagnosis of oral cancer, J. Am. Dent. Assoc. **90**:1262, 1975.

572 Pathology of oral mucosa, tongue, and salivary glands

Shafer, W. G.: Oral carcinoma in situ, Oral Surg. 39:227, 1975.

Shillitoe, E. J., and Silverman, S. Jr.: Oral cancer and herpes simplex virus: a review, Oral Surg. 48:216, 1979.

Silverman, S. Jr., and Griffith, M.: Smoking characteristics of patients with oral carcinoma and the risk for second oral primary carcinomas, J. Am. Dent. Assoc. 85:637, 1972.

Solomon, M. P.: Intraoral submucosal pseudosarcomatous fibromatosis, Oral Surg. 38:264, 1974.

Solomon, M. P., and Sutton, A. L.: Malignant fibrous histiocytoma of the soft tissues of the mandible, Oral Surg. 35:653, 1973.

Soman, C. S., and Sirat, M. V.: Primary malignant melanoma of the oral cavity in Indians, Oral Surg. 38:426, 1974.

Someren, A., Karcioglu, Z., and Clairmont, A. A., Jr.: Polypoid spindle-cell carcinoma (pleomorphic carcinoma), Oral Surg. 42:474, 1976.

Soule, E. H., and Enriquez, P.: Atypical fibrous histiocytoma, malignant fibrous histiocytoma, malignant histiocytoma, and epitheloid sarcoma: a comparative study of 65 tumors, CA 30:128, 1972.

Spiro, R. H., and Strong, E. W.: Epidermoid carcinoma of oral cavity and oropharynx: elective vs. therapeutic radical neck dissection as treatment, Arch. Surg. 107:382, 1973.

Stern, M. H., Turner, J. E., and Coburn, T. P.: Oral involvement in neuroblastoma, J. Am. Dent. Assoc. 88:346, 1974.

Stout, A. P.: Pseudosarcomatous fasciitis in children, CA 14:1216, 1961.

Stout, A. P., and Kenney, F. R.: Primary plasma-cell tumors of the upper air passages and oral cavity, CA 2:261, 1949.

Takagi, M., Ishikawa, G., and Mori, W.: Primary malignant melanoma of the oral cavity in Japan: with special reference to mucosal melanosis, CA 34:358, 1974.

Teisberg, P., and Enger, E.: Immunosuppressive therapy in Wegener's granulomatosis, Acta Med. Scand. 187:7, 1970.

Tomich, C. E., and Shafer, W. G.: Squamous acanthoma of the oral mucosa, Oral Surg. 38:755, 1974.

Tomich, C. E., and Shafer, W. G.: Lymphoproliferative disease of the hard palate, Oral Surg. 39:754, 1975.

Tsukada, Y., and Pickren, J. W.: Rhabdomyoma of sublingual region, Oral Surg. 20:640, 1965.

Turner, H., and Snitzer, J.: Carcinoma of the tongue in a child, Oral Surg. 37:663, 1974.

Wedgwood, D., Rusen, D., and Balk, S.: Gingival metastasis from primary hepatocellular carcinoma, Oral Surg. 47:263, 1979.

Weissfeld, B., and Shosheim, A. M.: Lethal midline granuloma: report of a case, J. Oral Surg. 27:206, 1969.

Weitzner, S.: Adenoid squamous-cell carcinoma of vermilion mucosa of lower lip, Oral Surg. 37:589, 1974.

Weitzner, S.: Clear-cell acanthoma of vermilion mucosa of lower lip, Oral Surg. **37:**911, 1974.

Weitzner, S.: Basal-cell carcinoma of the vermilion mucosa and skin of the lip, Oral Surg. **39:**634, 1975.

Weitzner, S., Lockey, M. W., and Lockard, V. G.: Adult rhabdomyoma of soft palate, Oral Surg. **47:**70, 1979.

Werning, J. T.: Nodular fasciitis of the orofacial region, Oral Surg. **48:**441, 1979.

Zegarelli, D. J., Tsukada, Y., Pickren, J. W., and Greene, G. W.: Metastatic tumor to the tongue, Oral Surg. **35:**202, 1973.

CHAPTER 17

Lesions of salivary glands

Nonneoplastic enlargements

1. Mumps (infectious parotitis)
2. Cat-scratch disease
3. Sarcoidosis (Besnier-Boeck-Schaumann disease)
   a. Heerfordt's syndrome (uveo-parotitis; uveoparotid fever)
4. Mikulicz's disease (benign lymphoepithelial lesion)
5. Mikulicz's syndrome
6. Sjögren's syndrome (sicca syndrome)
7. Fatty infiltration
8. Hypertrophy
9. Sialadenitis
10. Ranula and mucocele
11. Lymphoepithelial cyst
12. Cheilitis glandularis apostematosa
13. Cytomegalic inclusion disease
14. Necrotizing sialometaplasia
15. Miscellaneous enlargements

Neoplastic enlargements

1. Adenoma (monomorphic adenoma)
2. Oncocytoma
3. Warthin's tumor (papillary cystadenoma lymphomatosum)
4. Mixed tumor (pleomorphic adenoma)
5. Mucoepidermoid tumor
6. Acinic cell carcinoma
7. Adenocystic carcinoma (cylindroma; basaloid mixed tumor)
8. Adenocarcinoma
9. Juvenile hemangioma
10. Lymphangioma, schwannoma, and xanthoma

There are three major and from 400 to 500 minor salivary glands that empty their secretions in the oral cavity. During development, the invagination of the oral epithelium leads to their formation. Therefore, both developmentally and functionally, they are a part of the oral mucous membrane. Their secretions are mucous or serous or mixed, but the cells that line their ducts have the potential of differentiating into either a mucous or a serous type. The location, name, type, and other features of the major and minor salivary glands are given in Table 18.

574

Table 18. Major and minor salivary glands

Gland(s)	Type of secretory cell
Parotid	Serous
Submaxillary	Mainly serous but few mucous
Sublingual	Mainly mucous but few serous
Minor sublingual (Rivinus')	Mixed but mainly mucous
Of lip	Mixed but mainly mucous
Of cheek	Mixed but mainly mucous
Glossopalatine	Pure mucous
Anterior lingual (Blandin and Nuhn's)	Mixed
Of Ebner (associated with circum- vallate papillae	Serous
Of root of tongue	Mucous
Of posterior half of hard palate	Mucous
Of soft palate and uvula	Mucous
Of retromolar pad	Mucous

Besides these glands, salivary gland tissue may be included within the retromolar area of the mandible.

The parotid gland empties its secretion into the oral cavity through Stensen's duct, the submaxillary gland through Whartton's duct, and the sublingual gland through Bartholin's duct. The minor sublingual glands (Rivinus' glands) empty into the oral cavity by a number of small independent ducts (Rivinus' ducts). All other minor salivary glands have independent duct systems and independent small orifices on the mucosal surface.

It is apparent from Table 18 that salivary glands are present everywhere in the oral cavity with the exception of the gingiva and the anterior half of the hard palate.

The parotid and, to a lesser degree, the submaxillary glands are closely associated with true lymph nodes. The supraparotid, intraparotid, and subparotid lymph nodes lie on, within, or medial to the parotid gland (Fig. 17-1, A). These lymph nodes drain the skin of the anterior temporal region, the lateral parts of the forehead and eyelids, the posterior part of the cheek, part of the outer ear, the parotid gland, and the lateral wall of the pharynx. Since the parotid gland and the cervical lymph nodes,

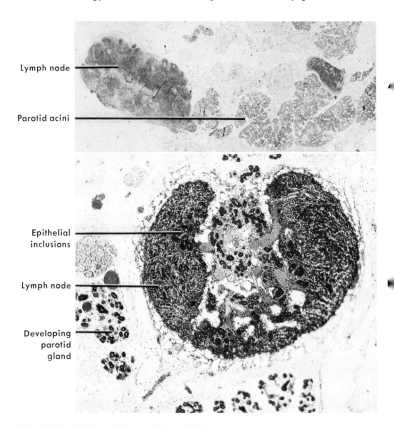

Lymph node

Parotid acini

Epithelial
inclusions

Lymph node

Developing
parotid
gland

Fig. 17-1. A, Part of the parotid gland showing two small lymph nodes among the glandular acini. **B,** Section from the cervical area of a fetus. Note the epithelial inclusions in the developing lymph node.

including the parotid nodes, develop simultaneously and within the same area in the fetus, cervical lymph nodes contain inclusions of glandular epithelium (Fig. 17-1, *B*). This relationship is of importance in understanding some of the salivary gland lesions.

The earliest stage in the development of the salivary glands consists of the invagination of oral epithelium and the formation of the duct system. Later the acini differentiate from the epithelial lining of these ducts. The duct cells maintain this potential throughout life and are the source of most if not all of the neoplasms.

NONNEOPLASTIC ENLARGEMENTS

Mumps (infectious parotitis). This higly infectious viral disease is transmitted through the patient's saliva.

It occurs most often in children (5 to 15 years), in whom it usually affects the parotid glands. Other salivary glands, the gonads, the pancreas, or the breast may also be affected; but these complications generally occur in older patients.

The disease has an incubation period of about 2 to 3 weeks and starts with fever, malaise, and pain in the parotid area, following which the parotid glands become swollen. The patient complains of bad taste and loss of appetite. The disease regresses in a week or 10 days. In rare cases (usually in adults) orchitis followed by sterility may result.

Microscopic sections show degenerative changes in the epithelium of the ducts, interstitial infiltration of the glandular lobules by lymphocytes and mononuclear cells, a few areas of acinar atrophy, and in cases of secondary bacterial infection the presence of polymorphonuclear leukocytes.

Mumps, like many viral diseases, requires only symptomatic treatment. Healing is usually uneventful and without any residual effects. One contact with the disease affords lifelong immunity.

Cat-scratch disease. This affliction, caused by the *Bedsonia* group of organisms (obligate intracellular parasites between the rickettsiae and viruses), primarily affects the lymph nodes. When it involves the parotid or submaxillary lymph nodes, it appears clinically as a submaxillary or parotid "tumor"; and for this reason it is described in the present chapter.

Cat-scratch disease is an inflammatory process associated with a cat scratch, and it has an incubation period of from 1 to 3 weeks. Patients are usually under 30 years of age, and the disease is most common during the fall and winter months. The regional nodes enlarge and become painful. The most common nodes involved are the axillary, followed by those in the cervical, preauricular, submandibular, and inguinal areas. The patient complains of malaise, fever, nausea, chills, and headache.

The disease is self-limiting, most cases regressing within 6 weeks. However, sometimes lymphadenopathy persists for as long as 6 months. A skin sensitivity test with the cat-scratch antigen (the Hanger-Rose test) is diagnostic.

Microscopic sections show hyperplastic lymph nodes with multiple abscesses. The abscesses have a central area of necrosis surrounded by a dense aggregate of neutrophils. Around the neutrophils is a zone of histiocytes (Fig. 17-2). The salivary gland appears normal.

Treatment of cat-scratch disease is only symptomatic, and lesions heal without complication.

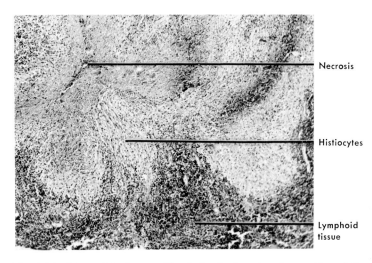

Necrosis

Histiocytes

Lymphoid tissue

Fig. 17-2. Cat-scratch disease. The lesion had produced a swelling of the parotid gland.

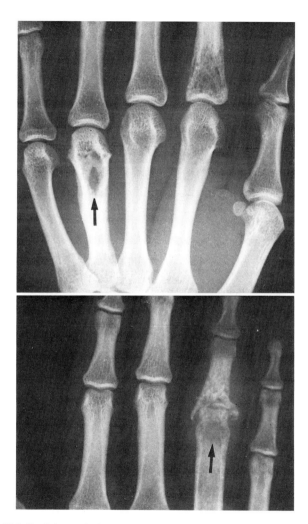

Fig. 17-3. Radiolucent lesions in the phalanges in a patient with sarcoidosis.

Occasionally the portal of entry is the conjunctiva, and in these cases conjunctivitis is associated with the enlargement of a parotid lymph node. This has been called *Parinaud's oculo-glandular syndrome*.

Sarcoidosis (Besnier-Boeck-Schaumann disease). This chronic granulomatous disease is believed to be related to tuberculosis.

Sarcoidosis usually affects young adults, involving the lungs, spleen, lymph nodes, skin, parotid glands, and bones of the hand (Fig. 17-3). Lesions may be asymptomatic and discovered accidentally, or the patient may complain of fever, malaise, and respiratory symptoms. A diagnostic skin sensitivity test (the *Kveim test*, or Nickerson-Kveim test) is positive in about 85% of active cases, but an immunoglobulin test is more reliable.

Oral lesions involve the parotid gland or the oral mucosa (e.g., the soft palate). In about half the cases the parotid glands are unilaterally enlarged, and in about half a bilateral enlargement is the first clinical manifestation (Figs. 17-4 and 17-5, *A*). Facial paralysis may be associated with the parotid involvement. Mucosal lesions appear as multiple granular areas or granulomatous masses (p. 676).

Microscopic sections of the parotid gland show a few or many small, circumscribed granulomas that replace the glandular parenchyma (Fig. 17-5, *B*). These consist of one or more giant cells and a syncytium of histiocytes. The latter superficially resemble epithelium and are therefore called epithelioid

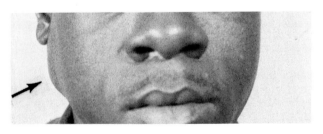

Fig. 17-4. Sarcoidosis of the parotid gland (arrow).

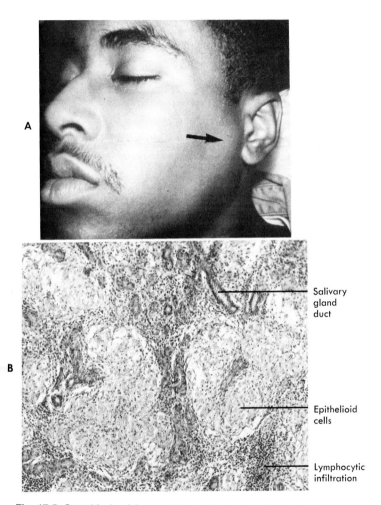

A

B

Salivary
gland
duct

Epithelioid
cells

Lymphocytic
infiltration

Fig. 17-5. Sarcoidosis of the parotid gland. In **A,** note the glandular enlargement (arrow). **B** shows how nodules of epithelioid cells have replaced the
glandular tissue.

cells. The giant cells may contain basophilic (Schaumann) or star-shaped (asteroid) bodies. There is no necrosis. The periphery of the granulomas shows very mild lymphocytic infiltration. The microscopic appearance of lesions of the mucosa is identical to that described for lesions of the parotid gland.

There is no local treatment for sarcoidosis of the parotid gland or oral mucosa.

Heerfordt's syndrome (uveoparotitis; uveoparotid fever). Sarcoidosis (or sarcoidosis-like lesions) and enlargement of the parotid gland associated with fever and inflammation of the uveal tract of the eye are called Heerfordt's syndrome. (The uveal tract consists of the choroid, iris, and ciliary body.) In addition to these features, malaise and facial paralysis may be present.

The disease usually regresses spontaneously. Microscopic sections through the enlarged gland show sarcoidosis.

Mikulicz's disease (benign lymphoepithelial lesion). This swelling of the salivary and lacrimal glands has had a somewhat long and mysterious history.

The lesions consist of unilateral, bilateral, or multiple involvement of the salivary glands; in the majority of cases (about 90%) one or both parotid glands are affected, and in the remaining cases the submaxillary glands are affected (Fig. 17-6). The parotid enlargement may be accompanied by enlargement of minor salivary glands (e.g., salivary glands of the tongue and palate) and of the lacrimal gland (Figs. 17-6 and 17-7).

Mikulicz's disease presents usually as asymptomatic swellings with a duration of a few months to many years. The swellings may be diffuse and involve the major part of the gland, or they may present as single or multiple nodules. The size of the swellings varies from time to time. The majority of lesions occur between the ages of 20 and 60 years, and males are afflicted about twice as frequently as females. Some patients have a history of local inflammatory lesions (e.g., abscessed tooth, upper respiratory tract infection).

Mikulicz's disease may appear in one of two forms: diffuse and nodular. In the *diffuse* form the gland lobules are replaced

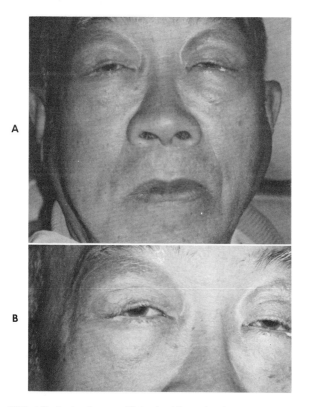

Fig. 17-6. Mikulicz's disease. Note the bilateral enlargement of the parotid glands **(A)** and lacrimal glands **(B).**

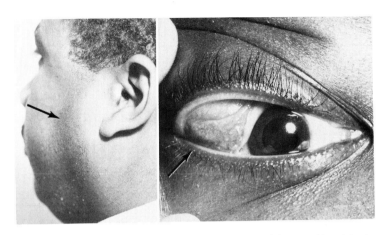

Fig. 17-7. Mikulicz's disease. Note the enlargement of the parotid and lacrimal glands (arrows).

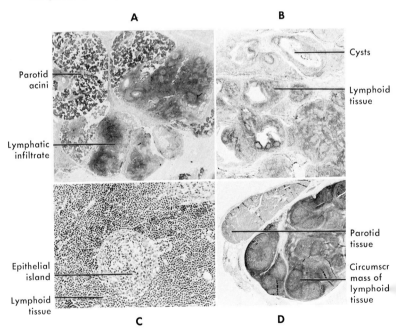

Fig. 17-8. Mikulicz's disease. **A** to **C,** Diffuse type. **D,** Nodular type. The epithelial islands in **B** are sometimes referred to as the *epimyoepithelial* islands.

by a sea of lymphocytes in which islands of squamous epithelium can be seen (Fig. 17-8, *A* and *B*). The acini in the affected lobules disappear, but some of the ducts enlarge to form microcysts (Fig. 17-8, *C*). In the *nodular* form of the disease, microscopic sections show a normal salivary gland with one or more clearly demarcated but hyperplastic lymph nodes (Fig. 17-8, *D*).

Mikulicz's disease represents a hyperplasia of the lymph nodes that are normally embedded in the parotid gland (or submaxillary gland). The lesion is inflammatory and, unless dictated by other circumstances, should be left untreated. Spontaneous regressions occur.

Mikulicz's syndrome. When the parotid or other salivary glands become enlarged due to leukemic infiltration, lymphosarcoma, or tuberculosis, the condition is referred to as Mikulicz's syndrome.

Sjögren's syndrome (sicca syndrome). Sjögren's syndrome consists of enlargement of the salivary glands (Fig. 17-9); dry mouth (xerostomia); dryness of the conjunctiva and pharyngeal, nasal, and laryngeal mucosae (conjunctivitis sicca, rhinitis sicca, pharyngolaryngitis sicca); and arthritis.

The disease is seen most frequently in middle-aged and elderly women. Although its cause is not established, it probably represents and autoimmune phenomenon. Because of the dryness of the mucous membranes, there is secondary inflammation of these areas. The parotid, submaxillary, and minor salivary glands of the lip are most often affected and show infiltration by lymphocytes and atrophy of acini.

Treatment of Sjögren's syndrome is empirical and usually consists of hormonal, vitamin, or antibiotic therapy.

Fatty infiltration. On rare occasion, a unilateral or bilateral enlargement of the major salivary glands, particularly the parotid gland, results from fatty infiltration. It is of unknown cause but may be seen in a variety of conditions, such as protein deficiency (kwashiorkor), alcoholism, cirrhosis of the liver, tuberculosis, pregnancy, lactation, and menopausal states. It occurs among underprivileged peoples in poor countries.

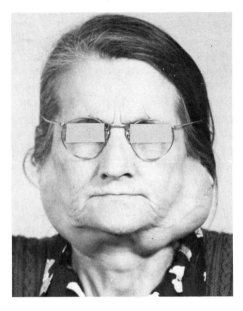

Fig. 17-9. Advanced Sjögren's syndrome. Note the bilateral enlargement of the parotid glands.

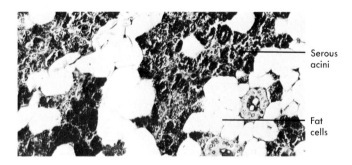

Serous
acini

Fat
cells

Fig. 17-10. Fatty infiltration of the parotid gland.

Microscopic sections reveal infiltration of the lobules with normal fat cells (Fig. 17-10). No treatment is indicated.

Hypertrophy. Hypertrophy occurs more often in the minor than in the major salivary glands. Of the major glands, the parotid is usually affected and hypertrophy occurs under the same conditions as described for fatty infiltration. Clinically the gland shows an asymptomatic, diffuse enlargement.

As stated above, hypertrophy most commonly affects the minor salivary glands (Fig. 17-11). Clinically it presents as a diffuse or small sessile elevation of the oral mucosa or tongue. Lesions are usually excised, and microscopic examination reveals an overabundance of normal salivary gland tissue (usually mucous).

The lesion is, of course, benign and harmless. In some in-

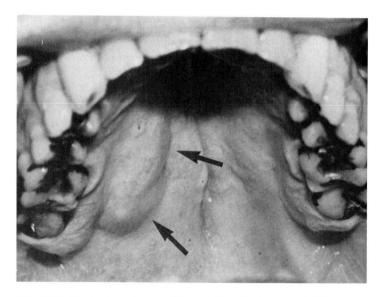

Fig. 17-11. Benign hypertrophy of the palatine glands (arrows). Biopsy was needed to make the correct diagnosis.

stances a diffuse enlargement of oral mucosa, such as the lip, will be due to hypertrophy of the salivary glands.

Sialadenitis. The term sialadenitis means inflammation of the salivary glands. It may be classified into *bacterial* and *obstructive* types.

Bacterial sialadenitis occurs in children or the aged and produces recurrent, acute, painful enlargement of the involved gland. The overlying skin may be red, and milking or compressing the gland will yield a purulent discharge at the duct orifice (Fig. 17-12). Pain and swelling are not related to eating. *Streptococcus viridans* has been associated with the lesions in children, and *Staphylococcus aureus* with lesions in geriatric patients. Treatment consists of heat application, pain-relieving drugs, and antibiotics. Elderly patients usually have some other systemic disability (malnutrition, cancer, dehydration); and in addition to antibiotics, their treatment should consist of hydration and elimination of the associated disability. On rare occasion, bacterial sialadenitis may follow the hematogenous route.

Microscopic sections of bacterial sialadenitis show edema and infiltration of the ducts and lobules by polymorphonuclear leukocytes.

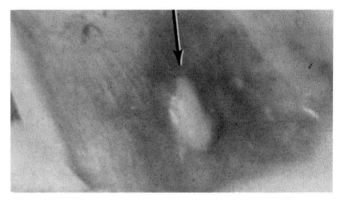

Fig. 17-12. Discharge of pus (arrow) at the orifice of Stensen's duct in a patient with acute parotitis.

Obstructive sialadenitis, the more common form, is associated with salivary stones (sialolithiasis) or mucus plugs. In these cases the duct of the gland is also inflamed (sialodochitis). Obstructive sialadenitis occurs in middle age, and males are afflicted more frequently than females. In order of frequency, the glands involved are the submaxillary (75%) (Fig. 17-13), parotid (20%), and major sublingual (5%). The involved gland is enlarged and painful; but these symptoms are especially prominent before, during, and soon after meals. In sialadenitis that has persisted for a long time, the gland becomes firm, permanently enlarged, and painless.

Clinical examination and manipulation may reveal the presence of a stone in the excretory duct. In rare cases obstructive sialadenitis may also follow stricture or stenosis of the duct due to scarring or surrounding pathology (tumors).

Radiographs of the area may reveal a salivary stone in either the major or the minor duct (Fig. 17-14). After the injection of

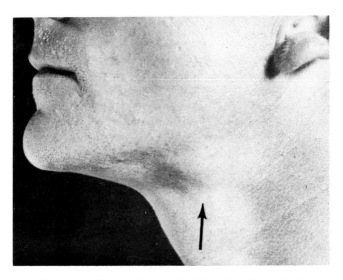

Fig. 17-13. Sialadenitis (arrow) of the submaxillary gland.

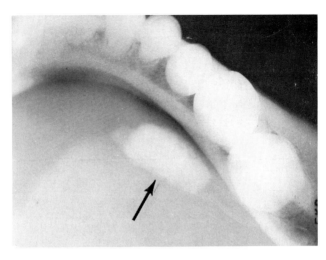

Fig. 17-14. Sialolith (arrow) obstructing Wharton's duct in sialadenitis of the submaxillary gland.

radiopaque material, an irregular pattern of the duct system of the gland as well as the presence of numerous small dilatations in the ducts can be visualized (Fig. 17-15).

Sections through the appropriate area reveal salivary stones that appear as concentric pink and blue bodies with varying degrees of calcification (Fig. 17-16). The major ducts of the gland are dilated. The duct containing the calculus or mucous plug shows squamous metaplasia of its lining. The interstitial tissue of the gland lobules shows edema and infiltration by plasma cells, neutrophils, and lymphocytes. Depending on the duration of the disease process, there is some atrophy of the acini (Fig. 17-17). In long-standing disease a considerable amount of fibrosis and atrophy can lead to replacement of the entire gland by connective tissue so that only the ducts of the original gland can be seen (Fig. 17-17).

Treatment varies with circumstances. Stones that lie near the duct orifice can be removed manually. In deep-seated ob-

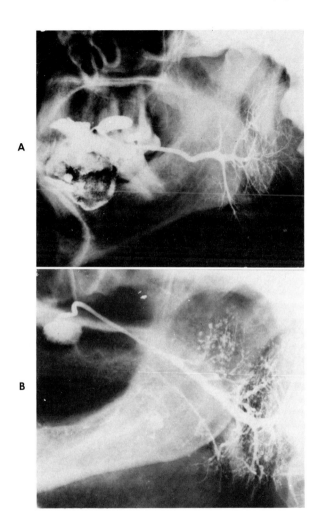

Fig. 17-15. Salivary duct system in a normal patient **(A)** and in a patient with sialadenitis **(B)** after an intraductal injection of radiopaque material. In **A,** note the treelike duct pattern. In **B,** note irregularities in the overall pattern as well as constrictions and dilatations of the individual ducts.

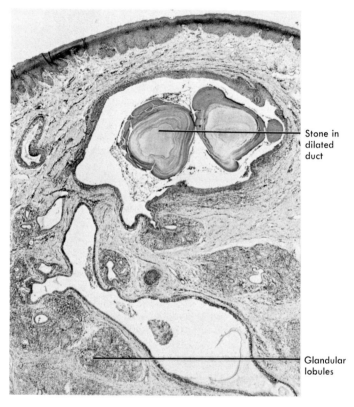

Stone in
dilated
duct

Glandular
lobules

Fig. 17-16. Obstructive sialadenitis. The gland lobules show atrophy of acini
and fibrosis. The duct contains a sialolith.

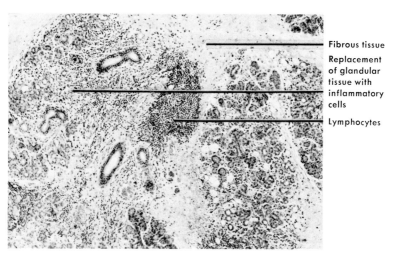

Fibrous tissue

Replacement of glandular tissue with inflammatory cells

Lymphocytes

Fig. 17-17. Sialadenitis is characterized by atrophy of acini and infiltration of the gland by plasma cells, neutrophils, and lymphocytes.

struction, sialagogues have been tried. In acute nonobstructive sialadenitis, antibiotics eliminate the process. In chronic, long-standing obstructive disease, surgical excision is often necessary. Sometimes ligation of the duct, with accompanying total atrophy of the gland, is the best treatment.

Lesions resembling those seen in sialadenitis have been described in the submaxillary, sublingual, and labial glands of children with cystic fibrosis of the pancreas. Biopsy of the lip has therefore been suggested as a diagnostic tool for this disease.

Salivary calculi and accompanying sialadenitis can occur in the minor salivary glands. The lesions appear as solitary, freely movable, firm masses and occur most often in the upper lip and buccal mucosa of adults. Microscopic findings are similar to those described for the major glands.

Ranula and mucocele. Ranulas and mucoceles are usually seen in the mucous membrane. Rarely, however, they arise within the major glands, where they produce an ill-defined enlargement. In these areas their microscopic appearance and mechanism of development are identical to those described earlier (mucocele, p. 461; ranula, p. 463).

Lymphoepithelial cyst. This relatively rare lesion occurs in the parotid gland and produces a clinically discernable enlargement.

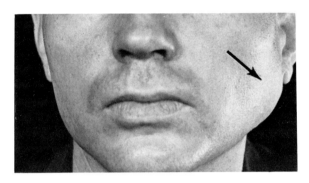

Fig. 17-18. Lymphoepithelial cyst of the parotid gland (arrow).

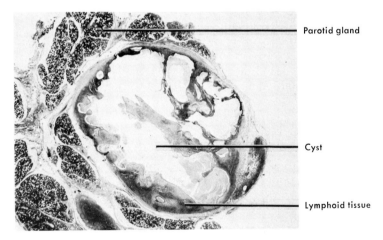

Fig. 17-19. Lymphoepithelial cyst of the parotid gland showing the glandular tissue and a cystic lesion that is lined by lymphocytes.

The lesion is freely movable, painless, and asymptomatic (Fig. 17-18). It develops as a result of a cystic change in the epithelial inclusions that are invariably seen in the parotid lymph nodes. It is therefore identical to the branchial cyst and similar to the lymphoepithelial cyst of the soft oral tissues.

Microscopic features are those of an epithelium-lined cystic cavity surrounded by lymphoid tissue (Fig. 17-19).

Because these cysts mimic tumors, they are usually excised, following which they do not recur.

Cheilitis glandularis apostematosa. This disease is characterized by a chronic enlargement and eversion of one or both lips. The lower lip is more often involved by the process. It is hardened, and its exposed mucosal surface is studded with numerous red openings that exude viscous mucus. Because of this secretion, the lips may stick together. The condition occurs more often in males and usually in whites.

Microscopic sections show hyperplasia of the mucous glands and infiltration by plasma cells and lymphocytes. The cause of this condition is unknown; but heredity and exposure to wind, sun, dust, and tobacco have been implicated.

The use of protective ointments or lip pomades is the treatment of choice.

Cytomegalic inclusion disease. The ductal epithelium of the salivary glands of some infants contains a virus that may cause serious generalized involvement of many organs such as the spleen, liver, bone marrow, and lungs.

This virus belongs to the herpes group of viruses and is characterized by marked enlargement of the cells in which it grows; it is therefore called the cytomegalovirus (Greek, *kytos,* "vessel" [i.e., cell]; *megal-,* "great"), and the disease it produces is cytomegalic inclusion disease. The salivary glands serve primarily as a habitat for this virus, and its presence in this organ does not always signify the clinical manifestation of the disease.

Necrotizing sialometaplasia. This benign lesion is a nonneoplastic, inflammatory, ulcerative disease of the salivary glands. It usually occurs in the minor salivary glands of the palate

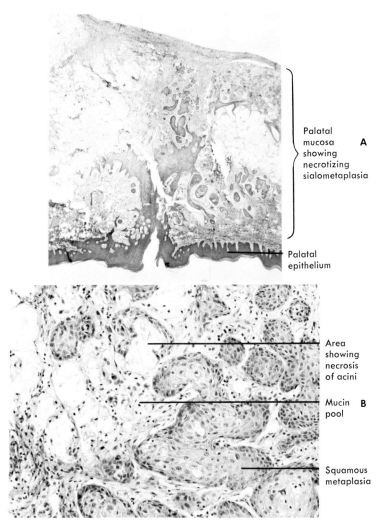

Palatal mucosa showing necrotizing sialometaplasia **A**

Palatal epithelium

Area showing necrosis of acini

Mucin pool **B**

Squamous metaplasia

Fig. 17-20. Histologic features of necrotizing sialometaplasia consist of changes that superficially mimic those of a neoplasm. **B** is a higher magnification of an area in **A**.

(88%), usually in the adult (fifth and sixth decades, average age 46 years), and is more common in the male than in the female (2.7:1). It involves whites more than blacks. Although primarily a lesion of the palate, it may occur in other areas of the oral cavity (retromolar pad, nasopharynx, parotid gland).

The lesion appears as an ulcer 1 to 2 cm in size, is of a few weeks' to months' duration, and clinically mimics salivary gland or squamous cell carcinoma. Its cause is not known, but trauma and infarction are probably contributing factors. The importance of this lesion lies in the fact that microscopically it mimics a mucoepidermoid carcinoma of the salivary glands. It actually is a response of the minor salivary glands to an overlying mucosal ulcer.

Histologic features consist of ulceration, necrosis of gland acini, pools of mucin, edema, neutrophilic infiltration, and prominent squamous metaplasia of ducts and acini (Fig. 17-20). This last feature mimics the mucoepidermoid carcinoma. The lobular morphology of the gland is retained.

This lesion is benign and self-limiting, and heals spontaneously.

Miscellaneous enlargements. Numerous systemic conditions are known to cause enlargement of major salivary glands. Some of these have been described and cause fatty infiltration or hypertrophy. Also, nonspecific enlargements can occur in patients with malnutrition, protein deficiency, vitamin A and vitamin B deficiencies, pellagra, beriberi, inadequate diet, alcoholism, diabetes mellitus, decreased endocrine pancreatic function, hypoglycemia and hyperglycemia, obesity, liver disease, cardiospasm, thyroid diseases, pregnancy, lactation, and menopause.

NEOPLASTIC ENLARGEMENTS

The tumors that arise in salivary glands have been the subject of numerous classifications. The number and variety of these classifications attest to the fact that these tumors are interesting but poorly understood. Although the literature on these tumors is extensive, the classification and incidence given in Table 19 represent a practical and pertinent summary.

Clinically tumors of the salivary glands usually fall into two distinct groups: benign and malignant. To avoid unnecessary repetition, therefore, these features are described prior to the discussion of the individual tumors.

Benign tumors are usually of long duration (years). They present as single nodules that are not fixed to the overlying skin or mucous membrane. However, recurrent lesions may be multinodular.

Benign tumors grow slowly and are usually asymptomatic. Unlike the inflammatory lesions, they do not fluctuate in size. Benign tumors of the palate do not, as a rule, produce diffuse radiolucencies or loosening of the teeth.

Table 19. Classification and incidence of tumors of salivary glands

Type	Approximate frequency (%)
Epithelial tumors	
Benign	
Adenoma	<0.5
Oncocytoma	<0.5
Warthin's tumor (papillary cystadenoma lymphomatosum)	4 to 5
Mixed tumor (pleomorphic adenoma)	75
Malignant	
Mucoepidermoid tumor	4 to 5
Acinic cell carcinoma	<0.5
Adenocystic carcinoma (cylindroma; basaloid mixed tumor)	4
All types of adenocarcinomas and malignant mixed tumor	8.5
Mesenchymal tumors	
Benign	
Juvenile hemangioma	<1
Lymphangioma, schwannoma, and xanthoma	<1
Malignant	
None	

Malignant tumors are usually of shorter duration than benign tumors (weeks to months). They grow rapidly or have a history of slow growth with sudden rapid activity. They are fixed to the surrounding tissues. The overlying skin or mucous membrane may be ulcerated and inflamed. Patients with a cancer of the major salivary glands are seven times more likely to develop cancer of the breast than is the general population.

Malignant tumors of the parotid gland may be associated with facial nerve paralysis or other neurologic symptoms. The regional lymph nodes may be enlarged. Tumors of the palate and retromolar glands infiltrate the underlying bone early and produce diffuse radiolucencies and loosening of the teeth.

Adenoma (monomorphic adenoma). This relatively rare tumor of salivary gland origin occurs more frequently in the minor than in the major glands, presents as a small, freely movable, circumscribed nodule (Fig. 17-21), and usually occurs after the

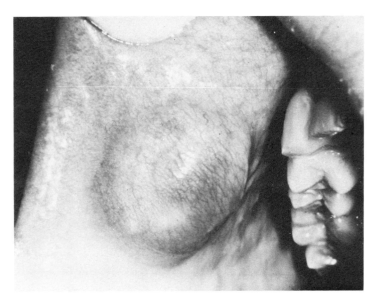

Fig. 17-21. Adenoma of the minor salivary glands of the cheek.

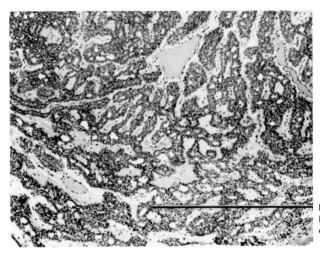
Ductlike structures
lined by
epithelium

Fig. 17-22. Adenoma of a palatal salivary gland. Note the uniform field of ductlike structures.

age of 30 years. Adenomas are the smallest and least aggressive of the epithelial salivary gland tumors.

Microscopic sections show an encapsulated lesion composed of a monotonous succession of ducts. These are lined by cuboidal or columnar epithelium (Fig. 17-22). It is extremely rare for adenomas to consist exlusively of mucous or serous cells.

Treatment consists of excision, and the lesion rarely recurs.

Oncocytoma. This rare benign tumor of old age usually occurs after the age of 55 years. Females are affected more often than males. The tumor is almost always seen in the parotid gland. Its clinical features are the same as those previously described for benign tumors in general (p. 598).

Microscopic sections show an encapsulated tumor that consists exclusively of a single cell type, the oncocyte (Greek, *onkos*, "bulk"). This is a large, clearly outlined, eosinophilic cell with a small dark, centrally located nucleus. The oncocytes occur in sheets and columns (Fig. 17-23).

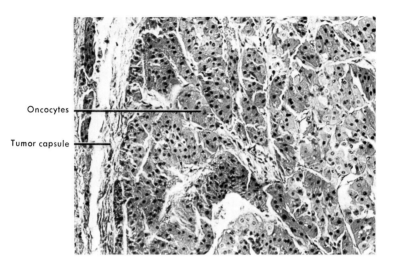

Oncocytes

Tumor capsule

Fig. 17-23. An oncocytoma consists of large eosinophilic cells called onco-cytes.

An oncocytoma is treated by excision. It does not recur. A malignant variant of this tumor has been described but is extremely rare.

Warthin's tumor (papillary cystadenoma lymphomatosum). Warthin's tumor constitutes about 4% of all salivary gland tumors (Table 19). It usually occurs between the ages of 40 and 70 years, with the greatest incidence between 50 and 60 years.

Almost 90% of patients are males. The majority of the lesions affect the parotid gland (Fig. 17-24), but the tumor may arise in the submaxillary gland or in the neck. Other clinical features of this tumor are the same as those described for benign tumors in general (p. 598). Gross specimens are encapsulated, and their cut surface shows cystic spaces that exude thick mucus.

Warthin's tumor is an encapsulated tumor consisting of numerous cystic spaces whose walls are thrown into papillae and

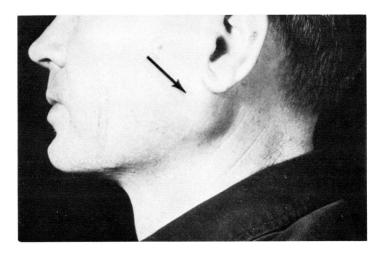

Fig. 17-24. Warthin's tumor (papillary cystadenoma lymphomatosum) (arrow).

folds. These are lined by a double layer of cells; the inner layer is columnar, the outer is cuboidal, and both are eosinophilic (Fig. 17-25). The cystic spaces contain homogeneous eosinophilic material. All cysts lie in a sea of lymphocytes that show follicles as well as sinusoids. The tumors arise from epithelial (glandular) inclusions within the parotid and cervical lymph nodes (p. 576).

Excision is the treatment of choice. If the tumor is completely excised, recurrences are rare. An extremely rare malignant form of this tumor has been described.

Mixed tumor (pleomorphic adenoma). In addition to the features described for benign tumors generally (p. 598), mixed tumor has the following clinical characteristics.

It constitutes 75% of all salivary gland tumors. Of the mixed tumors affecting the major salivary glands, 90% occur in the parotid gland, with the tail of the gland as the favored site (Fig. 17-26); 9% occur in the submaxillary gland; and 1% occur in the sublingual gland. The sites of origin of tumors of the minor sal-

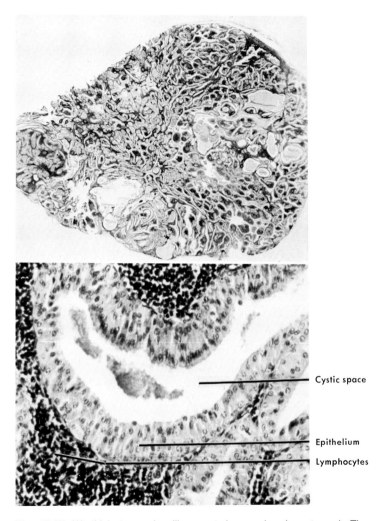

Fig. 17-25. Warthin's tumor (papillary cystadenoma lymphomatosum). The lesion consists of many epithelium-lined cystic spaces in a stroma of lympho-cytes.

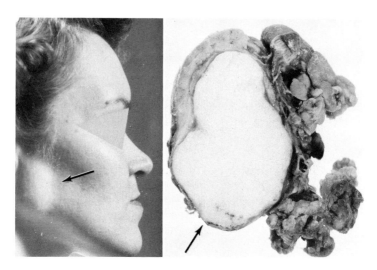

Fig. 17-26. Mixed tumor of the parotid gland (arrows).

ivary glands (in descending order of frequency) are the palate, lip, tongue, cheek, and floor of the mouth (Fig. 17-27). Mixed tumors occur after the age of 30 years and are slightly more common in females than in males. Grossly the tumors are solid, encapsulated, mucoid, pale yellow masses (Fig. 17-26).

As the name indicates, mixed tumor is a tumor with a varied (pleomorphic) microscopic picture. It contains areas resembling hyaline cartilage (i.e., homogeneous basophilic matrix in which numerous cells are seen). Although these areas resemble cartilage, they actually are mucoid material with embedded epithelial tumor cells (Fig. 17-28).

Microscopic features include myxomatous areas of loosely and sparsely arranged epithelial cells with overabundant intercellular substance (Fig. 17-28), ducts, islands, cords, and clusters of cuboidal, columnar, and squamosal epithelium, as well as rare areas of bone and keratin formation. A recurrent lesion is multinodular and nonencapsulated.

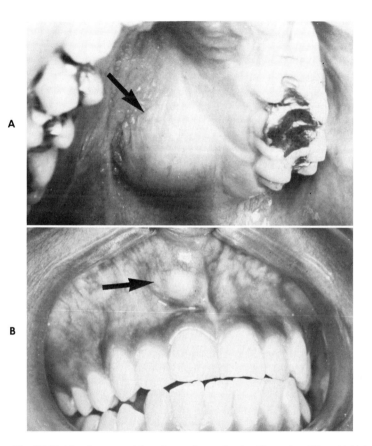

Fig. 17-27. Mixed tumors of the minor salivary glands of the palate **(A)** and labial anterior vestibule **(B).**

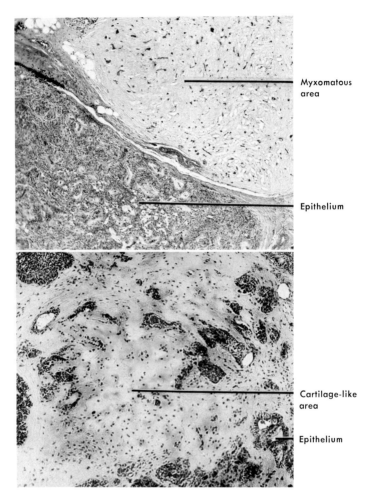

Fig. 17-28. Mixed tumor. Note the epithelial cords and sheets and the myxomatous and cartilage-like areas.

A wide surgical excision of the tumor is the recommended treatment. Mixed tumors are the most persistent of all benign salivary gland neoplasms, with a recurrence rate of 5% to 30%. Since recurrences are multinodular and therefore more difficult to eradicate than the primary lesion, wide excision of the primary lesion is indicated. The tumor does not metastasize, but on rare occasion it will terminate in a malignant mixed tumor that behaves like an adenocarcinoma (p. 615). A sudden spurt of growth in a slowly growing mixed tumor is thus an ominous sign.

Mucoepidermoid tumor. Between 4% and 5% of all salivary gland tumors belong to the group of mucoepidermoid tumors. About 69% of these occur in the parotid gland, 15% in the palate, 7% in the submaxillary gland, 5% in the cheek, and the remaining 4% in the lips, floor of the mouth (Figs. 17-29 and 17-30), and retromolar area.

Tumors of the major salivary glands are usually larger than those of the minor glands. Mucoepidermoid tumors are more common in males than in females. The average duration is two years. More than half the tumors occur between the ages of 20 and 40 years, with the remainder occuring in both younger and older patients.

Clinically some of these lesions resemble benign tumors, whereas others have the characteristics of malignant tumors. These features have already been described (p. 599). The cut surface of the tumor presents a slimy, semitranslucent, solid or cystic appearance (Fig. 17-29).

Microscopically mucoepidermoid tumors are composed of three cell types: mucous, epidermoid, and clear (Fig. 17-31). The *mucous* cells are essentially like those seen in the mucous glands (i.e., they are large, vacuolated, and light staining, and they contain mucin). The *epidermoid* cells are of various shapes and forms and resemble the cells in different layers of the oral epithelium. The *clear* cells are large, and their cytoplasm appears empty.

Electron microscopic studies show the mucus-secreting cells

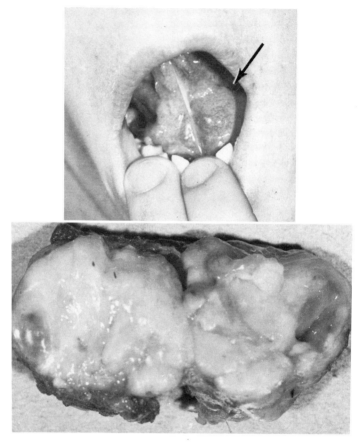

Fig. 17-29. Mucoepidermoid tumor of the floor of the mouth (arrow). The bisected gross specimen is shown below.

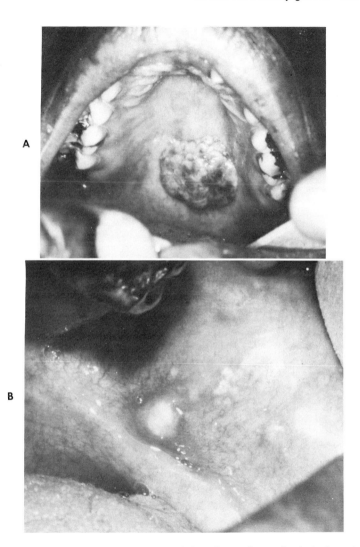

Fig. 17-30. Mucoepidermoid tumor of the minor salivary glands (palate, **A**, and cheek, **B**). Because of their location, intraoral lesions have a better prognosis than do lesions of the major salivary glands.

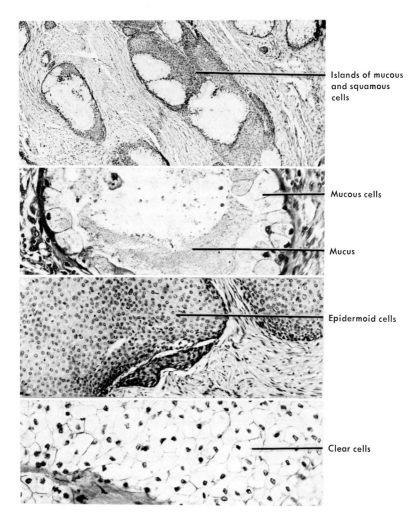

Islands of mucous and squamous cells

Mucous cells

Mucus

Epidermoid cells

Clear cells

Fig. 17-31. A mucoepidermoid tumor is composed of epidermoid, mucous, and clear cell types.

to have numerous mucous globules and bundles of fine cytoplasmic filaments. Epidermoid cells contain a moderate amount of tonofilaments and various organelles. Mucus-secreting and epidermoid cells surrounding cystic spaces show microvilli. The clear cells are rich in glycogen.

These three types of cells appear in varying proportions and in various morphologic arrangements. Large and small cysts containing mucus and lined by the cells described may be seen, or the three cell types may be in sheets. Small and large pools of mucus are often seen in the tumor stroma.

Wide surgical excision is the treatment of choice. Although some authors consider all mucoepidermoid tumors to be malignant, this in fact is not true. Benign and malignant forms exist. A detailed discussion of the problem is beyond the scope of the present text; but briefly, only those tumors which present some or many features of adenocarcinomas (i.e., absence or a minimum of mucoid features, anaplasia, hyperchromatism) are malignant. Malignant types metastasize to the lymph nodes, lungs, bone, or brain and cause death within two years. The benign form does not metastasize; but unless widely excised, it recurs frequently. Wide local excision gives a five-year cure rate of better than 92%.

Acinic cell carcinoma. This tumor occurs primarily in the parotid gland and clinically resembles a benign neoplasm (p. 598). On rare occasion lesions of minor salivary glands of the tongue, palate, and floor of mouth may be seen. It usually occurs in the third decade, is more common in males than in females, and has an average duration of three years.

Microscopic features are characteristic. The tumor consists of a single cell type (a very large cell with a round dark nucleus and deeply basophilic granular cytoplasm) that resembles the acinar cell of the serous glands. The cells are arranged in broad sheets (Fig. 17-32). The tumor is of a low-grade malignancy and may metastasize to regional nodes, but distant metastases are rare.

Surgical excision is the treatment of choice. If the lesion is widely excised, prognosis is good.

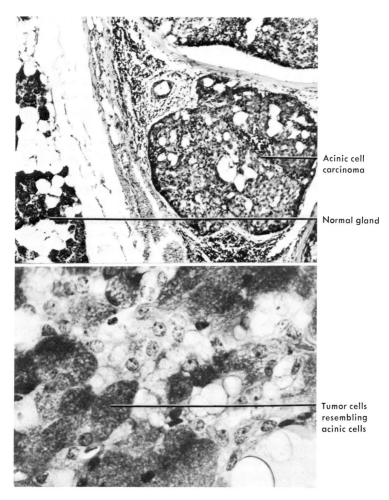

Acinic cell
carcinoma

Normal gland

Tumor cells
resembling
acinic cells

Fig. 17-32. Acinic cell carcinoma of the parotid gland. The prominent feature is a large granular cell that resembles the acinar cells of serous glands.

Adenocystic carcinoma (cylindroma; basaloid mixed tumor).
The adenocystic carcinoma has the following clinical features: it
constitutes about 4% of all salivary gland tumors; there is no
sexual predilection, and the tumor usually occurs after the age
of 50 years; the parotid gland is the favored site, with the palatal
glands (Fig. 17-33) and the submaxillary glands next most frequently affected.

In the major glands the tumor may present the clinical features of benign tumors (p. 598) or be associated with pain, neurologic symptoms, and fixation to surrounding tissues. Lesions
of the palate are accompanied by toothache, loosening of the
teeth, radiolucencies, and, if teeth are extracted, a failure of the
socket to heal. Adenocystic carcinoma is a relatively slow-grow-
ing tumor.

Microscopic sections show a characteristic picture. The tumor consists of small dark-staining epithelial cells that resemble
basal cells of the mucous membrane (Fig. 17-34). Because of
this feature, it is sometimes called basaloid mixed tumor. The

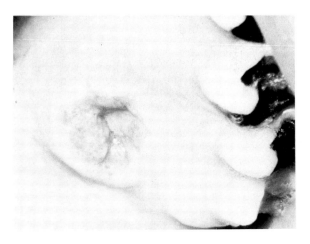

Fig. 17-33. Adenocystic carcinoma of the palatal glands. (Courtesy Milton
Knapp, D.D.S., Portland, Ore.)

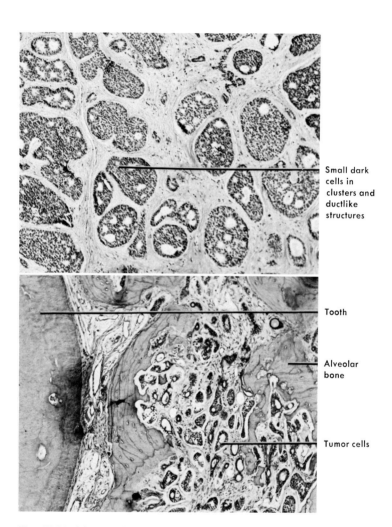

Small dark
cells in
clusters and
ductlike
structures

Tooth

Alveolar
bone

Tumor cells

Fig. 17-34. Adenocystic carcinoma of the maxilla. Note the "Swiss cheese"
appearance of the tumor (top).

epithelial cells are arranged in tubes, islands, columns, and acini. The tubes and acini are empty or contain a homogeneous material that may be basophilic or eosinophilic. In areas where empty tubes and acini predominate, the microscopic field looks like Swiss cheese (Fig. 17-34). The tumor is nonencapsulated, and it infiltrates the surrounding structures. Tumor cells are frequently seen in the perineural lymphatics.

Although adenocystic carcinoma is malignant, it does not metatasize until late in its life history—when it spreads to the regional lymph nodes, lungs, bones, and other viscera. However, the tumor is locally aggressive and may cause death only by local extension—for example, tumors of the palate extend through the cranial base and cause fatal complications.

Wide excision is the only treatment.

Adenocarcinoma. There are numerous varieties of adenocarcinoma that have been segregated from each other because of their morphology (e.g., anaplastic, transitional, squamous cell, trabecular, papillary, solid, malignant mixed). Except for their microscopic features, however, they resemble each other closely and will be considered as a group.

Besides the clinical features of malignant tumors in general (p. 599), the adenocarcinomas have the following characteristics: they constitute about 8.5% of all salivary gland tumors and are the most rapidly growing of all salivary gland neoplasms; on an average, they occur at a later age than do other types of salivary gland tumors; ulceration and fixation (Fig. 17-35), neurologic symptoms, and lymph node and distant metastases (Fig. 17-36) are common.

The microscopic pictures vary with the different types. Squamous cell carcinoma of the salivary glands resembles or is identical to the squamous cell carcinoma seen elsewhere. Some tumors show cords, tubes, islands, and acini of anaplastic glandular epithelium (adenocarcinoma). In a few tumors anaplastic, hyperchromatic, bizarre cells form large sheets of trabeculae without an attempt at gland formation (trabecular adenocarcinoma). One portion of a lesion may resemble a mixed tumor,

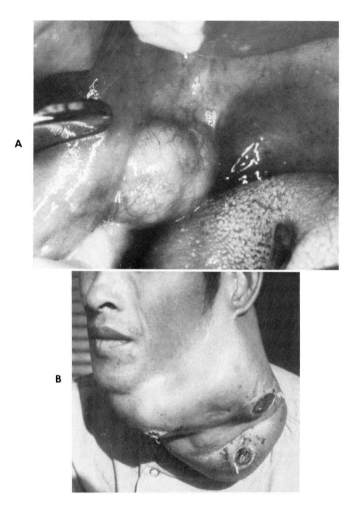

Fig. 17-35. Adenocarcinoma of the minor **(A)** and major **(B)** salivary glands.

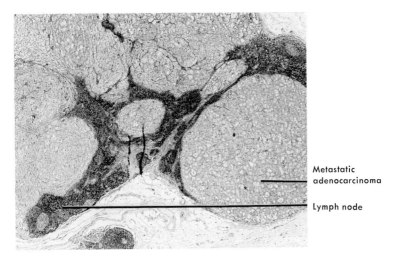

Metastatic
adenocarcinoma

Lymph node

Fig. 17-36. Adenocarcinoma of the salivary glands metastatic to a cervical lymph node.

whereas another will show the features of one of the adenocarcinoma types (malignant mixed tumor). In certain malignant tumors there are broad sheets of cells with ill-defined borders and absence of gland formation. The microscopic picture of these is almost identical to that of the transitional cell carcinoma, and they are so designated. In papillary or papillary cystic adenocarcinomas the projections of tumor cells extend fingerlike into the cystic cavity.

Radical surgical procedures constitute the only treatment of the adenocarcinomas. In inoperable cases, of course, radiation is used as a palliative procedure. The prognosis is grave.

Juvenile hemangioma. The most common salivary gland tumor of infancy, the juvenile hemangioma, is a mesenchymal tumor that usually occurs in the parotid gland. However, the submaxillary gland, lip, or sublingual gland is sometimes involved.

The vast majority of patients are under 6 months of age, and all of them are under 5 years. Females are afflicted almost three

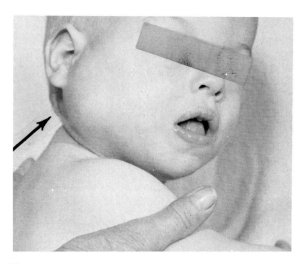

Fig. 17-37. Juvenile hemangioma (arrow) of the parotid gland.

times more frequently than males. The tumor presents as a diffuse, progressively enlarging mass (Fig. 17-37).

Microscopic sections reveal the infiltration and replacement of the glandular lobules by numerous small endothelium-lined blood vessels (Fig. 17-38).

The tumor is benign and can be treated by excision. Some lesions undergo spontaneous regression. Radiation or radical surgery is contraindicated.

Lymphangioma, schwannoma, and xanthoma. Lymphangiomas of the neck or cheek may extend to and involve the parotid gland or other major salivary glands (Fig. 17-39). They replace the glandular tissue and, in their histology and behavior, are identical to those seen in other areas of the oral cavity.

Schwannomas and xanthomas of the salivary glands are rare. Clinically and microscopically they resemble their counterparts elsewhere in the oral cavity (schwannoma, p. 512; xanthoma or xanthogranuloma p. 524).

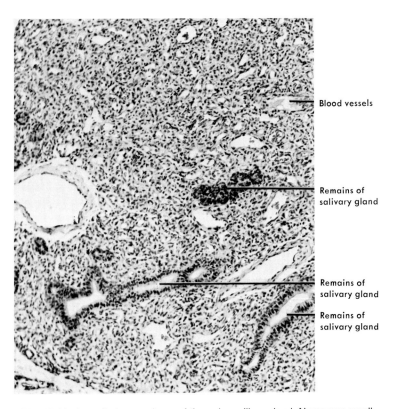

Blood vessels

Remains of
salivary gland

Remains of
salivary gland

Remains of
salivary gland

Fig. 17-38. Juvenile hemangioma of the submaxillary gland. Numerous small
blood vessels have replaced glandular acini.

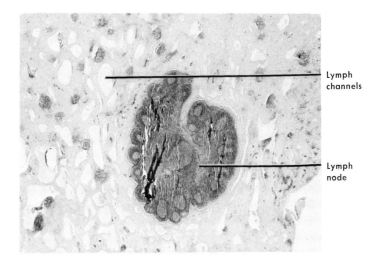

Fig. 17-39. Lymphangioma. Lymph channels have completely replaced the parotid gland. Only an intraparotid lymph node has remained unaffected.

REFERENCES

Abrams, A. M., Cornyn, J., Schofield, H. H., and Hansen, L. S.: Acinic cell adenocarcinoma of the major salivary glands, CA **18:**1145, 1965.

Abrams, A. M., and Melrose, R. J.: Acinic cell tumors of minor salivary gland origin, Oral Surg. **46:**220, 1978.

Abrams, A. M., Melrose, R. J., and Howell, F. V.: Necrotizing sialometaplasia, a disease simulating malignancy, CA **32:**130, 1973.

Adkins, K. F., and Daley, T. J.: Elastic tissues in adenoid cystic carcinomas, Oral Surg. **38:**562, 1974.

Anderson, L. G., and Talal, N.: The spectrum of benign to malignant lymphoproliferation in Sjögren's syndrome, Clin. Exp. Immunol. **9:**199, 1971.

Appel, B. N., El Attar, A. M., Paladino, T. R., and Verbin, R. S.: Multifocal adenoid cystic carcinoma of the lip, Oral Surg. **41:**764, 1976.

Arguelles, M. T., Viloria, J. B., Jr., Talens, M. C., and McCrory, T. P.: Necrotizing sialometaplasia, Oral Surg. **42:**86, 1976.

Batsakis, J. G.: Salivary gland neoplasia: an outcome of modified morphogenesis and cytodifferentiation, Oral Surg. **49:**229, 1980.

Berg, J. W., Hutter, R. V. P., and Foote, F. W., Jr.: The unique association between salivary gland cancer and breast cancer, J.A.M.A. **204:**771, 1968.

Bernier, J. L., and Bhaskar, S. N.: Lymphoepithelial lesions of salivary glands: histogenesis and classification based on 186 cases, CA **11:**1156, 1958.

Bhaskar, S. N.: Acinic-cell carcinoma of salivary glands, Oral Surg. **17:**62, 1964.

Bhaskar, S. N., and Bernier, J. L.: Histogenesis of branchial cysts: a report of 468 cases, Am. J. Pathol. **35:**407, 1959.

Bhaskar, S. N., and Bernier, J. L.: Milkulicz's disease: clinical features, histology, and histogenesis; report of seventy-three cases, Oral Surg. **11:**1387, 1960.

Bhaskar, S. N., Bolden, T. E., and Weinmann, J. P.: Experimental obstructive adenitis in the mouse, J. Dent. Res. **35:**852, 1956.

Bhaskar, S. N., and Lilly, G. E.: Salivary gland tumors of infancy, J. Oral Surg. **21:**307, 1963.

Bhaskar, S. N., and Weinmann, J. P.: Tumors of minor salivary glands: a study of 23 cases, Oral Surg. **8:**1278, 1955.

Bluestone, R., Gumpel, J. M., Goldberg, L. S., and Holborow, E. J.: Salivary immunoglobulins in Sjögren's syndrome, Int. Arch. Allergy Appl. Immunol. **42:**686, 1972.

Briggs, J., and Evans, J. N. G.: Malignant oxyphilic granular-cell tumor (oncocytoma) of the palate, Oral Surg. **23:**796, 1967.

Buchner, A., and David, R.: Pigmented cells in adenolymphoma (Warthin's tumor), J. Oral Pathol. **6:**106, 1977.

Buchner, A., and Sreebny, L. M.: Enlargement of salivary glands, Oral Surg. **34:**209, 1972.

Calman, H. I., and Reifman, S.: Sjögren's syndrome, Oral Surg. **21:**158, 1966.

Catone, G., Merrill, R. G., and Henny, F. A.: Sublingual mucous retention phenomena, J. Oral Surg. **27:**774, 1969.

Chaudhry, A. P., Vickers, R. A., and Gorlin, R. J.: Intraoral minor salivary gland tumors, Oral Surg. **14:**1194, 1961.

Chen, S. Y.: Adenoid cystic carcinoma of minor salivary gland, Oral Surg. **42:**606, 1976.

Chen, S. Y.: Ultrastructure of mucoepidermoid carcinoma in minor salivary glands, Oral Surg. **47:**247, 1979.

Chisholm, D. M., Beeley, J. A., and Mason, D. K.: Salivary proteins in Sjögren's syndrome: separation by isoelectric focusing in acrylamide gels, Oral Surg. **35:**620, 1973.

Chisholm, D. M., Blair, G. S., Low, P. S., and Whaley, K.: Hydrostatic sialography as an index of salivary gland disease in Sjögren's syndrome, Acta Radiol. [Diagn.] **11:**577, 1971.

Chisholm, D. M., and Mason, D. K.: Salivary gland function in Sjögren's syndrome, Br. Dent. J. **135:**393, 1973.

Chisholm, D. M., Waterhouse, J. P., Kraucunas, E., and Sciubba, J. J.: A qualitative and quantitative electro microscopic study of the structure of the adenoid cystic carcinoma of human minor salivary glands, J. Oral Pathol. **4:**103, 1975.

Daniels, T. E., Silverman, S., Michalski, J. P., Greenspan, J. S., Sylvester, R. A., and Talal, N.: The oral component of Sjögren's syndrome Oral Surg. **39:**875, 1975.

Daniels, W. B., and MacMurray, F. G.: Cat-scratch disease, J.A.M.A. **154:**1247, 1954.

Devildos, L. R., and Langlois, C. C.: Minor salivary gland lesion presenting clinically as tumor, Oral Surg. **41:**657, 1976.

Doku, H. C., Shklar, G., and McCarthy, P. L.: Cheilitis glandularis, Oral Surg. **20:**563, 1965.

Drummond, J. F., Giansanti, J. S., Sabes, W. R., and Smith, C. R.: Sialadenoma papilliferum of the oral cavity, Oral Surg. **45:**72, 1978.

Dunlap, C. L., and Barker, B. F.: Necrotizing sialometaplasia, Oral Surg. **37:**722, 1974.

Dunley, R. F., and Jacoway, J. R.: Necrotizing sialometaplasia, Oral Surg. **47:**169, 1979.

Einstein, R. A. J.: Sialography in the differential diagnosis of parotid masses, Surg. Gynecol. Obstet. **122:**1079, 1966.

Eisenbud, L., Hymowitz, S. S., and Shapiro, R.: Cheilitis granulomatosa: report of case treated with injection of trianicinolone acetonide aqueous suspension, Oral Surg. **32:**384, 1971.

Epker, B. N.: Obstructive and inflammatory diseases of the major salivary glands, Oral Surg. **33:**2, 1972.

Fechner, R. E.: Necrotizing sialometaplasia: a source of confusion with carcinoma of the palate, Am. J. Clin. Pathol. **67:**315, 1977.

Forney, S. K., Foley, J. M., Sugg, W. E., Jr., and Oatis, G. W., Jr.: Necrotizing sialometaplasia of the mandible, Oral Surg. **43:**720, 1977.

Freedman, P. D., and Lumerman, H.: Sialadenoma papilliferum, Oral Surg. **45:**88, 1978.

Frommer, J.: The human accessory parotid gland: its incidence, nature, and significance, Oral Surg. **43:**671, 1977.

Gadient, S. E., and Kalfayan, B.: Mucoepidermoid carcinoma arising within a Warthin's tumor, Oral Surg. **40:**391, 1975.

Goldberg, M. H., and Harrigan, W. F.: Acute suppurative parotitis, Oral Surg. **20:**281, 1965.

Gray, J. M., Hendrix, R. C., and French, A. J.: Mucoepidermoid tumors of salivary glands, CA **16:**183, 1963.

Greenspan, J. S., Daniels, T. E., Talal, N., and Sylvester, R. A.: The histopathology of Sjögren's syndrome in labial salivary gland biopsies, Oral Surg. **37:**217, 1974.

Gross, B. D., and Case, D.: Cat scratch disease, Oral Surg. **43:**698, 1977.

Hall, H. D.: Diagnosis of diseases of the salivary glands, J. Oral Surg. **27:**15, 1969.

Harrison, J. D., and Garrett, J. R.: An ultrastructural and histochemical study of a naturally occurring salivary mucocele in a cat, J. Comp. Pathol. **85:**411, 1975.

Harrison, J. D., and Garrett, J. R.: The effects of ductal ligation on the parenchyma of salivary glands of the cat studied by enzyme histochemical methods, Histochem. J. **8**:35, 1976.

Herzberg, S. M., White, C., and Wolf, R. O.: Characterization of salivary proteins in patients with Sjögren's syndrome, Oral Surg. **36**:814, 1973.

Hettwer, K. J., and Tyler, C. F.: The normal sialogram, Oral Surg. **26**:790, 1968.

Hovinga, J., and De Jager, H.: A patient with necrotizing sialometaplasia, Int. J. Oral Surg. **6**:280, 1977.

Jacobson, F. L.: Xerostomia (Sjögren's syndrome) associated with unusual dental caries, Oral Surg. **21**:34, 1966.

Jensen, J. L., Howell, F. V., Rick, G. M., and Correll, R. W.: Minor salivary gland calculi, Oral Surg. **47**:44, 1979.

Jensen, J. L., and Reingold, I. M.: Sialadenoma papilliferum of the oral cavity, Oral Surg. **35**:521, 1973.

Keller, A. Z.: Residence, age, race and related factors in the survival and associations with salivary tumors, Am J. Epidemiol. **90**:269, 1969.

Kenny, F. E., and Long, J. E.: Sjögren's syndrome: review of literature and report of a case, J.A.M.A. **155**:435, 1954.

Kerpel, S. M., Freedman, P. D., and Lumerman, H.: The papillary cystadenoma of minor salivary gland origin, Oral Surg. **46**:820, 1978.

Kessler, R., Koznizky, I. L., and Schindel, J.: Malignant Warthin's tumor, Oral Surg. **43**:111, 1977.

Krolls, S. O., and Hicks, J. L.: Mixed tumors of the lower lip, Oral Surg. **35**:212, 1973.

Landrsis, P. H.: Notes on certain anatomical and clinical aspects of parotid lithiasis: therapeutic inferences in 6 cases, Rev. Stomatol. **68**:650, 1967.

Leake, D. L., Krakowiak, F. J., and Leake, R. C.: Suppurative parotitis in children, Oral Surg. **31**:174, 1971.

Leban, S. G., and Stratigos, G. T.: Benign lymphoepithelial sialoadenopathies, Oral Surg. **38**:735, 1974.

LiVolsi, V. A.: Prostatic carcinoma presenting as a primary parotid tumor, Oral Surg. **48**:447, 1979.

Lumerman, H., Freedman, P., Caracciolo, P., and Remigio, P. S.: Synchronous malignant mucoepidermoid tumor of the parotid gland and Warthin's tumor in adjacent lymph node, Oral Surg. **39**:953, 1975.

Lynch, D. P., Crago, C. A., and Martinez, M. G., Jr.: Necrotizing sialometaplasia, Oral Surg. **47**:63, 1979.

Maisel, R. H., Johnston, W. H., Anderson, H. A., and Cantrell, R. W.: Necrotizing sialometaplasia involving the nasal cavity, Laryngoscope **87**:429, 1977.

Mandel, I. D., and Baurmash, H.: Sialochemistry in Sjögren's syndrome, Oral Surg. **41**:182, 1976.

Matilla, A., Flores, T., Nogales, F. F., Jr., and Galera, H.: Necrotizing sialometaplasia affecting the minor labial glands, Oral Surg. **47**:161, 1979.

Matteson, S., and Herman, P. A.: Warthin's tumor, Oral Surg. **41:**129, 1976.

Nicolatou, O., Harwick, R. D., Putong, P., and Leifer, C.: Ultrastructural characterization of intermediate cells of mucoepidermoid carcinoma of the parotid, Oral Surg. **48:**324, 1979.

Pitdar, G. G., and Paymaster, J. C.: Tumors of minor salivary glands, Oral Surg. **28:**310, 1969.

Pullon, P. A., and Miller, A. S.: Sialolithiasis of accessory salivary glands: review of 55 cases, J. Oral Surg. **30:**832, 1972.

Rickles, N. H.: Cat-scratch disease, Oral Surg. **13:**282, 1960.

Russell, E. A., Jr., and Nelson, J. F.: Adenocarcinoma of the palate—diagnosis and management, Oral Surg. **45:**528, 1978.

Rye, L. A., Calhoun, N. R., and Redman, R. S.: Necrotizing sialometaplasia in a patient with Buerger's disease and Raynaud's phenomenon, Oral Surg. **49:**223, 1980.

Sage, H.: Duct ligation and small-dose x-radiation: a new treatment for Mikulicz's disease, Oral Surg. **20:**287, 1965.

Sapiro, S. M., and Eisenberg, E.: Sjögren's syndrome (sicca complex), Oral Surg. **45:**591, 1978.

Sigala, J. L., Silverman, S., Brody, A. B., and Kushner, J. H.: Dental involvement in histiocytosis, Oral Surg. **33:**42, 1972.

Solomon, M. P., Rosen, Y., and Gardner, B.: Metastatic malignancy in the submandibular gland, Oral Surg. **39:**469, 1975.

Stene, T., and Pedersen, K. N.: Aberrant salivary gland tissue in the anterior mandible, Oral Surg. **44:**72, 1977.

Strader, R. J.: Review of a technique in the treatment of mucoceles, Oral Surg. **37:**695, 1974.

Talal, N.: Sjögren's syndrome, lymphoproliferation and renal tubular acidosis, Ann. Intern. Med. **74:**633, 1971.

Talal, N., Asofsky, R., and Lightbody, P.: Immunoglobulin synthesis by salivary gland lymphoid cells in Sjögren's syndrome, J. Clin. Invest. **49:**49, 1970.

Tarpley, T. M., Jr., Anderson, L., Lightbody, P., and Sheagren, J. N.: Minor salivary gland involvement in sarcoidosis, Oral Surg. **33:**755, 1972.

Tarpley, T. M., Jr., Anderson, L. G., and White, C. L.: Minor salivary gland involvement in Sjögren's syndrome, Oral Surg. **37:**64, 1974.

Tarpley, T. M., Jr., and Giansanti, J. S.: Adenoid cystic carcinoma, Oral Surg. **41:**484, 1976.

Thompson, J.: Parotid duct calculus, Proc. R. Soc. Med. **66:**352, 1973.

Warwich, W. J., Bernard, B., and Meskin, L. H.: The involvement of the labial mucous salivary gland in patients with cystic fibrosis, Pediatrics **34:**621, 1964.

Whaley, K., Glen, A. C. A., Deodhar, S. D., Dick, W. C., Nuki, G., and Buchanan, W. W.: Cellular immune mechanisms in rheumatoid arthritis and Sjögren's syndrome, Ann. Rheum. Dis. **30:**332, 1971.

Whaley, K., Glen, A. C. A., MacSween, R. N. M., Deodhar, S. D., Dick, W. C., Nuki, G., Williamson, J., and Buchanan, W. W.: Immunological responses in Sjögren's syndrome and rheumatoid arthritis, Clin. Exp. Immunol. **9**:721, 1971.

White, N. S.: Sjögren's syndrome, Oral Surg. **22**:163, 1966.

Youngberg, G., and Rao, M. S.: Ultrastructural features of monomorphic adenoma of the parotid gland, Oral Surg. **47**:458, 1979.

PART V

SPECIAL ORAL PATHOLOGY

CHAPTER 18

Developmental malformations

Abnormalities resulting from disturbances of growth and development are referred to as developmental malformations. They may be apparent at birth, termed *congenital* (e.g., cleft palate, pyloric stenosis), or they may not be clinically evident until much later in life (e.g., diabetes, certain hereditary degenerations of the central nervous system, dentinogenesis imperfecta). However, the defect or its "seed" is always present at birth.

At conception a fetus may receive a defective hereditary character from one or both of its parents or, having been conceived normally and being of normal "genetic potential," may acquire a defect while it undergoes intrauterine development. Developmental malformations therefore may be *hereditary* in nature or be *acquired* in utero. The hereditary malformations are a result of a recessive or a dominant mutation and are transmitted by the germ cells. The acquired malformations are the result of some damage acquired in utero (e.g., congenital syphilis).

The following diseases and disturbances belong in the category of developmental malformations. Many of these have been described elsewhere in the book. Those that have not been described previously are included in the present chapter.

Malformations affecting jaws

1. Cleidocranial dysostosis (p. 99)
2. Craniofacial dysostosis (p. 100)
3. Mandibulofacial dysostosis (p. 100)
4. Macrognathia, micrognathia, and agnathia (pp. 100, 101)
5. Cleft palate (p. 101)
6. Pierre Robin syndrome (p. 103)
7. Cleft mandible (p. 104)
8. Cherubism (p. 306)
9. Osteopetrosis (p. 344)
10. Osteogenesis imperfecta (p. 346)

Malformations affecting teeth

1. Ectodermal dysplasia (p. 104)
2. Anodontia (p. 104)
3. Accessory teeth (p. 106)
4. Supernumerary teeth (p. 106)
5. Predeciduous dentition (p. 107)
6. Postpermanent teeth (p. 107)
7. Hutchinson's incisors (p. 108)
8. Mulberry molars (p. 108)
9. Macrodontia and microdontia (p. 109)
10. Dens in dente (p. 109)
11. Gemination (p. 114)
12. Taurodontism (p. 116)
13. Amelogenesis imperfecta (p. 119)
14. Dentinogenesis imperfecta (p. 119)
15. Shell teeth (p. 123)
16. Odontodysplasia (p. 124)
17. Enamel hypocalcification (hereditary) (p. 127)
18. Concrescence (p. 128)

Malformations affecting soft tissues

1. Cleft upper lip
2. Congenital pits or fistula of lip
3. Macrostomia
4. Macrocheilia
5. Double lip
6. Macroglossia
7. Microglossia and aglossia
8. Ankyloglossia
9. Lingual thyroid
10. Thyroglossal duct cyst
11. Median rhomboid glossitis
12. Cleft tongue
13. Midline fistula of tongue
14. Fissured tongue (scrotal tongue)
15. Epstein's pearl (Bohn's nodule; dental lamina cyst)
16. Dermoid cyst
17. White sponge nevus (p. 380)
18. Fordyce's disease (p. 397)
19. Branchial cyst (p. 469)
20. Branchial sinus
21. Congenital epulis (p. 523)

MALFORMATIONS AFFECTING JAWS

Malformations affecting the jaws have been described previously (see the preceding classification for page references).

MALFORMATIONS AFFECTING TEETH

Malformations affecting the teeth have been described previously (see the preceding classification for page references).

MALFORMATIONS AFFECTING SOFT TISSUES

The malformations affecting soft tissues that have not been described previously are included in this discussion. For page references to those described earlier, see the preceding classification.

Cleft upper lip. The etiology and incidence of cleft upper lip are identical to the etiology and incidence of cleft palate.

Cleft upper lip is a result of failure of fusion between the maxillary, the lateral nasal, and the median nasal processes. The defect runs between the area of the canine and the lateral incisor. It may be unilateral or bilateral (harelip), is seen more often in male infants than in female infants.

Congenital pits or fistula of lip. This rare condition is characterized by one or more unilateral or bilateral pits in the lip mucosa. It is most common in the lower lip (Fig. 18-1).

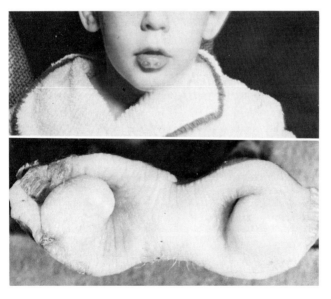

Fig. 18-1. Congenital pits of the lower lip.

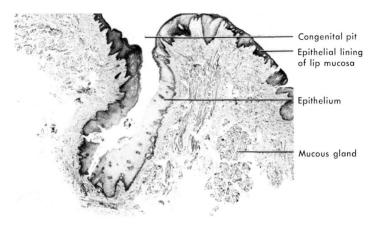

Fig. 18-2. Congenital pits of the lip. Note the cryptlike defect lined by epithelium.

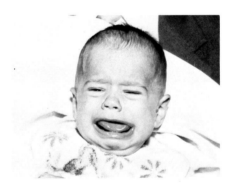

Fig. 18-3. Macrostomia is produced by the incomplete fusion of the maxillary and mandibular processes.

The pits usually are connected with one or more mucous glands and therefore may exude saliva. Due to impaction of debris, they may be sources of repeated episodes of inflammation.

Microscopic sections show a depression or a crypt of the lip mucosa lined by stratified squamous epithelium. The latter may

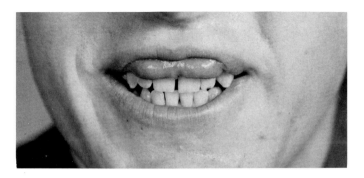

Fig. 18-4. Double lip is characterized by an overabundance of tissue.

be keratinized. The bottom of the pit of crypt may show the opening of one or more mucous glands (Fig. 18-2).

The exact cause of this developmental disturbance is unknown. Treatment consists of excision.

Macrostomia. Large mouth, a rare deformity, is produced by an incomplete fusion of the maxillary and mandibular processes of the developing face (Fig. 18-3).

Macrocheilia. This term refers to a large lip.

Double lip. In double lip there is an overabundance of tissue on the lingual aspect of the lip. The upper lip is usually affected. When the patient smiles, the excess tissue appears as a double lip (Fig. 18-4). The condition may be congenital or acquired. Its occurrence with blepharochalasis (redundant skin of the eyelids) and nontoxic thyroid enlargement is called *Ascher's syndrome*.

Macroglossia. Enlargement of the tongue may be of developmental origin. As a result of crowding, the lateral borders of the tongue show indentations caused by the teeth.

In addition to developmental or hereditary macroglossia, enlargement of the tongue may be acquired—as in amyloidosis, cretinism, hyperpituitarism, and tumors (hemangioma, lymphangioma, neurofibroma).

Microglossia and aglossia. Microglossia refers to a small

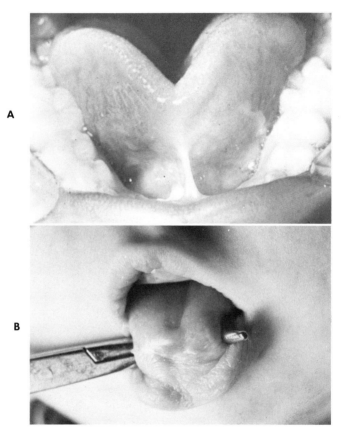

Fig. 18-5. Ankyloglossia. In **B,** the deformity is severe and consists of fusion of the tongue to the mandibular ridge and lip mucosa.

tongue, and aglossia refers to absence of the tongue. Although these conditions are sometimes seen in malformed fetuses, they are rarely seen in liveborn infants.

Ankyloglossia. The condition in which the ventral surface of the tongue is partially or completely attached to the oral floor is called ankyloglossia (tonguetie) (Fig. 18-5). The fixation is due to the fact that the lingual frenum is attached too far forward toward the tip of the tongue.

Treatment of ankyloglossia is surgery.

Lingual thyroid. The thyroid gland develops as an endothermal downgrowth from an area that is represented in the adult tongue by the foramen cecum. Part or all of this thyroid anlage may remain in the base of the tongue. When it does so, its presence is referred to as the lingual thyroid. It may be asymptomatic, or it may present as a tumorlike growth (Fig. 18-6).

Lingual thyroid is seen far more frequently in females than in males and may be clinically apparent either at birth or at any time in later life. Microscopic sections reveal thyroid follicles in the tongue musculature (Fig. 18-7).

Treatment is excision, but care must be exercised to make certain the patient has normal thyroid tissue in the neck.

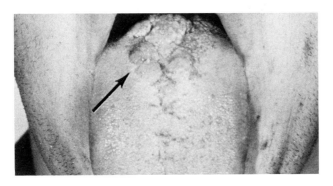

Fig. 18-6. Lingual thyroid. Note the masses of tissue on the dorsum of the tongue (arrow).

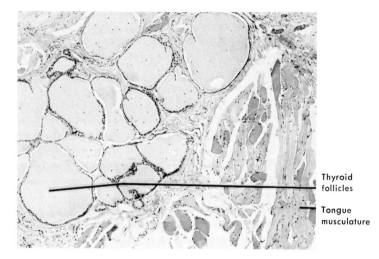

Thyroid
follicles

Tongue
musculature

Fig. 18-7. Lingual thyroid. Note the presence of thyroid tissue in the tongue musculature.

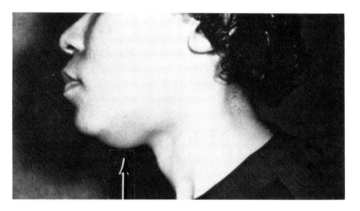

Fig. 18-8. Thyroglossal cyst. Note the enlargement in the midline of the submandibular area (arrow).

Thyroglossal duct cyst. The blind epithelial duct that descends from the tongue to the location of the future thyroid gland is called the thyroglossal duct. After the descent and differentiation of the thyroid gland, the duct degenerates; but numerous epithelial remnants are left in its wake. These remnants may undergo cystic degeneration and give rise to the thyroglossal cyst.

Clinically this cyst may be located anywhere in the midline from the foramen cecum to the thyroid gland (Fig. 18-8). Microscopic sections reveal a cyst lined by ciliated columnar epithelium.

Median rhomboid glossitis. This condition appears as a smooth, flat, depressed or elevated nodular area just anterior to the circumvallate papillae. It may be rhomboid, diamond shaped, or irregular in outline (Fig. 18-9). Since the area is de-

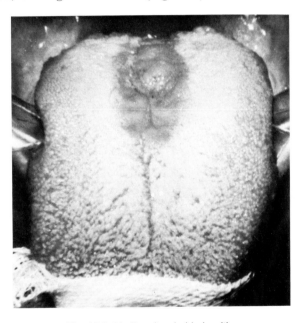

Fig. 18-9. Median rhomboid glossitis.

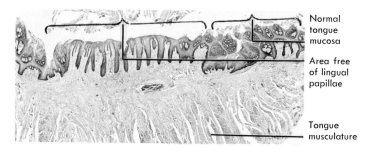

Fig. 18-10. Median rhomboid glossitis. Note the area that is devoid of papillae.

void of papillae, it contrasts strikingly with the remainder of the tongue.

Median rhomboid glossitis was believed to be a developmental anomaly caused by the persistence of the tuberculum impar. However, it has not been observed in children, and a developmental origin is now considered doubtful. Although its cause is as yet obscure, the possibility that it is a chronic lesion produced by *Candida albicans* has been proposed. It occurs in about 0.1% of the adult population and is more common in males. When the area is slightly depressed, it may accumulate debris and become a source of inflammation.

Microscopic sections reveal a covering of stratified squamous epithelium that is free of lingual papillae (Fig. 18-10). The epithelium shows hyperplasia, parakeratosis, and elongation of rete ridges; and in many instances it contains hyphae of *C. albicans*. The connective tissue under the epithelium is infiltrated by plasma cells and lymphocytes. Degeneration and hyalinization of muscle fibers underneath the lesion may be seen.

If the lesion is elevated and interferes with function or if it is depressed and becomes a constant source of inflammation (as a result of the accumulation of food), it should be excised.

Cleft tongue. A midline cleft in the tongue is extremely rare.

Midline fistula of tongue. This uncommon anomaly consists

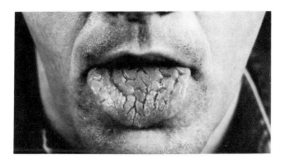

Fig. 18-11. Fissured tongue is characterized by deep or shallow fissures on the dorsum of the tongue.

of an epithelium-lined tract in the midline of the anterior part of the tongue.

Fissured tongue (scrotal tongue). Deep fissures on the tongue may be of developmental origin. Such a condition is called fissured or scrotal tongue (Fig. 18-11).

Since the incidence of fissured tongue increases with age, it is believed to be an acquired lesion. Although it is usually asymptomatic, food debris may accumulate in the fissures and give rise to inflammation and pain.

Fissured tongue is seen in about 5% of the population and affects both sexes equally. Daily brushing of the tongue will prevent secondary inflammation. Fissuring of the tongue sometimes occurs in conjunction with recurrent facial swellings that subsequently become permanent and with recurrent paralysis of the facial nerve. Some cases also show chronic, edematous, painless swelling of the attached gingiva. This symptom complex is called the *Melkersson-Rosenthal syndrome*. Related to this syndrome is the *cheilitis granulomatosa of Miescher*, which is an oligosymptomatic or milder form of this syndrome. Histologically in both of these conditions the affected tissues are characterized by perivascular accumulation of plasma cells, lymphocytes, histiocytes, and noncaseating granulomatous areas of epithelioid and giant cells.

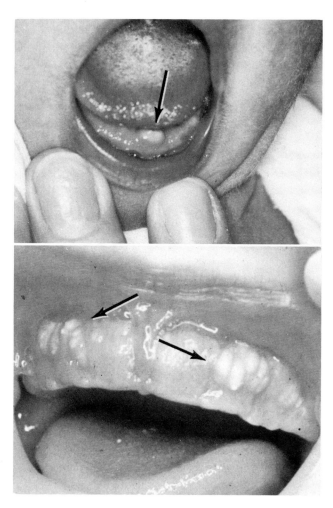

Fig. 18-12. Epstein's pearls (arrows) of the mandibular and maxillary alveolar mucosa in two newborn infants. (Courtesy Joe Frisch, D.D.S., Beverly Hills, Calif.)

Epstein's pearl (Bohn's nodule; dental lamina cyst). In about 80% of newborn infants, small firm white or grayish white lesions are seen on the palatal or alveolar mucosa (Fig. 18-12). They may be located along the midline of the palate, along the alveolar crest of the maxilla or mandible, or on the buccal and lingual aspects of the maxillary and mandibular ridges. The term *Epstein's pearl* is sometimes used when the lesions are along the midline of the palate; *dental lamina cyst*, when they are on the crest of the ridges; and *Bohn's nodule*, when they lie along the buccal and lingual aspects of the ridges. This classification, however, is artificial.

The lesions are usually multiple, do not increase in size, and require no treatment.

Microscopic sections reveal that the nodules are small, superficial, keratin-containing cysts lined by stratified squamous epithelium (Fig. 18-13). Because of their superficial location, they are spontaneously "shed" within a few weeks.

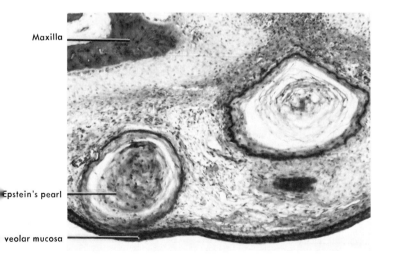

Fig. 18-13. Epstein's pearls consist of keratin-containing cysts.

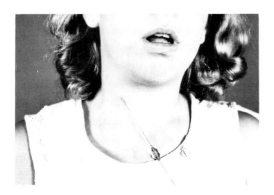

Fig. 18-14. A branchial sinus is an epithelium-lined tract of varying depth in the cervical area.

Dermoid cyst. Although the term dermoid cyst has been used loosely for cysts lined by dermal structures, in reality these are true benign tumors and belong to the group of teratomas (neoplasms composed of multiple tissues foreign to the part in which they arise).

Dermoids occur most commonly in the ovaries, but the floor of the oral cavity may be affected.

Microscopic sections reveal cysts that contain hair and teeth and that are lined by stratified squamous, ciliated, or alimentary epithelium. The walls of the cysts contain all types of tissue (nerve, thyroid, salivary gland, bone, cartilage, muscle, etc.).

Surgical excision is the treatment of choice.

Branchial sinus. This rare defect of the cervical area results from an incomplete fusion of the branchial arches (Fig. 18-14). It is an epithelium-lined tract of varying depth and should not be confused with a branchial cyst (p. 469).

REFERENCES

Aboyans, V., and Ghaemmaghami, A.: The incidence of fissured tongue among 4,009 Iranian dental outpatients, Oral Surg. **36:**34, 1973.

Ashley, D. J. B.: Origin of teratomas, CA **32:**390, 1973.

Baker, B. R.: Pits of the lip commissures in Caucasoid males, Oral. Surg. **21:**56, 1966.

Barnett, M. L., Bosshardt, L. L., and Morgan, A. F.: Double lip and double lip with blepharochalasis (Ascher's syndrome), Oral Surg. **34**:727, 1972.

Baughman, R. A.: Lingual thyroid and lingual thyroglossal tract remnants, Oral Surg. **34**:781, 1972.

Burkes, E. J., and Lewis, J. R.: Carcinoma arising in the area of median rhomboid glossitis, Oral Surg. **41**:649, 1976.

Delemarre, J. F. M., and van der Waal, I.: Clinical and histopathologic aspects of median rhomboid glossitis, Int. J. Oral Surg. **2**:203, 1973.

Encyclopedia of medical syndromes, New York, 1960, Hoeber Medical Division, Harper & Row, Publishers.

Fromm, A.: Epstein's pearls, Bohn's nodules and inclusion-cysts of the oral cavity, J. Dent. Child. **34**:275, 1967.

Gorlin, R. J., and Pindborg, J. J.: Syndromes of the head and neck, New York, 1964, McGraw-Hill Book Co.

Leider, A. S., Lucas, J. W., and Eversole, L. R.: Sebaceous choristoma of the thyroglossal duct, Oral Surg. **44**:261, 1977.

Lewis, M. I., and Hollerman, W. M.: Ectopic thyroid gland in children, Am. J. Surg. **115**:688, 1968.

McGinnis, J. P., Jr., and Parham, D. M.: Mandible-like structure with teeth in an ovarian cystic teratoma, Oral Surg. **45**:104, 1978.

Papanayotou, P. H., and Hatziotis, J. C.: Ascher's syndrome, Oral Surg. **35**:467, 1973.

Pullon, P. A., and Child, P. L.: An unusual dental variant of ovarian teratoma, Oral Surg. **34**:800, 1972.

Reaume, C. E., and Sofie, V. L.: Lingual thyroid, Oral Surg. **45**:841, 1978.

Sauk, J. J.: Ectopic lingual thyroid, J. Pathol. **102**:239, 1971.

Sharp, G. S., and Bullock, W. K.: Carcinoma arising in glossitis rhombica mediana, CA **11**:148, 1958.

Small, E. W.: The lingual thyroid, Oral Surg. **37**:692, 1974.

Strickland, A. L., Macfie, J. A., van Wyk, J. J., and French, F. S.: Ectopic thyroid glands simulating thyroglossal duct cysts, J.A.M.A. **208**:307, 1969.

van der Waal, I., Beemster, G., and van der Kwast, W. A. M.: Median rhomboid glossitis caused by candida? Oral Surg. **47**:31, 1979.

Wampler, H. W., Krolls, S. O., and Johnson, R. P.: Thyroglossal-tract cyst, Oral Surg. **45**:32, 1978.

Widstrom, A., Magnusson, P., Hellqvist, H., Hallberg, O., and Ruben, H.: Adenocarcinoma originating in thyroglossal ducts, Ann. Otol. Rhinol. Laryngol. **85**:286, 1976.

Worsaae, N., and Pindborg, J. J.: Granulomatous gingival manifestations of Melkersson-Rosenthal syndrome, Oral Surg. **49**:131, 1980.

Wright, B. A.: Median rhomboid glossitis: not a misnomer, Oral Surg. **46**:806, 1978.

Zecha, J. J., van Dijk, L., and Hadders, H. N.: Cheilitis granulomatosa (Melkersson-Rosenthal syndrome), Oral Surg. **42**:454, 1976.

CHAPTER 19

Oral manifestations of generalized diseases

The oral manifestations of the following generalized diseases are discussed in this chapter:

1. Vitamin deficiencies
2. Blood dyscrasias
3. Metabolic disturbances
4. Poisoning due to metals
5. Endocrine disturbances
6. Chronic granulomatous diseases
7. Diseases of the skin and mucous membranes
8. Diseases of bone
9. Miscellaneous diseases

Lesions in the oral cavity may be divided into three main groups:

1. *Group A* includes those diseases the occur exclusively in the oral tissues. To this group belong caries, odontogenic cysts, odontogenic tumors, periodontal diseases, salivary gland tumors, etc.

2. *Group B* includes those diseases that are generalized but become manifest in the oral cavity before anywhere else. To this group belong *some* cases of lichen planus, pemphigus, erythema multiforme, leukemias, lymphomas, multiple myeloma, Hand-Schüller-Christian disease, eosinophilic granuloma, Paget's disease, etc.

3. *Group C* includes those diseases that are generalized but become apparent in the mouth only in a late stage of their development. To this group belong certain cases of lymphomas, anemias, fungous infections, metastatic tumors, tuberculosis, etc.

It is apparent, therefore, that a dentist should not only be acquainted with the lesions classified as group A but should also be able to recognize the oral manifestations of generalized diseases, particularly those belonging to group B.

Diseases belonging to group C are no diagnostic problem to the dentist; by the time they manifest themselves in the oral cavity, their diagnosis either has been established or is quite apparent. Nevertheless, they deserve brief consideration.

In the following discussion of the oral features of the generalized diseases, emphasis has been placed only on the oral lesions. It is presumed that the reader has acquired detailed information on the extraoral manifestations of these diseases in a course of general pathology.

VITAMIN DEFICIENCIES

1. Vitamin A deficiency
2. Vitamin B deficiency
3. Vitamin C deficiency
4. Vitamin D deficiency

Vitamin A deficiency. Vitimin A is a fat-soluble, colorless alcohol derived from the carotenes (plant pigments). It is found in fish oil, butter, and eggs. Transformation of the majority of carotenes to vitamin A and the absorption of vitamin A take place in the small intestines. The vitamin is then stored in large quantities in the liver, and in small amounts in the skin and kidneys. Vitamin A is essential for the maintenance of function and structure of specialized epithelium, for the production (after combination with a protein) of photosensitive pigments (visual purple, visual violet) utilized by the rods and cones of the eye, and for the maintenance of normal skeletal growth.

In man, because of tremendous reserves, lesions produced by a deficiency of vitamin A are rare. These are (1) night blindness, which results from a lack of the photosensitive pigments; (2) a gray, triangular, elevated area on the conjunctiva called Bitot's spot; (3) xerophthalmia (dry conjunctiva); (4) multiple firm papules 1 to 5 mm in size on the skin of the shoulders, back, and buttocks called toad skin or follicular keratosis; and (5) squamous metaphasia in the epithelia of the respiratory and urogenital systems with subsequent secondary infections (e.g., bronchopneumonia).

Oral lesions are not common. However, in severe vitamin A

deficiency there may be a reduction in salivary flow. Hyperkeratotic areas on the oral mucosa have been described. Because of this observation, the administration of vitamin A has been suggested as a treatment for white patches on the oral mucosa. It is of no value, however.

Vitamin B deficiency. There are more than twenty members of a heterogeneous group of substances occurring abundantly in foodstuffs such as liver, yeast, milk, and leafy green vegetables that are referred to as the vitamin B complex. They generally fall into two groups: (1) those related to the intracellular metabolism of carbohydrates, fats, and proteins and (2) those related to blood cell production. The first group includes thiamine, niacin, riboflavin, pantothenic acid, and biotin. These are the energy-releasing vitamins. Members of the second group are the hematopoietic vitamins and include vitamin B_{12} (cobalamin) and folic acid. Only in deficiencies of thiamine, niacin, and riboflavin have oral changes been described.

Thiamine (vitamin B₁) deficiency. Thiamine is important in carbohydrate metabolism and is found in cereals, nuts, yeast, etc. Its deficiency produces beriberi.

There are two types of beriberi: a *wet form*, characterized by chronic passive congestion, edema, enlargement of the right side of the heart, hydrothorax, and hydropericardium, and a *dry form*, characterized by degenerative changes in nerves that lead to polyneuritis.

The oral manifestations of beriberi consists of edema of the tongue, loss of papillae, and pain.

Niacin (nicotinic acid; pellagra-preventive or P-P factor) deficiency. Niacin is important in intracellular oxidation and is found in meat, liver, yeast, milk, and vegetables. Its deficiency produces pellagra.

Characteristics of pellagra include rough, scaly keratotic lesions on the exposed areas of the skin (dermatitis); oral lesions that consist essentially of swelling, redness, and ulceration of the mucosa; inflammation of the colon leading to diarrhea; and demyelinization in the central nervous system leading to dementia, weakness, fears, insomnia, irritability, numbness, headaches, etc. Changes in pellagra may be summarized as the four D's (dementia, dermatitis, diarrhea, and death).

The oral mucous membrane is inflamed and bleeds easily. The tongue is red and enlarged; its papillae disappear, giving it a bald appearance *(Sandwith's bald tongue)*. The lateral margins of the tongue show indentations by the teeth. The tongue lesions are of great importance, because in some patients they are the only symptoms present and may precede other manifestations of pellagra by months or years. Microscopic sections reveal edema, atrophy of the papillae, and infiltration by plasma cells and lymphocytes.

Riboflavin (vitamin B₂; vitamin G) deficiency. Riboflavin is found in eggs and green leaves. In humans its deficiency produces vascularization of the cornea, keratitis, and later corneal ulceration, cheilosis, circumoral pallor, and seborrheic (greasy) dermatitis of the nasolabial fold and the ear.

The oral changes in riboflavin deficiency are seen in the tongue and lips. The tongue is red and inflamed, loses its papil-

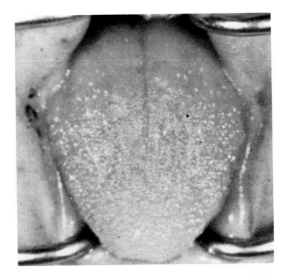

Fig. 19-1. Glossitis and angular cheilosis in riboflavin deficiency.

lae, and may show ulceration and appear cyanotic. Because of the cyanosis, the condition is called *magenta glossitis*. The lips show fissures, painful cracks, scaling, and maceration. These changes are particularly marked at the angles of the mouth *(angular cheilosis)* (Fig. 19-1).

Microscopic sections through these lesions show ulceration, edema, and infiltration by plasma cells and lymphocytes. In addition to these features, the tongue lesions show loss of the filiform papillae.

• • •

Since vitamin B deficiency is usually a multiple B complex deficiency, the oral changes related to it may be summarized as follows:

1. Reddening, ulceration, and erosions of the oral mucosa, particularly the tongue
2. Reddening of the tongue (sometimes magenta)
3. Loss of lingual papillae
4. Swelling of the tongue and indentation of its lateral borders (Fig. 19-2)

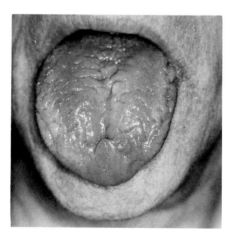

Fig. 19-2. Enlarged tongue with surface devoid of papillae in vitamin B complex deficiency.

5. Crusting, fissuring, and erosions of the lips and angles of the mouth
6. Microscopic sections nonspecific but showing edema and infiltration by plasma cells and lymphocytes*

Vitamin C deficiency. Vitamin C is a water-soluble substance essential to the production and maintenance of ground substance of all connective tissues (connective tissue proper, bone, cartilage, blood vessels, etc.). In severe deficiency it produces scurvy.

The general manifestations of vitamin C deficiency are petechial or massive hemorrhages into the skin, muscles, joints, etc.; resorption of bone leading to osteoporosity; marked reduc-

---

*In addition to vitamin B deficiency, other conditions leading to changes in the tongue that are essentially the same as those described are anemias (macrocytic and microcytic) and gastrointestinal disturbances (sprue and stricture).

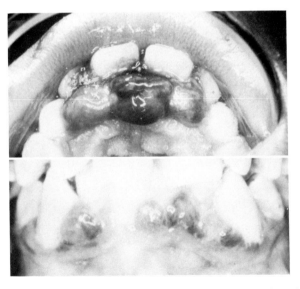

Fig. 19-3. Vitamin C deficiency is characterized by enlarged, bleeding gingiva. Illustrated are the palatal gingiva and labial mandibular gingiva of the same patient. (Courtesy John Nabers, D.D.S., Wichita Falls, Texas.)

tion in resistance to infections; and slow wound healing or failure of wound healing.

Oral changes in vitamin C deficiency are striking. These are petechiae and ecchymoses in the mucous membrane; hyperemia, edema, and enlargement of the gingiva with an increased bleeding tendency (Fig. 19-3); mild to marked loosening of the teeth; loss of teeth; secondary fusospirochetosis or Vincent's infection; and failure of wound healing.

Microscopic sections prepared from the involved oral tissues show edema, hemorrhages, and infiltration by plasma cells and lymphocytes. The most striking picture, however, is seen in sections specially stained for connective tissue (e.g., Mallory's connective tissue stain). In these the tissue from a patient with vitamin C deficiency, such as a gingival biopsy, shows a striking reduction in the amount of collagen.

Vitamin D deficiency. Vitamin D is believed to aid in the absorption of calcium and phosphorus through the mucous membranes of the intestines, to promote the calcification of bone and cartilage, and to be antagonistic to parathormone.

Deficiency of vitamin D produces *rickets* in the growing child and *osteomalacia* in the adult. These two diseases are characterized by a failure of calcification of cartilage and bone. Although there are no oral manifestations in osteomalacia, children with rickets may show severe disturbances in the teeth and jaws, such as retardation of tooth eruption, malpositioning of the teeth, retardation of the growth of the mandible, and class II malocclusion.

BLOOD DYSCRASIAS

Diseases affecting leukocytes

1. Leukemias (p. 561)
2. Agranulocytosis

Diseases affecting erythrocytes

1. Primary and secondary polycythemia
2. Anemias

Hemorrhagic disorders

1. Platelet deficiency
2. Prothrombin deficiency
3. Fibrinogen deficiency
4. Deficiency of specific proteins
5. Increased capillary fragility

Oral manifestations are seen in all severe blood dyscrasias. As a general rule, these changes are most apparent in the soft oral tissues and consist of enlargements, ulcerations, and bleeding. In some leukemias (especially monocytic) and anemias, the oral manifestations appear early and lead to the final diagnosis. However, in most other blood dyscrasias the oral lesions accompany or follow the generalized manifestations of the disease.

The literature on blood dyscrasias is extensive. As far as the oral manifestations are concerned, however, the pertinent information is summarized in the following paragraphs.

Diseases affecting leukocytes

Leukemias. The oral manifestations of the acute and chronic forms of the leukemias were discussed earlier in the book (p. 561).

Agranulocytosis. Characterized by a marked reduction in the granular leukocytes, this disorder usually occurs in adults; and females are afflicted more frequently than males.

The majority of cases are due to the toxic effect of drugs (antihistamines, sulfonamides, chloramphenicol, streptomycin, some tetracyclines). However, cases may result also from hypersensitivity to drugs (aminopyrine).

Oral lesions—which are almost always present—consist of gangrenous ulceration of the gingiva, tonsils, soft palate, lips, pharynx, and buccal mucosa (Fig. 19-4). Ulcers have yellow or gray membrane but lack the red halo. The absence of the red halo is due to the absence of the inflammatory response. Ulceration of the pharnyx are sometimes referred to as *agranulocytic angina*. Microscopic sections show an ulcer surrounded by connective tissue that reveals few if any granular leukocytes.

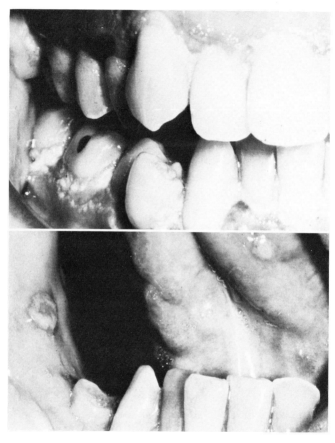

Fig. 19-4. Agranulocytosis with necrosis and multiple ulcerations of the gingiva, cheek, and tongue (two cases). (Courtesy Milton J. Knapp, D.D.S., Portland, Ore.)

Diseases affecting erythrocytes

Primary and secondary polycythemia. Primary polycythemia (also called erythremia, polycythemia vera, or polycythemia rubra) is a disease in which there is an increase in red blood cells (up to 10 million per cubic millimeter) due to some unknown cause. By contrast, secondary polycythemia—or erythrocytosis—is an increase in erythrocytes due to a known cause, such as high altitude or congenital heart disease. In both primary and secondary forms the oral mucous membrane may be deep raspberry or purple in color, and spontaneous gingival bleeding may occur.

Anemias. Deficiency of erythrocytes and hemoglobin is the characteristic of anemias. Although there are numerous forms of anemia, the following types present oral lesions:

1. Iron-deficiency anemia, which is due to deficiency of iron
2. Pernicious anemia, which is due to deficiency of the antipernicious anemia factor (vitamin B_{12})
3. Anemias caused by diseases of the gastrointestinal tract, such as sprue, celiac disease, strictures, and fish tapeworm infestation
4. Anemias caused by aplasia or obliteration of red bone marrow, as in drug sensitivity or marrow-replacing tumors
5. Hemolytic anemias, in which there is excessive destruction of red cells, particularly erythroblastosis fetalis, thalassemia (Cooley's anemia), and sickle cell anemia

Iron-deficiency anemia. Due to a deficiency of iron in the diet, this anemia is characterized by erythrocytes that are smaller than normal (microcytic) and have little hemoglobin (hypochromic).

It can occur under a variety of conditions such as pregnancy, infancy, nutritional deficiencies, and excessive bleeding; or it may be idiopathic. It is seen at all ages and in both sexes. Clinically symptoms are fatigue, pallor, and weakness.

The oral cavity may show atrophy of the papillae and bald spots on the tongue, pain in the tongue and oral mucosa, diffi-

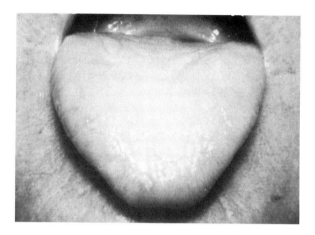

Fig. 19-5. Atrophic tongue in Plummer-Vinson syndrome.

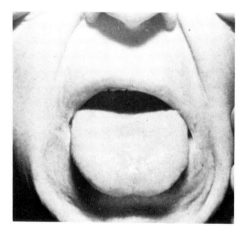

Fig. 19-6. Atrophic tongue in pernicious anemia.

culty in swallowing (dysphagia), a feeling of food sticking in the throat, and leukoplakia of the esophagus. This symptom complex is called the *Plummer-Vinson syndrome* and is seen most frequently in middle-aged women (Fig. 19-5). These patients may develop carcinoma of the esophageal mucosa.

Pernicious anemia. This disease, also known as Addison's anemia, is often associated with oral lesions. The tongue is sore, has a burning sensation, and shows atrophy of the papillae (Fig. 19-6). Due to inflammation, it appears glazed and beefy red. Ulcerations may also occur.

The entire symptom complex of the tongue in pernicious anemia is referred to as *Hunter's glossitis*. Besides tongue lesions, pernicious anemia is often associated with nonspecific stomatitis.

Anemias caused by gastrointestinal disturbances. In anemias caused by gastrointestinal disturbances, the oral changes are similar to those in pernicious anemia and consist of glossitis, atrophy of the papillae, ulcerations, and pain (glossodynia).

Anemias caused by aplasia or obliteration of red bone marrow. Anemias produced by suppression of red bone marrow (*aplastic*) are severe and rapidly fatal. The oral cavity shows bleeding, ulceration, and necrosis.

Hemolytic anemias. In these anemias there is destruction of erythrocytes.

Erythroblastosis fetalis is a congenital and familial disease and is produced as follows: The red blood cells of the majority of the population (85%) have a factor, called Rh factor, that is transmitted as a dominant character; thus the father or the mother can transmit the Rh factor to the fetus; if the mother is Rh negative but the fetus is not, the mother's blood develops antibodies against the Rh factor of the fetus; these antibodies pass to the fetus and destroy its red blood cells. Due to hemolysis, jaundice and anemia result. Oral manifestations consist of black, brown, or bluish pigmentation of the teeth (Fig. 4-30).

Thalassemia (Mediterranean anemia or Cooley's anemia) is also a congenital familial disease that is predominant among per-

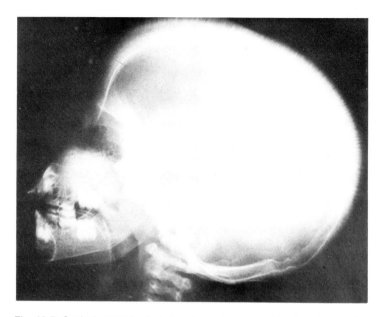

Fig. 19-7. Cooley's anemia. A skull radiograph shows thickening of the diploe and the "hair on end" appearance.

sons of Mediterranean origin and is caused by a defect in the rate of synthesis of hemoglobin A. It is characterized by anemia, yellow coloration of the skin, a mongoloid appearance, spleno-megaly, fever, and malaise. The head is enlarged, and radiographs show thickening of the diploe and a "hair on end" appearance (Fig. 19-7). The latter is due to the formation of bone trabeculae at right angles to the cranial vault. Oral manifestations are protrusion of the upper anterior teeth. Radiographs of the jaws show osteoporosis accompanied by peculiar coarsening of some trabeculae (Fig. 19-8). In its severe form the disease is usually fatal.

Sickle cell anemia is seen in Negroes and is characterized by sickle-shaped or distorted erythrocytes. Sickling of the cells is due to an abnormal type of hemoglobin (hemoglobin S). These

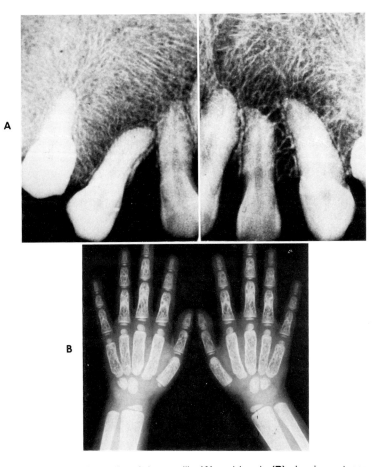

Fig. 19-8. Radiographs of the maxilla **(A)** and hands **(B)** showing osteoporosis and coarse bone trabeculation.

cells are destroyed in the spleen, liver, and bone marrow with resultant anemia (hemolytic). Oral manifestations, seen only on radiographs, consist of the presence of a coarse trabecular pattern, osteoporosis, and the appearance of large irregular areas of radiolucency that represent marrow spaces. The alveolar bone proper (lamina dura) is not affected.

Hemorrhagic disorders

The mechanisms of blood coagulation may be summarized in the following three steps:

1. Platelets + Calcium + Thromboplastin precursors* → Thromboplastin
2. Prothrombin (source, vitamin K) + Thromboplastin + Accessory factors† → Thrombin
3. Fibrinogen + Thrombin → Fibrin

It is thus apparent that disturbances in blood coagulation can occur if there is a deficiency in platelets, plasma proteins, vitamin K, calcium, or any one of the factors mentioned. Furthermore, an increased hemorrhagic tendency can result from the increased fragility of vessel walls.

In all these diseases or deficiencies the overall oral picture is of spontaneous bleeding around the teeth, petechiae and/or ecchymoses, and profuse and prolonged bleeding following even minor oral surgical procedures. These conditions are therefore of interest to the dentist.

Platelet deficiency. Although platelet deficiency may occur secondary to other blood dyscrasias or as a result of the ingestion of poisons, the most common cause is an idiopathic deficiency of platelets called *Werlhof's disease* or *thrombocytopenic purpura*. It usually occurs before the age of 20 years and is more common in females.

---

*Thromboplastin precursors are present in plasma. These are antihemophilic globulin (factor VIII), plasma thromboplastin component (PTC or factor IX), Stuart-Prower factor (factor X), plasma thromboplastin antecedent (PTA or factor XI), Hageman factor (factor XII), and Laki-Lorand or fibrin stabilizing factor (factor XIII).

†Accessory factors are labile factor (factor V), stable factor (factor VII), and antihemophilic globulin (AHG or factor VIII).

The lesions are most prominent in the oral cavity (also the skin and other mucous membranes) and consist of bleeding gingiva, petechiae, and ecchymoses. The ecchymoses may enlarge to form submucosal hematomas that present as large dark tumors (Fig. 19-9).

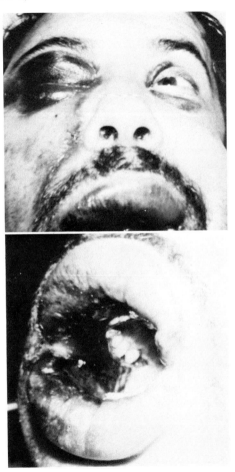

Fig. 19-9. Massive hematomas in a patient with thrombocytopenia purpura. (Courtesy Milton J. Knapp, D.D.S., Portland, Ore.)

Prothrombin deficiency. Vitamin K is the source of prothrombin, and the liver is the site of prothrombin production. Prothrombin deficiency therefore occurs in either vitamin K deficiency or liver diseases.

Fibrinogen deficiency. Fibrinogen deficiency occurs in severe protein shortage in the diet, in liver damage, or in diseases of the blood-forming organs.

Deficiency of specific proteins. Deficiency of the thromboplastin precursors as well as of the accessory factors (p. 656) leads to hemorrhagic diseases of varying severity.

Lack of antihemophilic globulin (factor VIII) produces the classic hemophilia, or hemophilia A; lack of plasma thromboplastin component (factor IX) leads to hemophilia B, or Christmas disease; lack of plasma thromboplastin antecedent (PTA, or factor XI) produces mild or pseudohemophilia that affects both sexes; lack of labile factor (factor V) causes parahemophilia; and a deficiency of stable factor, Stuart-Prower factor, and Hageman factor (factors VII, X, and XII respectively) produces hemorrhagic disorders in neonates.

The oral manifestation of all these disorders is spontaneous bleeding or persistent bleeding following minor trauma.

Increased capillary fragility. Increased capillary fragility is seen in vitamin C deficiency and in allergic reactions.

Oral manifestations are rare. When present, however, they consist of petechiae and bleeding.

Commonly used laboratory tests in hemostasis include the following:

clotting time Normal range is 4 to 10 minutes. Roughly measures the overall intrinsic clotting mechanism. However, slight deficiencies of the various factors may not be detected, because only a small amount of thrombin is needed to produce a fibrin clot. Few normal platelets are required for clotting, which explains the normal clotting time in thrombocytopenia.

bleeding time Normal range for Duke's method is 1 to 3 minutes, and 2 to 6 minutes for the Ivy method. Normal contraction of capillaries and the presence of sufficient numbers of normal platelets are tested. Thus hemophiliacs have normal bleeding time.

clot retraction Normal retraction is about 50%. Measures the amount of fibrin and the number and quality of the platelets.

tourniquet test (Rumpel-Leede test) Measures capillary integrity and adequate platelet function.

prothrombin time Normal range is 12 to 15 seconds. Tests the extrinsic system by supplying excess preformed extrinsic thromboplastin and thus bypasses the intrinsic system (platelets; factors VIII, IX, XI, XII). The test depends on the presence of fibrinogen, prothrombin, and factors V, VII, and X.

partial thromboplastin time Normal activated time is 25 to 45 seconds. Tests for an intact intrinsic clotting system by adding a platelet substitute. Deficiencies of almost all coagulation factors except factor VII and platelets are picked up.

Bleeding problems associated with coagulation disorders such as hemophilia can generally be clinically differentiated from disorders due to platelet or blood vessel deficiencies. Coagulation disorders characteristically demonstrate hemarthroses, rarely display petechiae, are commonly associated with a positive family history, usually afflict males, and manifest a delayed onset of bleeding from trauma. However, platelet and vessel defects rarely demonstrate bleeding into the joints but characteristically display petechiae, are rarely associated with a family history, more often afflict females, and are manifested by immediate oozing following trauma.

METABOLIC DISTURBANCES

The metabolic diseases are believed to be associated with a deficiency, an excess, or a disturbance in the metabolism of some constituent of the diet. Under this heading, therefore, fall a heterogeneous group of diseases. However, only those disturbances that present oral manifestations are included in this book. With the exception of diabetes, amyloidosis, and mucopolysaccharidoses, these diseases have been described previously (see the following classification for page references).

1. Diabetes
2. Amyloidosis
3. Mucopolysaccharidoses (Hurler's and Hunter's syndromes)
4. Eosinophilic granuloma (p. 356)
5. Hand-Schüller-Christian disease (p. 360)
6. Letterer-Siwe disease (p. 361)
7. Gaucher's disease (p. 362)
8. Neimann-Pick disease (p. 362)
9. Vitamin deficiencies (p. 643)

Diabetes. Carbohydrate metabolism is controlled essentially by the pancreas, adrenal cortex, and pituitary gland.

Insulin, secreted by the islets of Langerhans, converts blood sugar into glycogen, which is stored in the liver and depolymerized to form glucose; epinephrine, secreted by the adrenal medulla, mobilizes sugar from liver glycogen; and adrenocortical hormones (S or sugar group) convert amino acids into sugar instead of protein. Also, there is a diabetogenic hormone secreted by the anterior pituitary gland that is antagonistic to insulin (i.e., elevates the blood sugar).

Diabetes mellitus, however, is most often a result of insulin insufficiency. This means that blood sugar is neither stored nor utilized; and it rises markedly (hyperglycemia) and is excreted in the urine (glycosuria). Excessive urination (polyurea) is due to a lack of urine concentration and leads to excessive thirst (polydipsia). Since carbohydrates are not available to the body, fats are utilized. Therefore, ketone bodies are produced and accumulate, causing acidosis and leading to coma and death.

The oral manifestations of uncontrolled diabetes are severe and consist of the following: marked destruction of the supporting bone of the teeth leading to periodontosis-like lesions, periodontitis complex, loosening and loss of teeth, gingivitis and painful gingivae, xerostomia, pulpitis in which the affected tooth may appear free of caries (the pain is believed to be due to arteritis), ulcerations of the oral mucous membrane, acetone breath, and lowered tissue resistance leading to markedly delayed healing of oral tissues.

Amyloidosis. In this disturbance a peculiar homogeneous translucent material of unknown chemical nature, but probably a protein-carbohydrate complex called amyloid, is deposited in the tissues.

The clinical manifestations of the disease depend on the organs affected. The condition would accordingly vary from being completely harmless to a fatal involvement of most internal organs. There are four types of amyloidosis: *primary, secondary, tumor amyloid,* and *amyloidosis associated with multiple myeloma.*

A   B

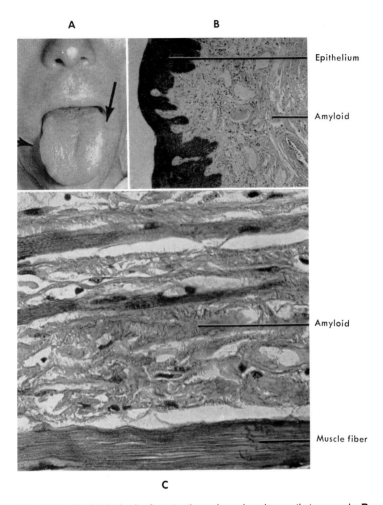

Epithelium

Amyloid

Amyloid

Muscle fiber

C

Fig. 19-10. Amyloidosis. In **A,** note the enlarged and smooth tongue. In **B** and **C,** note the homogeneous material (amyloid) between the muscle fibers.

In *primary amyloidosis*, deposits of amyloid occur without any apparent cause. The usual sites affected are the tongue, gingiva, gastrointestinal tract, heart, and skin. The tongue is involved in almost 50% of cases, and the gingiva in almost 80%. The tongue is enlarged (macroglossia) and smooth and may show ulcerations (Fig. 19-10, *A*). The gingiva may also appear enlarged. Microscopic sections reveal the presence of a homogeneous eosinophilic material between the muscle fibers and collagen bundles (Fig. 19-10, *B* and *C*).

Secondary amyloidosis occurs as a result of some long-continued tissue-destroying process such as tuberculosis or osteomyelitis. In this form the deposition of amyloid occurs in parenchymatous organs such as the liver, spleen, and kidneys. Amyloid deposits also occur in the gingiva; and a gingival biopsy, among other tests, may be used as an aid in diagnosis.

In *tumor amyloid*, tumorlike localized deposits of amyloid occur in various tissues, such as the neck, heart, larynx, gingiva, and tongue. Indeed, the oral tissues are common sites. The tongue and gingiva appear enlarged and smooth, and microscopic sections reveal masses of homogeneous material surrounded by foreign body giant cells.

In a small percentage (about 7%) of patients with *multiple myeloma*, amyloidosis is an associated finding. In both distribution and staining properties, the amyloid deposit in this type is the same as in primary amyloidosis. When present, therefore, it frequently involves the tongue and gingiva.

Staining qualities of amyloid. Amyloid gives a number of reactions that aid in its recognition. In sections stained with crystal violet, amyloid appears as a purplish violet material, whereas everything else stains blue.

In sections stained with hematoxylin and eosin, amyloid appears as a homogeneous, amorphous, light pink material. Congo red stains it pink or red. If Congo red is injected intravenously, 90% or more of the dye is absorbed in patients with amyloidosis. All these reactions are far more consistent in *secondary* amyloidosis than in other forms.

Mucopolysaccharidoses (Hurler's and Hunter's syndromes).
These are a group of genetic disorders that lead to increased
storage of mucopolysaccharides in the tissues.

Hurler's syndrome is fatal before 10 years of life and is characterized by mental retardation, dwarfism, and a deformed head
and face. Death results from cardiac or lung involvement.
Hunter's syndrome is a less severe form in which patients may
live to 20 years of age.

Oral changes are characterized by a short and broad mandible, coarse lips, lack of tooth eruption, and radiolucencies
around the crowns of unerupted teeth. These radiolucencies are
caused by accumulation of mucopolysaccharides in the tissues.

POISONING DUE TO METALS

1. Arsenic
2. Lead
3. Bismuth
4. Mercury
5. Silver
6. Phosphorus

A number of metallic salts act as systemic poisons. The most
prominent among these are arsenic, lead, bismuth, mercury,
silver, and phosphorus.

Arsenic. Oral lesions in arsenic poisoning consist of gingivitis
and stomatitis. Other clinical features include vomiting, diarrhea, hyperkeratosis, hyperpigmentation, and neurologic disturbances.

Lead. Lead poisoning manifests itself in the oral cavity as
excessive salivation, metallic taste, swelling of the salivary
glands, and a dark line (lead line) along the gingival margin
(Fig. 19-11).

Microscopically the lead line consists of a granular pigment
deposit in the perivascular areas of the submucosa and the basement membrane (Fig. 19-12). The pigment is lead sulfide. The
presence of a lead line is especially pronounced in patients
whose oral hygiene is poor.

Other manifestations of lead poisoning are gastrointestinal
upset, convulsive seizures, neuritis, anemia, a peculiar baso-

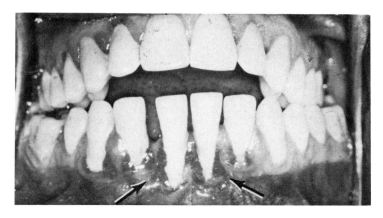

Fig. 19-11. Lead line. Note the dark granular areas along the free marginal gingiva of the anterior mandibular teeth (arrows).

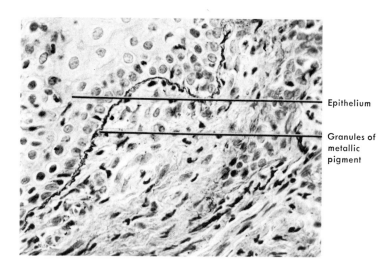

Epithelium

Granules of metallic pigment

Fig. 19-12. Lead line. Note the deposition of dark metallic pigment in the basement membrane.

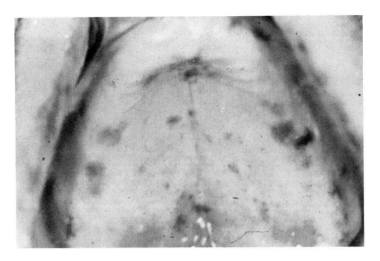

Fig. 19-13. Pigmented patches in bismuth poisoning.

philic stippling of erythrocytes, and osteosclerotic lines in the metaphyses of long bones.

Bismuth. Bismuth poisoning was common when this metal was used in the treatment of syphilis.

The oral manifestations consist of a metallic taste, burning sensations of the oral mucosa, and a bismuth line (which is similar to the lead line and occurs along the gingival margin in patients with poor oral hygiene). Sometimes other areas of the oral mucosa show pigmented patches (Fig. 19-13).

Microscopically granular deposits of a black pigment (bismuth sulfide) are seen in the submucosa. The bismuth salt is believed to react with hydrogen sulfide that is produced from the degradation of food debris in the mouth and to produce bismuth sulfide, which, in turn, deposits as an insoluble precipitate.

Mercury. Acute and chronic poisoning with metallic mercury leads to disturbances in the central nervous system (tremors, emotional instability) and gastrointestinal tract. Oral manifestations consist of increased salivation, stomatitis and glossitis, swelling of the salivary glands, and sometimes a dark line on the gingiva similar to that seen in bismuth poisoning.

Silver. Prolonged contact with organic or inorganic silver compounds produces argyria. The skin and oral mucous membrane acquire an ashen gray hue. Microscopic sections show a deposit of fine black granular pigment in the subepithelial connective tissue. The granules are an insoluble albuminate of silver and give a permanent pigmentation to the tissues.

Phosphorus. Chronic poisoning follows prolonged inhalation of phosphorus compounds, and the most remarkable oral manifestation is persistent and progressive osteomyelitis of the maxilla and mandible.

ENDOCRINE DISTURBANCES

Excessive or deficient endocrine gland function can produce dramatic alterations in the body. Endocrine disturbances and imbalances in which the oral lesions can be seen are as follows:

1. Hypopituitary dwarfism
2. Gigantism
3. Acromegaly
4. Hyperparathyroidism (primary)
5. Hyperparathyroidism (secondary)
6. Hypoparathyroidism
7. Imbalance of sex hormones
8. Addison's disease
9. Hyperthyroidism
10. Hypothyroidism
11. Diabetes (p. 660)

Hypopituitary dwarfism. Hypofunction of the pituitary gland in infancy leads to dwarfism. In pituitary dwarfism there is a delayed shedding of deciduous teeth, delayed eruption of permanent teeth, absence of third molars, and under development of the maxilla and mandible.

Gigantism. Growth hormone, of the anterior lobe of the pituitary gland, is produced by eosinophilic cells. It promotes the growth of cartilage and connective tissue. Thus, when it acts on the cartilaginous epiphyseal plates of tubular bones and on connective tissue sutures of flat bones, it stimulates growth of the skull and skeleton.

At the time of sexual maturity, sex hormones act antagonistically toward growth hormone, the cartilaginous plates disappear, and the dramatic phase of the growth period comes to a close. If an adenoma of the eosinophilic cells should occur before the cessation of the normal growth period, a giant (or gigantism) is the result.

The oral manifestations of gigantism are an enlarged maxilla and mandible, a marked increase in vertical dimension, early eruption of teeth, an enlarged tongue, hypercementosis, and macrodontia in patients in whom the tumor starts early in life.

Acromegaly. If a pituitary adenoma or hyperplasia of the eosinophilic cells develops after the normal growth period of the patient has ceased, acromegaly results.

Since all epiphyseal plates have disappeared by the end of the normal growth period, the patient's height does not increase in acromegaly. However, the sutures of the skull, cartilage of the mandibular condyle, periosteum, and connective tissue everywhere are all reactivated. Consequently the patient develops thick bones, large hands, and a large skull. The enlarged pituitary gland may, by intracranial pressure, produce neurologic symptoms and visual disturbances.

Orally both the mandible and the maxilla enlarge; but the former grows faster, producing a class III malocclusion. There are diastemas, periodontitis and gingivitis, hypercementosis, and osteoporosis.

Hyperparathyroidism (primary). The primary function of parathormone is to maintain the calcium and phosphorus levels of the blood.

Parathormone does this by producing destruction of bone and thus liberating calcium salts and by regulating the renal excretion of phosphorus. In cases of excessive secretion of parathormone (tumor or hyperplasia of the parathyroid glands), the most striking changes occur in the skeleton.

Hyperparathyroidism is also referred to as *osteitis fibrosa cystica generalisata* or *von Recklinghausen's disease*.The condition usually occurs in middle age and is twice as common in females as in males. The general systemic manifestations consist of weakness, fatigue, constipation, polydipsia, polyuria, sponta- neous fractures, marked resorption of bone, increased blood cal- cium (more than 11 mg per 100 ml), low blood phosphorus (less than 2.5 mg per 100 ml), and increased urine calcium and phos- phorus. Due to increased urine calcium, urinary stones are seen in 3% to 12% of patients with hyperparathyroidism.

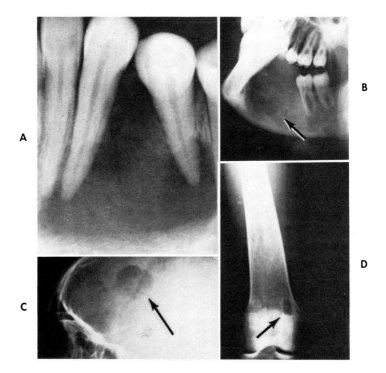

Fig. 19-14. Hyperparathyroidism in a 27-year-old woman. **A,** Radiolucent area in the mandible. The area was swollen and painful and had been present for one and one half years. Results of a biopsy showed a giant cell granu- loma—like lesion. **B,** The teeth in the area were extracted. **C** and **D,** Five months later lesions were evident in the skull and long bones. Blood studies indicated hyperparathyroidism. At surgery a parathyroid adenoma was re- moved.

Since oral lesions are usually present in hyperparathyroidism and sometimes precede all other symptoms by many months (Fig. 19-14), they are of great importance to the dentist. They consist of diffuse bone loss in the jaws, loosening of the teeth, loss of the lamina dura, and central radiolucent lesions of the maxilla or mandible that at microscopic examination resemble giant cell granuloma of the jaws (p. 295). These lesions are called *brown nodes* or *giant cell nodes*—the former because they almost always contain areas of hemorrhage and therefore appear brown, the latter because they contain giant cells. Unlike the giant cell granuloma of the jaws, however, they recur. Treatment consists of removal of the diseased parathyroid gland.

Hyperparathyroidism (secondary). Secondary hyperplasia of the parathyroid glands is a common accompaniment of renal disease, rickets, osteomalacia, and extensive tumors of bone (e.g., multiple myeloma). Since symptoms of hyperparathyroidism occur secondarily, the symptom complex is called secondary hyperparathyroidism.

Hypoparathyroidism. Deficiencies in parathormone production cause metabolic disturbances leading to hypocalcemia and increased neuromuscular excitability. This condition most commonly occurs as a postsurgical sequel to thyroidectomy or radical neck dissection for oral cancer.

Idiopathic hypoparathyroidism can also contribute to changes affecting structures of ectodermal origin such as enamel hypoplasia (Fig. 19-15). The *Di George syndrome* is caused by agenesis of both the parathyroid and the thymus glands with subsequent extensive hypoclacemia and cellular immune deficiency.

Imbalance of sex hormones. During certain periods of life, there is a physiologic change in the quantity of sex hormones in the body. These periods are puberty, menstruation, pregnancy, and menopause.

During these periods oral manifestations may occur. *Puberty* is associated with hyperplastic gingivitis, *pregnancy* with preg-

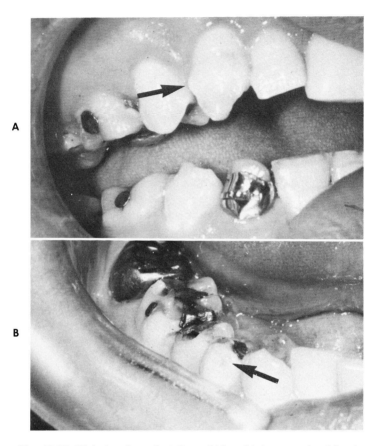

Fig. 19-15. Clinical oral manifestations of idiopathic hypoparathyroidism in a brother and sister. In **A**, note morphologic defect of the maxillary canine (arrow). In **B**, the arrow points to enamel pits on one of the affected teeth. (Courtesy P. Tsaknis, D.D.S., Washington, D.C.)

nancy gingivitis and pregnancy tumors, *menstruation* with transitory gingivitis, and *menopause* with desquamative gingivitis and glossodynia. These lesions have been discussed in Chapter 8.

Addison's disease. Chronic insufficiency of the adrenal cortex produces Addison's disease.

Although usually due to tuberculosis, the disease may be produced by other conditions such as amyloidosis and parasitic infections of the adrenal gland. It occurs in adults, and its general symptoms consist of weakness, low blood pressure, pigmentation of the skin, nausea, and vomiting. The oral lesions are represented by yellowish to brown pigmentation of the mucous membrane. The most commonly affected areas are the lips, buccal mucous membrane, gingiva, and tongue (Fig. 19-16).

Microscopic sections reveal an excessive amount of melanin in the basal layers of the epithelium. Since melanin and epi-

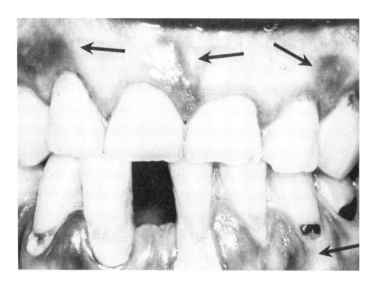

Fig. 19-16. Multiple pigmented areas of the gingiva in Addison's disease. (Courtesy Milton J. Knapp, D.D.S., Portland, Ore.)

nephrine (secreted by the adrenal medulla) have a common precursor substance, the theory has been suggested that in patients with Addison's disease the adrenal medulla is damaged, epinephrine cannot be produced in normal amounts, and there is an excess of the precursor substance in the body. This excess leads to an excessive production and deposition of melanin.

Hyperthyroidism. Excessive production of the thyroid hormone thyroxine produces symptoms of hyperthyroidism.

The primary role of thyroxine is to stimulate cellular metabolism, growth, and differentiation of all tissues. In excess, therefore, it leads to a high basal metabolic rate, weight loss, excitability, elevated temperature, and generalized osteoporosis.

Oral manifestations are not too remarkable. If the disturbance begins in the early years of life, premature eruption of the teeth and loss of the deciduous dentition are common findings. However, hyperthyroidism is usually seen in adults, and the only alteration in the oral region may be a generalized osteoporosis of the mandible and maxilla.

Hypothyroidism. In contradistinction to hyperthyroidism, hypothyroidism is marked by a lowered metabolism and retardation of growth, differentiation, and body activities in general. If the deficiency begins in childhood, cretinism develops. If it begins in adulthood, myxedema results.

Cretinism. This form of hypothyroidism occurs in childhood and is characterized by a short, mentally retarded, poorly developed child in whom all developmental processes, such as speaking and learning to walk, are considerably slowed.

The head appears relatively large for the small stature, the skin is coarse, the hair is brittle, and the blood pressure is below normal.

Oral manifestations are retarded eruption of the teeth, delayed exfoliation of the deciduous teeth, malocclusion, a large protruding tongue, drooling of saliva because of poor control, and large lips (Fig. 19-17).

Myxedema. Occurring more frequently in females than in males and usually in the middle-age group, the adult form of

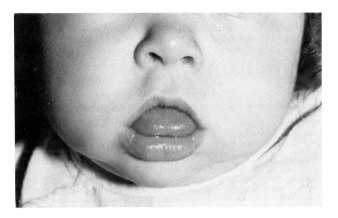

Fig. 19-17. Macroglossia in a cretin.

hypothyroidism is characterized by fatigue, lethargy, low blood pressure, coarse edematous skin, and retarded mental processes. Oral manifestations consist of thickened lips and an enlarged tongue.

Diabetes. Diabetes has been described previously in the discussion of metabolic disturbances (p. 660).

CHRONIC GRANULOMATOUS DISEASES

When living tissues are exposed to an irritant or to injury, they respond in various ways. They may, for example, undergo rapid proliferation (as in regeneration of damaged epithelium); produce a response that is marked by edema and neutrophilic migration (as in acute inflammation) or that shows plasma cell and lymphocytic infiltration with fibroblastic proliferation (as in chronic inflammation); or respond by an inflammatory process that, in addition to other features, is marked by a great deal of histiocytic proliferation. The last type of inflammatory response is the characteristic feature of the *chronic granulomatous diseases*.

Although in a sense the dental granuloma is a chronic granulomatous lesion, in this discussion only those diseases that are generalized in nature and present oral manifestation are considered. These may be classified into the following three groups:

Infective granulomas

1. Syphilis
2. Yaws (frambesia)
3. Bejel
4. Tuberculosis
5. Sarcoidosis
6. Histoplasmosis
7. Candidiasis (moniliasis) (p. 396)
8. Actinomycosis
9. South American blastomycosis

Granulomas of unknown nature

1. Histiocytosis X
   a. Eosinophilic granuloma (p. 356)
   b. Hand-Schüller-Christian disease (p. 360)
   c. Letterer-Siwe disease (p. 361)
2. Crohn's disease

Foreign body granulomas

Infective granulomas

Syphilis, yaws or frambesia, and bejel are caused by spirochetes. Tuberculosis and sarcoidosis are caused by bacteria. Histoplasmosis, candidiasis (moniliasis), actinomycosis, and South American blastomycosis are caused by fungi.

Syphilis. A spirochetal *(Treponema pallidum)* venereal disease, syphilis manifests itself in the acquired and congenital forms.

Acquired syphilis is divided into primary, secondary, and tertiary stages.

Primary syphilis commonly follows sexual intercourse with an infected person. Therefore, the primary lesion (chancre) is usually in the genital area. Depending on sites of exposure to the organism, however, the fingers, the lips, and rarely the tongue may be involved. The chancre appears about 3 weeks after exposure and starts as a macule that progressively becomes a papule and then an ulcer. The ulcer has indurated borders. The lips are the most common extragenital site for primary syphilis. The upper lip is affected more often than the lower lip, and the lesions are often in the middle third of the lip. The chancre spontaneously disappears in 4 to 6 weeks. Microscopic sections show an ulcer with edema and dense infiltration by plasma cells, macrophages, and lymphocytes.

Lesions of *secondary syphilis* begin 5 to 6 weeks after the disappearance of the chancres. This stage starts with a sore throat, malaise, fever, chills, and most prominently a macular cutaneous eruption. Oral lesions are multiple grayish erosions of the mucous membrane, called *mucous patches*, occurring anywhere on the oral mucosa; however, the tongue, lips, and tonsils are the most commonly affected sites. Although these lesions are usually associated with a skin eruption, *they may be the only manifestation of secondary syphilis*. They are highly infective, and the dentist with skin erosions or cuts on his fingers may acquire the disease while operating on such patients. Microscopically mucous patches show ulceration, an infiltrate of plasma cells and lymphocytes, and endarteritis.

In addition to mucous patches, secondary syphilis may also be attended by wartlike growths on the genital mucosa and, rarely, on the oral mucosa. These lesions are called *condylomas;* and under the microscope they appear as elevated masses of connective tissue with dense infiltration by plasma cells, macrophages, and lymphocytes and a covering of hyperplastic epithelium.

Tertiary syphilis manifests itself some years later and may involve the central nervous system, cardiovascular system, skeleton, joints, skin, and almosy any other part or organ of the body. The lesions, however, are essentially of two types. In one (the *gumma*) a circumscribed focus 2 to 10 cm in size, consisting of inflammation and rubberlike necrosis, occupies an organ or tissue. In the second there is a prolonged, smoldering inflammation of an organ or part, and the symptoms therefore vary depending on the site of involvement.

There are two types of oral lesions in tertiary syphilis: (1) gummas on the palate that produce palatal perforation and (2) chronic inflammation of the tongue (syphilitic glossitis) associated with arteritis. The arteritis leads to proliferation of the intima and narrowing or occlusion of the lumen with resultant ischemia. The lingual papillae therefore atrophy, leaving a bald, atrophic tongue. Severe cases are followed by fibrosis and fissuring of the tongue (scrotal tongue). Syphilitic glossitis is often associated with leukoplakia, and in these patients the incidence of squamous cell carcinoma is high.

Congenital syphilis is, of course, acquired in utero. Up to the eighteenth week the embryo is somehow protected against the infection and the development is unhampered. If the mother is treated successfully before this time, the child is normal. Congenital syphilis may have any of the manifestations of the secondary and tertiary acquired forms.

Oral lesions consist of Hutchinson's incisors (p. 108), Pflüger and mulberry molars (p. 108), gummas, glossitis, mucous patches, and fissuring and scarring of the corners of the mouth (*rhagades*).

Yaws (frambesia). Yaws is a spirochetal *(Treponema pertenue)* nonvenereal disease that is probably transmitted by the bite of a fly and occurs in damp tropical countries. Its systemic lesions closely mimic those occurring in the secondary and tertiary stages of syphilis. In the oral cavity gumma-like lesions destroy the palate and maxilla and are severely deforming.

Bejel. This nonvenereal spirochetal disease closely mimics syphilis and is seen mostly in the Arab countries. Its oral manifestations are important and consist of mucous patches and gummas of the palate. These lesions resemble those seen in syphilis.

Tuberculosis. Oral manifestations of tuberculosis are extremely rare. In terminal stages of the disease, however, self-inoculation may occur from the patient's sputum.

Oral lesions consist of persistent ulcers or granulomatous masses. Microscopic sections reveal an ulcer, the connective tissues under which show circumscribed nodules of epithelioid cells and giant cells.

Sarcoidosis. In the oral region sarcoidosis occurs most commonly in the parotid gland, where it presents as a tumor or enlargement of the gland (p. 580). Lesions may also occur in the soft palate, gingiva, floor of the mouth, and cheek and present

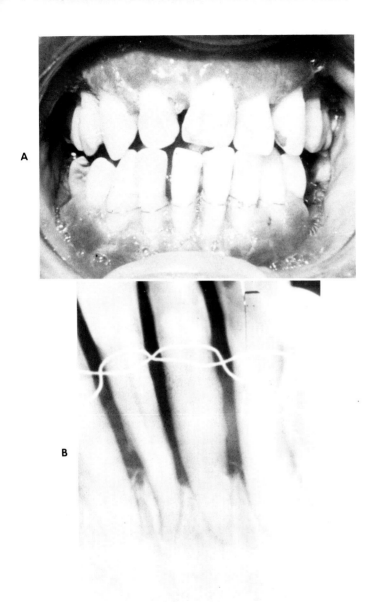

Fig. 19-18. A and **B,** Clinical and radiographic picture of a case of sarcoid-osis that had been mistaken for and treated as "periodontitis."

Continued.

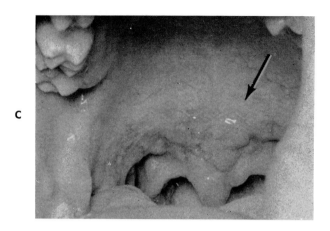

C

Fig. 19-18, cont'd. A second case, **C,** represents sarcoidosis of the palate (arrow).

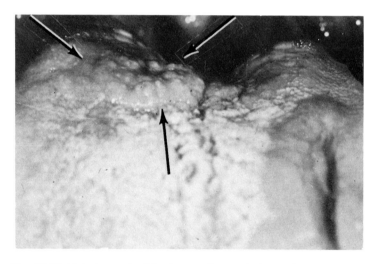

Fig. 19-19. Histoplasmosis of the tongue. Arrows designate the granular features of the lesion.

as submucosal circumscribed nodules or enlargements (Fig. 19-18). The microscopic picture is described on p. 580.

Lesions similar to sarcoidosis have been described as tissue reaction to the pine pollen.

Histoplasmosis. This generalized fungous infection is caused by *Histoplasma capsulatum*. It is seen most frequently in persons residing in the Mississippi basin and is characterized by fever, malaise, cough, loss of weight, and enlargement of the organs of the reticuloendothelial system (spleen, lymph nodes, and liver).

Oral lesions occur in at least 30% of patients and may be the first clinical manifestation of the disease. They consist of ulcerations and nodular elevations on the gingiva, tongue (Fig. 19-19), or palate and rarely appear elsewhere in the oral mucosa. Individual lesions may simulate carcinoma, but their multiple distribution aids in excluding malignant disease.

Microscopic sections show an almost monotonous picture of numerous large histiocytes whose cytoplasm is filled with small (about 1 μm), dotlike, encapsulated bodies (Fig. 19-20). These are spores of *Histoplasma capsulatum*. Treatment with amphotericin B is beneficial.

Candidiasis (moniliasis). Candidiasis was described previously with the surface lesions of the oral mucosa (p. 396).

Actinomycosis. Caused by bacteria-like fungi, the anaerobic *Actinomyces israelii* and the aerobic *Nocardia asteroides*, this disease occurs in one of three forms: cervicofacial, abdominal, and pulmonary.

Cervicofacial actinomycosis is the most common, constituting almost 50% of all cases. It involves the jaw and upper neck and supposedly follows some local trauma such as tooth extraction or fracture. This provides a portal of entry for the organisms, which are normal inhabitants of the mouth.

Clinically the disease starts as a swelling over the upper part of the neck, under the ear, or over the mandible (Fig. 19-21). The skin becomes red or bluish red and taut. Areas of the skin break down and discharge pus that often contains small yellow-

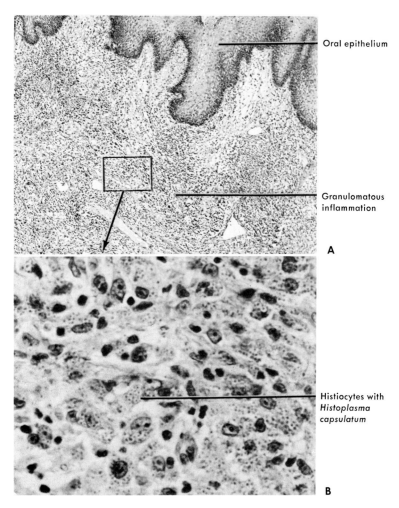

Fig. 19-20. Histoplasmosis. **A,** Inflammatory cells. **B,** Note the numerous dotlike bodies within the histiocytes.

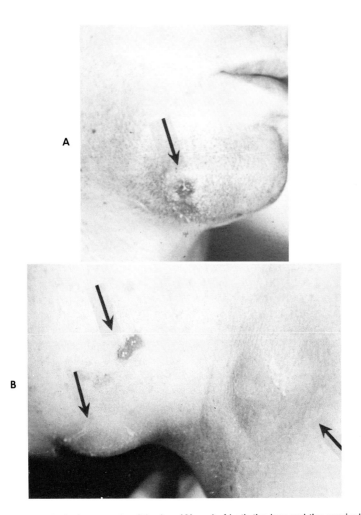

Fig. 19-21. Actinomycosis of the jaw **(A)** and of both the jaw and the cervical area **(B)**.

ish granules (sulfur granules), each of which represents a colony of the fungus. Pus-discharging sinuses heal, but new ones appear; and the process of breakdown and healing continues, so that the disease may persist for years and leave disfiguring scars.

The mandible, overlying soft tissues, and the parotid gland are most commonly affected. Radiographs therefore may show marked destruction of bone.

The microscopic picture of cervicofacial actinomycosis is usually diagnostic. There are numerous abscesses whose centers are typically occupied by colonies of the fungus (Fig. 19-22). The colonies consist of a dense mat of filaments that on the periphery form club-shaped swellings. Because of this appearance, the *Actinomyces* is also called the *ray fungus*. In addition to these abscesses, the involved tissues show scarring and infiltration by plasma cells, macrophages, and lymphocytes. Treatment consists of large doses of penicillin.

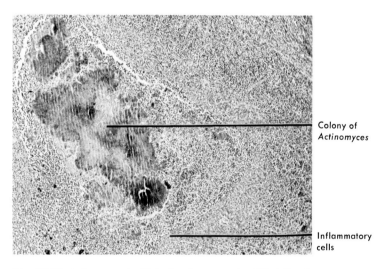

Colony of
Actinomyces

Inflammatory
cells

Fig. 19-22. Actinomycosis. Note the dense neutrophilic infiltration around a colony of the fungus (sulfur granule).

Abdominal actinomycosis involves the appendix or large bowel and the liver. *Pulmonary actinomycosis* involves the lungs and, like the abdominal form, is characterized by multiple abscesses.

South American blastomycosis. The fungous infection is caused by *Blastomyces brasiliensis*. Unlike the North American type, it produces prominent oral manifestations as chronic, progressive granulomatous inflammatory lesions of the lips, cheeks, floor of the mouth, tongue, and pharynx.

Granulomas of unknown nature

Histiocytosis X. Eosinophilic granuloma, Hand-Schuller-Christian disease, and Letterer-Siwe disease make up a group of diseases to which the term histiocytosis X is applied. They are considered by some authors to represent granulomatous inflammations of obscure cause and have been described earlier.

Crohn's disease. This granulomatous infection of unknown etiology usually involves the distal ileum, right colon, and stomach. Patients have chronic, intermittent diarrhea and abdominal cramps. However, oral, anal, and esophageal lesions may often be the first evidence of the disease. The appearance of oral lesions depends on the location. On the buccal mucosa lesions have a cobblestone appearance; in the vestibule linear hyperplastic folds and ulcers are seen; and the lips show diffuse swelling and induration. Lesions of the gingiva and alveolar mucosa reveal granular, erythematous swelling; and the palate shows multiple ulcers that resemble aphthae. The disease is more common in males than in females and is generally seen in the second and third decades of life.

Histologic features consist of noncaseating granulomatous inflammation. Treatment is systemic and empirical and consists of cortisone therapy. Oral lesions are treated symptomatically.

Foreign body granulomas

Although granulomatous inflammation of the oral tissues caused by foreign bodies such as sutures, sponges, or other materials do not constitute systemic diseases, they are mentioned here so that the list of chronic granulomatous inflammations of the oral cavity will be complete.

Clinically these lesions may appear as a radiolucency or, when they occur in soft tissues, as a mass of granulation tissue or a swelling. Microscopically the foreign body is surrounded by numerous giant cells. Also there is abundant connective tissue in which plasma cells, histiocytes, and lymphocytes can be seen.

DISEASES OF THE SKIN AND MUCOUS MEMBRANES

The following diseases of the skin and mucous membranes affect the oral cavity. Many of these have been described previously (see the classification for page references). Those not described earlier are included here.

1. Lichen planus (p. 387)
2. Erythema multiforme (p. 415)
3. Scleroderma
4. Psoriasis
5. Pemphigus (p. 418)
6. Smallpox and chickenpox (p. 422)
7. Measles (p. 422)
8. Lupus erythematosus
9. Darier's disease (keratosis follicularis)
10. Epidermolysis bullosa (p. 426)
11. Acanthosis nigricans

Scleroderma. Scleroderma is a skin disease that occurs in circumscribed (morphea) and generalized (diffuse) forms.

In the *morphea* type the lesions consist of one or more red or ivory-colored, smooth, hard patches on the skin. This condition is benign and does not present oral manifestations.

The *diffuse* type occurs usually in females and is a serious disease in which the skin becomes red and edematous and then undergoes atrophy and shrinkage and becomes fixed to underlying tissues and bones. Such fixation limits movements of all types, including respiration. In the late stages of the disease, calcifications occur in the skin. Also, scleroderma may affect the internal organs (e.g., the esophagus, leading to difficulty in swallowing). Death usually occurs as a result of secondary infections and debilitation.

Oral manifestations of generalized scleroderma are widening

of the periodontal space (which is striking on radiographs) and atrophy of the oral mucous membrane with hardening and fixation of the oral mucosa to underlying structures. The tongue may become indurated and painful. These changes lead to difficulty in speech, deglutition, and mastication.

Microscopic features of scleroderma are thinning of the epithelium and atrophy of the subepithelial connective tissue fibers and their replacement by hyalinized, structureless material that apparently represents altered collagen bundles. In skin lesions there is atrophy of the skin appendages.

Psoriasis. This skin disease of unknown cause affects about 2% of the white population.

Psoriasis is characterized by symmetric white scaly patches on the skin of the elbows, knees, scalp, and other areas (Fig. 19-23). The disease is chronic but presents remissions and exacerbations. Although it does not endanger life, it may be accompanied by arthritis.

Oral lesions of psoriasis are extremely rare and consist of erythematous patches with white scaly surfaces (Fig. 19-23, *A*). Lesions of the lip, palate, gingiva, and cheek have been reported. Since the microscopic features are not pathognomonic, a diagnosis of oral psoriasis should be made only when skin lesions are present.

Microscopically psoriasis shows hyperkeratosis and parakeratosis, elongation of epithelial redges and a club-shaped thickening of their tips, thinning of the epithelial covering over the connective tissue papillae, aggregates of neutrophilic leukocytes in the keratin layer (Munro's microabscesses), and rigid, tortuous venules in the connective tissue papillae (Fig. 19-24). Ultrastructurally the involved epithelium shows a marked increase in mitochondria, prominent, rough endoplasmic reticulum, and the Golgi complex. Immunologic studies reveal IgG in the keratinized layer.

Lupus erythematosus. This skin disease of unknown cause occurs in two forms: chronic (or discoid) and acute.

In the *chronic* form, discrete white scaly macules and

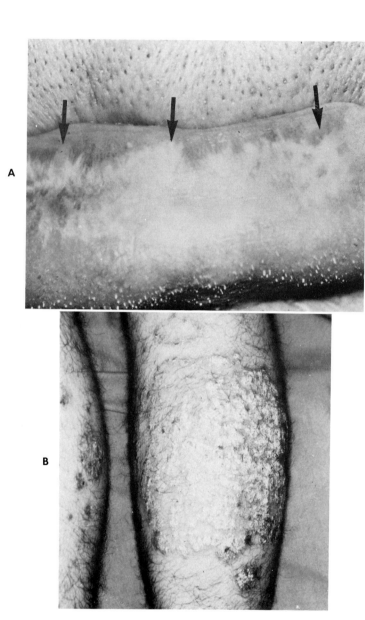

Fig. 19-23. White scaly lesions of psoriasis on the lower lip **(A)** and on the flexor surface of the leg **(B)**.

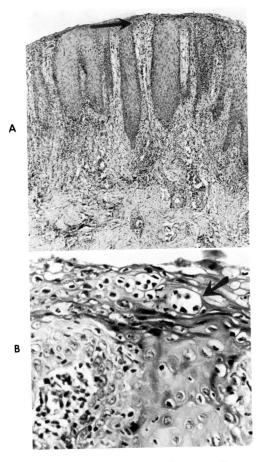

Fig. 19-24. Psoriasis. **A,** Thinning of epithelium over the connective tissue ridges (arrow), which appear club shaped. **B,** High-power magnification of the epithelial covering with microabscesses (arrow).

plaques occur, usually on the malar area and on the bridge of the nose in a butterfly configuration. They may regress spontaneously but are aggravated by sunlight.

Oral lesions may precede or follow the skin lesions and are seen in about 25% of patients. These consist of multiple white plaques with dark reddish purple margins and may clinically resemble leukoplakia or benign hyperkeratosis (pachyderma oris). In some patients, ulceration of the plaques may occur.

The microscopic picture of the skin lesions consists of hyperplasia and hyperkeratosis of the epithelium, liquefactive degeneration of the basal layer of epithelium, dense lymphocytic infiltration under the epithelium and around sebaceous and sweat glands, keratin plugging of hair follicles, and basophilic degeneration of collagen. The lesions of the oral mucous membrane have similar microscopic features: hyperkeratosis or parakeratosis, basophilic degeneration of collagen, liquefactive degeneration of the basal layer of epithelium, and perivascular lymphocytic infiltration in the subepithelial tissues.

The *acute* form of lupus erythematosus usually occurs in young females. It is characterized by red edematous macules, papules, vesicles, bullae, or scales on the malar areas as well as elsewhere on the skin. Patients also have fever, leukopenia, hyperglobulinemia, splenomegaly, vomiting, diarrhea, anorexia, dysphagia, vegetations on the heart valves (Libman-Sacks disease), and fibrinoid degeneration of glomerular capillaries of the kidneys.

Oral lesions of acute lupus erythematosus consist of hemorrhagic macules that may ulcerate and become secondarily infected.

The microscopic features of acute lupus erythematosus are not pathognomonic. These consist of liquefactive degeneration of the basal layer of the epithelium, edema of the subepithelial connective tissue, and fibrinoid degeneration of the collagen. The fibrinoid degeneration consists of shredding and swelling of collagen fibers.

One of the laboratory tests for acute lupus erythematosus is the so-called LE (for lupus erythematosus) phenomenon. This means that when the peripheral blood or bone marrow of the patient is incubated, LE cells are formed. The LE cell is a large, circular, homogeneous basophilic inclusion, probably a leukocyte, that is seen within a neutrophil. The formation of the LE cells is due to the presence of a so-called LE factor in the serum of the patient. The LE phenomenon or test is positive in about 80% of patients with acute lupus erythematosus; but false-positive results may be encountered in patients with rheumatoid arthritis, chronic hepatitis, and sometimes leukemia and multiple myeloma. The so-called hematoxylin body is a large, basophilic, deeply staining body lying in the tissues of patients with acute lupus erythematosus. It probably represents a damaged leukocyte nucleus and is a counterpart of the LE cell. Sometimes a cluster of polymorphonuclear leukocytes surround the hematoxylin body, and the resulting structure is called a rosette.

In the absence of skin lesions and on the basis of oral lesions alone, it is not possible to make a diagnosis of acute or chronic lupus erythematosus.

Darier's disease (keratosis follicularis). This hereditary skin disease is characterized by multiple crusted, greasy lesions that may present a foul odor.

Lesions occur usually on the face and neck but may be seen on other areas of the body. The disease afflicts young persons. Oral lesions are not uncommon and consist of small papules.

Microscopically Darier's disease is characterized by the formation of clefts and lacunae in the epithelial covering (Fig. 19-25). The clefts and lacunae contain thin, grainlike epithelial cells called *corps grains* and round eosinophilic cells called *corps ronds*. Both corps ronds and corps grains represent keratinized epithelial cells. The term benign dyskeratosis is sometimes applied to this type of keratinization. Benign dyskeratosis, in contradistinction to malignant dyskeratosis (p. 379), does not signify a premalignant change.

Vitamin A administration has been suggested as a treatment for Darier's disease.

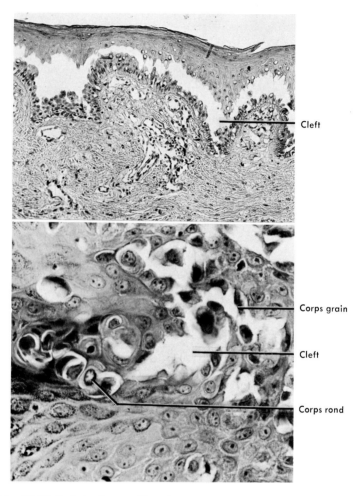

Cleft

Corps grain

Cleft

Corps rond

Fig. 19-25. Darier's disease. Note the presence of clefts in the epithelium. The clefts contain altered epithelial cells (corps grains and corps ronds).

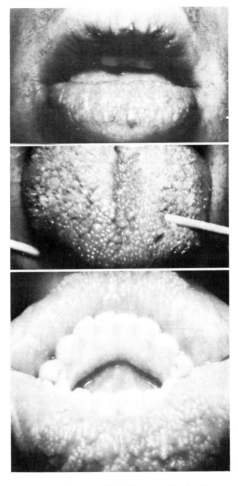

Fig. 19-26. Acanthosis nigricans with lesions on the lip, tongue, and gingiva.
(Courtesy Milton J. Knapp, D.D.S., Portland, Ore.)

On rare occasion, a single, isolated focus of Darier's disease occurs on the skin or in the oral cavity. Such a lesion is called a *warty dyskeratoma*. Oral lesions are rare but have been described on the palate and alveolar mucosa as small white areas with a central depression. Microscopic features are identical to those of Darier's disease.

Acanthosis nigricans. This skin disease is characterized by hyperpigmented, verrucous, velvety patches in the folds of the neck, axilla, and groin.

About 50% of patients have oral lesions. The tongue and lips are most often affected, but lesions may be elsewhere on the oral mucosa. The involved mucous membrane shows many papillary projections (Fig. 19-26).

There are two types of acanthosis nigricans: benign and malignant. The *benign* form is a genetic disorder limited to the skin and mucous membrane. The *malignant* form does not have a genetic basis but is associated with a malignant lesion of some internal organ. These patients usually have an adenocarcinoma of the gastrointestinal tract, and in 60% the primary site is the stomach.

Microscopic features of acanthosis nigricans consist of acanthosis, hyperkeratosis, and pigmentation of the basal layer.

Mycosis fungoides. Also known as granuloma fungoides, this is a fatal disease of skin that, in reality, represents Hodgkin's disease, reticulum cell sarcoma, or leukemia wherein the skin lesions predominate. Skin lesions occur in many forms and, depending on the stage of development, consist of eczematoid, pruritic, red, scaling patches; generalized reddening of skin; loss of hair, or multiple tumors (Fig. 19-27). Oral lesions correspond to those of the skin and may appear as tumors (Fig. 19-28, *A*) or areas of erythema (Fig. 19-28, *B*).

Microscopic sections of advanced cases of mycosis fungoides show an infiltration of the subepithelial connective tissue by abnormal lymphocytes, plasma cells (Marschalko plasma cells), eosinophils, and giant cells. The overlying epithelium contains "microabcesses," or accumulations of tumor cells. These are called the "microabcesses of Darier-Pautrier."

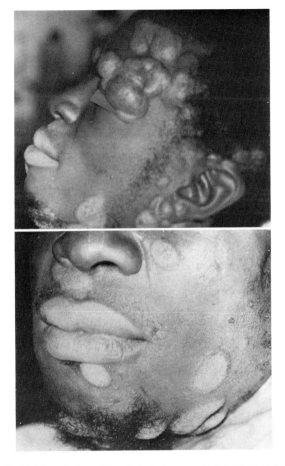

Fig. 19-27. Mycosis fungoides. Skin lesions are in the advanced stage.

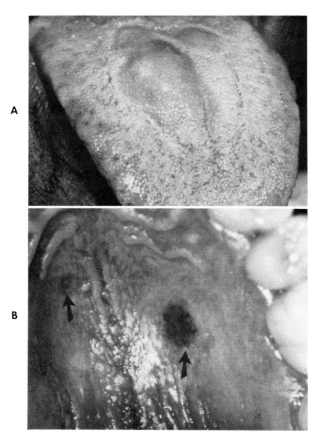

Fig. 19-28. Mycosis fungoides (same patient as seen in Fig. 19-27). Lesions on the dorsum of the tongue are in the form of a tumor **(A)**, while the palate **(B)** shows two erythematous areas.

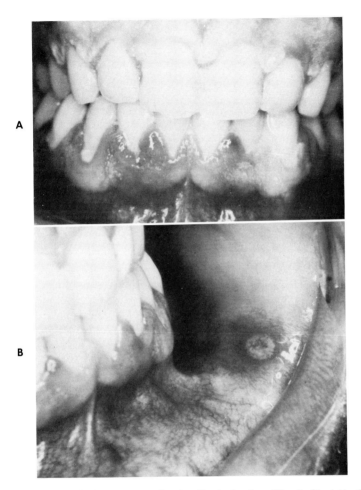

Fig. 19-29. Infectious mononucleosis with gingivostomatitis. **A,** Gingivitis. **B,** Ulceration of the oral mucosa.

Mycosis fungoides may terminate in leukemia, visceral lesions, lymphosarcoma, or various forms of leukemia. The prognosis is grave.

DISEASES OF BONE

The following diseases of the bone present oral manifestations. All have been described previously (see the classification for page references).

1. Paget's disease (p. 340)
2. Osteopetrosis (Albers-Schönberg disease) (p. 344)
3. Leontiasis ossea (p. 346)
4. Engelmann's disease (p. 346)
5. Osteogenesis imperfecta (p. 346)
6. Caffey's disease (p. 347)
7. Fibrous dysplasia (p. 354)

MISCELLANEOUS DISEASES

Infectious mononucleosis. This disease is probably caused by a herpeslike virus called the EB (Epstein-Barr) virus and occurs most frequently in the second and third decades. The incubation period is up to 7 weeks, and the disease lasts for about a month. Symptoms consist of fatigue, sore throat, malaise, headache, nausea, elevation of temperature, and enlargement of cervical lymph nodes.

Lesions of the oral cavity may be the first manifestation of the disease. These consist of gingivostomatitis, gingival bleeding, and multiple pinpoint petechiae at the junction of the hard and soft palates (Figs. 13-64, *B,* and 19-29). It is believed that in 80% of patients oral lesions appear 3 to 5 days before the glandular enlargement. A heterophil antibody test called the *Paul-Bunnell* test is diagnostic.

REFERENCES

Albers, D. D.: Conservative treatment of the oral bony lesions of hyperparathyroidism, Oral Surg. **38:**209, 1974.

Alexander, W. N., and Bechtold, W. A.: Alpha thalassemia minor trait accompanied by clinical oral signs, Oral Surg. **43:**892, 1977.

Archard, H. O., Roebuck, N. F., and Stanley, H. R.: Oral manifestations of chronic discoid lupus erythematosus, Oral Surg. **16:**696, 1963.

Aubrey, J. J., and Hibbard, E. D.: Congenital agranulocytosis, Oral Surg. **35:**526, 1973.

Beck, J. D.: Infectious mononucleosis: a current concept and treatment, J. Kans. Med. Soc. **70:**55, 1969.

Bell, W. A., Gamble, J., and Garrington, G. E.: North American blastomycosis with oral lesions, Oral Surg. **28:**914, 1969.

Bentley, K. C., and deVries, J.: Diagnosis and treatment of cervicofacial actinomycosis, J. Can Dent. Assoc. **39:**715, 1973.

Bernstein, M. L., and McDonald, J. S.: Oral lesions in Crohn's disease: report of two cases and update of the literature, Oral Surg. **46:**234, 1978.

Betten, B., and Koppang, H. S.: Sarcoidosis with mandibular involvement, Oral Surg. **42:**731, 1976.

Bhaskar, S. N., Bernier, J. L., and Godby, F.: Aneurysmal bone cyst and other giant cell lesions of the jaws: report of 104 cases, J. Oral Surg. **17:**30, 1959.

Bishop, R. P., Brewster, A. C., and Antonioli, D. A.: Crohn's disease of the mouth, Gastroenterology **62:**302, 1972.

Boden, R. A.: Disseminated histoplasmosis with an oral lesion, Oral Surg. **23:**549, 1967.

Bradlaw, R. V.: The dental stigmata of prenatal syphilis, Oral Surg. **6:**147, 1953.

Chue, P. W. Y.: Gonorrhea—its natural history, oral manifestations, diagnosis, treatment, and prevention, J. Am. Dent. Assoc. **90:**1297, 1975.

Currie, D. P.: Sickle-cell anemia in oral surgery, Ala. J. Med. Sci. **10:**171, 1973.

Diversi, H. L., Griffin, J. W., and Payne, T. F.: Correlation of cytologic nuclear changes to anemias, Oral Surg. **21:**341, 1966.

Eisenbud, L., Katzka, I., and Platt, N.: Oral manifestations in Crohn's disease, Oral Surg. **34:**770, 1972.

Ellis, J. P., and Truelove, S. C.: Crohn's disease with mouth involvement, Proc. R. Soc. Med. **65:**1080, 1972.

Farman, A. G., and Uys, P. B.: Oral Kaposi's sarcoma, Oral Surg. **39:**288, 1975.

Fischman, S. L., Barnett, M. L., and Nisengard, R. J.: Histopathologic, ultrastructural, and immunologic findings in an oral psoriatic lesion, Oral Surg. **44:**253, 1977.

Fiumara, N. J., Grande, D. J., and Giunta, J. L.: Papular secondary syphilis of the tongue, Oral Surg. **45:**540, 1978.

Franklin, E. C., and Franklin, D. Z.: Current concepts of amyloid, Adv. Immunol. **15:**249, 1972.

Gahrton, G., and Foley, G. E.: Leukemia-like pattern of the DNA, RNA, and protein content of the individual mononuclear cells in the peripheral blood of patients with infectious mononucleosis, Cancer Res. **29:**1076, 1969.

Gambardella, R. J.: Kaposi's sarcoma and its oral manifestations, Oral Surg. **38:**491, 1974.

Gardner, D. G.: The oral manifestations of Hurler's syndrome, Oral Surg. **32:**46, 1971.

Gerber, P., Hamre, D., Moy, R. A., and Rosenblum, E. N.: Infectious mononucleosis; complement-fixing antibodies to herpes-like virus associated with Burkitt lymphoma, Science **161:**173, 1968.

Gordon, N. C., Brown, S., Khosla, V. M., and Hansen, L. S.: Lead poisoning: a comprehensive review and report of a case, Oral Surg. **47**:500, 1979.

Gorlin, R. J., and Peterson, W. C., Jr.: Warty dyskeratoma: a note concerning its occurrence on the oral mucosa, Arch. Dermatol. **95**:292, 1967.

Gupta, R. M., and Gupta, O. P.: A clinico-pathological study of oral histoplasmosis, Laryngoscope **80**:472, 1970.

Hylton, R. P., Samuels, H. S., and Oatis, G. W., Jr.: Actinomycosis: is it really rare? Oral Surg. **29**:138, 1970.

Joseph, E. A., Mare, A., and Irving, W. R.: Oral South American blastomycosis in the United States of America, Oral Surg. **21**:732, 1966.

Kalnins, V.: Actinomycotic granuloma, Oral Surg. **32**:276, 1971.

Kaplan, M. E., and Tan, E. M.: Antinuclear antibodies in infectious mononucleosis, Lancet **1**:561, 1968.

Kerr, N. W.: Sarcoidosis, Oral Surg. **20**:166, 1965.

Knoblich, R.: Accessory thyroid in the lateral floor of the mouth, Oral Surg. **19**:234, 1965.

Kosowicz, J., and Rzymski, K.: Abnormalities of tooth development in pituitary dwarfism, Oral Surg. **44**:853, 1977.

Kraut, R. A., and Buhler, J. E.: Heroin-induced thrombocytopenic purpura, Oral Surg. **46**:637, 1978.

Langerlof, D., Martensson, G., and Wersall, J.: Tuberculosis lesions of the oral mucosa, Oral Surg. **18**:735, 1964.

Laskaris, G. C., Nicolis, G. D., and Capetanakis, J. P.: Mycosis fungoides with oral manifestations, Oral Surg. **46**:40, 1978.

Lautenbach, E., and Dockhorn, R.: Osteodystrophia fibrosa generalisata (Recklinghausen's disease; hyperparathyroidism) and its effects on the jaws, Oral Surg. **25**:479, 1968.

Lovett, D. W., Cross, K. R., and Allen, M. V.: The prevalence of amyloids in gingival tissues, Oral Surg. **20**:444, 1965.

Mace, M. C.: Oral African histoplasmosis resembling Burkitt's lymphoma, Oral Surg. **46**:407, 1978.

Massucco, R. L.: Sickle-cell anemia, Oral Surg. **21**:397, 1966.

Merchant, H. W., and Schuster, G. S.: Oral gonococcal infection, J. Am. Dent. Assoc. **95**:807, 1977.

Millard, H. D., and Gobetti, J. P.: Nonspecific stomatitis—a presenting sign in pernicious anemia, Oral Surg. **39**:562, 1975.

Miller, J.: Pigmentation of teeth due to rhesus factor, Br. Dent. J. **9**:121, 1951.

Mincer, H. H., and Oglesby, R. J.: Intraoral North American blastomycosis, Oral Surg. **22**:36, 1966.

Mishkin, D. J., Akers, J. O., and Darby, C. P.: Congenital neutropenia, Oral Surg. **42**:738, 1976.

Mourshed, F., and Tuckson, C. R.: A study of the radiographic features of the jaws in sickle-cell anemia, Oral Surg. **37**:812, 1974.

Murphy, J. B., Robinson, K., and Segelman, A.: PTA deficiency (factor XI deficiency), Oral Surg. **42:**26, 1976.

Murphy, N. C., and Bissada, N. F.: Iron deficiency: an overlooked predisposing factor in angular cheilitis, J. Am. Dent. Assoc. **99:**640, 1979.

Nealon, F. H.: Scleroderma: oral manifestations, Oral Surg. **24:**319, 1967.

Niederman, J. C., McCollum, E. W., Henle, G., and Henle, W.: Infectious mononucleosis; clinical manifestations in relation to EB virus antibodies, J.A.M.A. **203:**205, 1968.

Orlean, S. L., and O'Brien, J. J.: Sarcoidosis manifesting a soft lesion in the floor of the mouth, Oral Surg. **21:**819, 1966.

Orlian, A. I., and Birnbaum, M.: Intraoral localized sarcoid lesion, Oral Surg. **49:**341, 1980.

Perry, H. O.: Skin diseases with mucocutaneous involvement, Oral Surg. **24:**800, 1967.

Powell, E. A., and Januska, J. R.: Sickle cell anemia: chronology, natural history, and implications for dental practice, Q. Natl. Dent. Assoc. **31:**72, 1973.

Poyton, H. G., and Davey, K. W.: Thalassemia, Oral Surg. **25:**564, 1968.

Rappaport, J., Shiffman, M. A., and Greaney, E. M.: Parathyroid disease, Oral Surg. **17:**802, 1964.

Reddy, P., Sutaria, M. K., Christianson, C. S., and Brasher, C. A.: Oral lesions as presenting manifestation of disseminated histoplasmosis: report of five cases, Ann. Otol. Rhinol. Laryngol. **79:**389, 1970.

Reichart, P.: Pathologic changes in the soft palate in lepromatous leprosy, Oral Surg. **38:**898, 1974.

Ritchie, G. M., and Fletcher, A. M.: Angular inflammation, Oral Surg. **36:**358, 1973.

Robinson, I. B., and Sarnat, B. G.: Roentgen studies of the maxillae and mandible in sickle-cell anemia, Radiology **58:**517, 1952.

Rosenberg, E. H., and Guralnick, W. C.: Hyperparathyroidism: a review of 220 previous cases, with special emphasis on findings in the jaws, Oral Surg. **15**(suppl. 2):84, 1962.

Salman, S. J., Salman, L., and Salman, R. A.: Thrombocytopenic purpura secondary to quinidine hypersensitivity, Oral Surg. **44:**45, 1977.

Scopp, I. W., and Schlagel, E.: Scleroderma: its orofacial manifestations, Oral Surg. **15:**1510, 1962.

Shira, R. B., and Bhaskar, S. N.: Oral surgery-oral pathology conference 4 (oral histoplasmosis), Oral Surg. **16:**994, 1963.

Slavin, G., Cameron, H., Forbes, C., and Mitchell, R. M.: Kaposi's sarcoma in East African children—a report of 51 cases, J. Pathol. **100:**187, 1970.

Stankler, L., Ewen, S. W. B., and Kerr, N. W.: Crohn's disease of the mouth, Br. J. Dermatol. **87:**501, 1972.

Steiner, M., and Alexander, W. N.: Primary syphilis of the gingiva, Oral Surg. **21:**530, 1966.

Taylor, R. N., Donohoe, D. F., and Williams, A. C.: Parahemophilia (a case diagnosed after excessive postextraction bleeding), Oral Surg. **31**:180, 1971.

Taylor, V. E., and Smith, C. J.: Oral manifestations of Crohn's disease without demonstrable gastrointestinal lesions, Oral Surg. **39**:58, 1975.

Tiecke, R. W., Baron, H. J., and Casey, D. E.: Localized oral histoplasmosis, Oral Surg. **16**:441, 1963.

Tillman, H. H., Taylor, R. G., and Carchidi, J.: Sarcoidosis of the tongue, Oral Surg. **21**:190, 1966.

Timosca, G., and Iasi, L. G.: Primary localized amyloidosis of the palate, Oral Surg. **44**:76, 1977.

Ulmansky, M.: Primary amyloidosis of oral structures and pharynx, Oral Surg. **15**:800, 1962.

Uthman, A. A.: Plummer-Vinson syndrome, Oral Surg. **20**:449, 1965.

Weathers, D. R., and Driscoll, R. M.: Darier's disease of the oral mucosa, Oral Surg. **37**:711, 1974.

White, G. E.: Oral manifestations of leukemia in children, Oral Surg. **29**:420, 1970.

Witorsch, P., and Utz, J. P.: North American blastomycosis; a study of 40 patients, Medicine **47**:169, 1968.

Young, L. L.: Gingival lesions in histoplasmosis, J. Ky. Dent. Assoc. **25**:13, 1973.

Young, L. L., Dolan, C. T., Sheridan, P. J., and Reeve, C. M.: Oral manifestations of histoplasmosis, Oral Surg. **33**:191, 1972.

CHAPTER 20

General manifestations of oral diseases

Any disease involving an organ or an organ system must, in the last analysis, produce some effect, however small, in the body as a whole. Consequently every disturbance of the oral cavity has an effect on the total patient. This effect may be only psychologic (e.g., the traumatic loss of the anterior teeth in a young patient) or it may produce death (e.g., a malignant oral tumor or rare case of septicemia following a tooth extraction). In the present discussion, only those conditions that produce physical disturbances will be considered.

1. Cavernous sinus thrombosis and meningitis
2. Septicemia
3. Oral infections
4. Malignant oral tumor
5. Loss of teeth
6. Foci of infection
7. Extractions, scaling procedures, and vigorous massage of gingiva

Cavernous sinus thrombosis and meningitis. Cavernous sinus thrombosis and meningitis occur in rare instances in which an acute inflammatory process involving the maxilla extends to the cranial base and the meninges.

Septicemia. On rare occasion, particularly prior to the advent of antibiotics, single or multiple tooth extractions were followed by septicemia and death.

Oral infections. A dental abscess and osteomyelitis often are accompanied by fever, malaise, headache, joint pains, and leukocytosis.

Malignant oral tumor. Malignant oral tumors, such as carcinoma, lymphoepithelioma, osteogenic sarcoma, malignant salivary gland tumor, and primary oral lymphoma, metastasize and kill the patient. Even some benign tumors of the maxilla, such as chondroma, can prove fatal by local extension to the cranial base.

Loss of teeth. When the loss of teeth is not corrected by artificial dentures, the ability of the patient to select or masticate a nutritionally adequate diet is reduced and secondary deficiencies result.

Foci of infection. Infected dental pulps, dental granulomas, inflamed gingivae, and inflammatory periodontal lesions such as pockets are, in *some* instances, foci of infection. This means that they are a constant source of bacteria and/or bacterial products that get into the bloodstream. Once in the bloodstream, bacteria *may* set up secondary inflammatory or allergic lesions in distant parts of the body. The process has been called *focal infection;* and it has been much debated whether gastrointestinal and neurologic disturbances, various forms of arthritis, subacute bacterial endocarditis, and some skin diseases and ocular disturbances originate through this mechanism. Whatever the systemic implications of focal infection, all lesions in the oral cavity, inflammatory or otherwise, deserve attention and eradication.

Extractions, scaling procedures, and vigorous massage of gingiva. Extractions, scaling procedures, and even vigorous massage of the gingival tissue lead to a transitory bacteremia that usually lasts less than 30 minutes. This is usually caused by the alpha hemolytic streptococci. Irrigation of the gingival sulcus and a mouthwash of a few drops of phenol in warm water can markedly reduce the incidence of postextraction bacteremia (by almost 70%).

REFERENCES

Bender, I. D., Seltzer, S., and Yermish, M.: The incidence of bacteremia in endodontic manipulation, Oral Surg. **13:**353, 1960.

Cobe, H. M.: Transitory bacteremia, Oral Surg. **7:**609, 1954.

Haymaker, W.: Fatal infections of the central nervous system and meninges after tooth extraction, Am. J. Orthodont. [Sect. Oral Surg.] **31:**117, 1945.

Jones, J. C., Cutcher, J. L., Goldberg, J. R., and Lilly, G. E.: Control of bacteremia associated with extraction of teeth, Oral Surg. **30:**454, 1970.

Lantzman, E., and Michman, J.: Leukocyte counts in the saliva of adults before and after extraction of teeth, Oral Surg. **30:**766, 1970.

Lineberger, L. T., and De Marco, T. J.: Evaluation of transient bacteremia following routine periodontal procedures, J. Periodontol. **44:**757, 1973.

Mehrotra, M. C.: Cavernous sinus thrombosis with generalized septicemia, Oral Surg. **19:**715, 1965.

Robinson, L., Kraus, F. W., Lazansky, J. P., Wheeler, R. E., Gordon, S., and Johnson, V.: Bacteremias of dental origin. I. A review of the literature. II. A study of the factors influencing occurrence and detection, Oral Surg. **3:**519, 923, 1950.

Sconyers, J. R., Crawford, J. J., and Moriarty, J. D.: Relationship of bacteremia to toothbrushing in patients with periodontitis, J. Am. Dent. Assoc. **87:**616, 1973

CHAPTER 21

Neurologic disturbances involving oral regions

Only those neurologic disturbances that directly affect the oral region are included in this chapter. These conditions are as follows:

1. Myofacial pain dysfunction syndrome (MPD)
2. Trigeminal neuralgia (tic douloureux)
3. Glossodynia
4. Auriculotemporal syndrome (Frey's syndrome)
5. Sphenopalatine neuralgia (Sluder's neuralgia)
6. Glossopharyngeal neuralgia
7. Facial paralysis (Bell's palsy)
8. Causalgia
9. Eagle's syndrome

Myofacial pain dysfunction syndrome (MPD). This symptom complex is characterized primarily by pain and dysfunction around the temporomandibular joint and face.

Many names and theories of origin of this disease have been proposed over the past decades, but its true nature and terminology have only recently been described. Patients have four main groups of complaints: pain in the temporomandibular joint area, muscle tenderness, limited opening or deviation on opening of the jaw or both, and noise in the temporomandibular joint. Considered for many years as a syndrome produced by occlusal disharmonies, it is now generally believed to be a neuromuscular disorder. More than 80% of patients are female and in the third decade or older.

The disease is produced by masticatory muscle fatigue and spasm. The fatigue and spasm in most patients with MPD are caused primarily by emotional stress rather than mechanical factors such as occlusal disharmonies.

Since the MPD has been shown to be produced on a psychophysiologic basis, its treatment is conservative and consists of analgesics, muscle relaxing drugs, tranquilizers, psychologic counseling, a good patient-dentist relationship, placebos, and warm compresses. Occlusal grinding and reconstruction are not indicated as therapy for MPD.

Trigeminal neuralgia (tic douloureux). Trigeminal neuralgia is characterized by severe unilateral lancinating pain in the area of the face supplied by the trigeminal nerve. Pain is transitory, and the attacks may be precipitated by touching some area of the face—the so called trigger zone. There is some evidence that it is caused by the herpes simplex type 1 virus.

Tic douloureux usually occurs in middle age, and the right side of the face is affected more often than the left side. There is no permanent treatment for the disease. The injection of boiling water or alcohol into the gasserian ganglion has been tried.

Glossodynia. Glossodynia refers to pain or an unpleasant sensation (itching or burning) in the tongue. Numerous contributing factors may cause it. Some of these are nutritional deficiencies, anemias, xerostomia, cancerphobia, poisoning with heavy metals, and postmenopausal syndrome. It usually occurs in middle-aged or older women.

Auriculotemporal syndrome (Frey's syndrome). The auriculotemporal syndrome is the result of a defective repair of a damaged auriculotemporal nerve, so that the sweat glands become enervated by the parasympathetic salivary fibers. As a result of this anomalous repair, the patient sweats in the temporal area during eating. The condition usually follows surgical procedures in the area of the parotid gland and mandibular condyle.

Sphenopalatine neuralgia (Sluder's neuralgia). Sphenopalatine neuralgia is characterized by radiating pain in the regions of the maxilla, teeth, cheek, and ear. It affects only one side of the face. Pain is periodic and transitory.

Females are affected more often than males, and the condition occurs at any age. Pain may be associated with other symptoms such as sneezing and nasal discharge. Unlike trigeminal neuralgia, there is no trigger zone.

Glossopharyngeal neuralgia. Severe pain in the posterior part of the tongue and pharynx is characteristic of glossopharyngeal neuralgia. It occurs in older patients and is unilateral; its cause is unknown. Pain is similar to that experienced in trigeminal neuralgia.

Facial paralysis (Bell's palsy). This term refers to paralysis of the muscles supplied by the seventh cranial nerve. The cause may be unknown, may be associated with a malignant tumor of the parotid gland, or may follow surgical procedures in the parotid area. Some cases are believed to be caused by the herpes

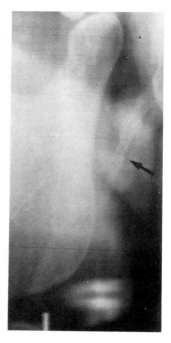

Fig. 21-1. Eagle's syndrome. Note the elongated styloid process.

simplex type I virus. The paralysis is unilateral and occurs in adults.

Females are affected more often than males. On the affected side the eye cannot be closed (which leads to eye infections), the mouth droops, and saliva escapes from the corner of the mouth. Because of paralysis of the facial muscles, the patient is expressionless and has difficulty with speech and mastication.

Causalgia. Causalgia referes to a burning pain in the area of a previous injury or surgical procedure. In the oral region it occurs following tooth extraction. A few days or weeks after extraction the socket is the site of intense burning pain although the wound is completely healed. Pain is transitory and may be precipitated by emotional, visual, auditory, or physical stimuli. Treatment is empirical.

Eagle's syndrome. A syndrome described by Eagle consists of a feeling of foreign bodies in the throat and pain in the throat, pharynx, ear, and side of the neck as well as difficulty in swallowing. In some cases these symptoms appear after tonsillectomy and persist for many years. They are believed to be caused by elongation of the styloid process, and most patients are over 30 years of age (Fig. 21-1).

REFERENCES

Al-Ubaidy, S. S., Bakeen, G., and Gossous, M.: The auriculotemporal syndrome (Frey's syndrome), J. Ir. Dent Assoc. **19:**190, 1973.

Ayer, W. A., Machen, J. B., and Getter, L.: Survey of myofacial pain-dysfunction syndrome and pathologic bruxing habits among dentists, J. Am. Dent. Assoc. **94:**730, 1977.

Baddour, H. M., McAnear, J. T., and Tilson, H. B.: Eagle's syndrome, Oral Surg. **46:**486, 1978.

Bayer, D. B., and Stenger, T. G.: Trigeminal neuralgia: an overview, Oral Surg. **48:**393, 1979.

Brooke, R. I., and Stenn, P. G.: Postinjury myofacial pain dysfunction syndrome: its etiology and prognosis, Oral Surgery **45:**846, 1978.

Brooke, R. I., Stenn, P. G., and Mothersill, K. J.: The diagnosis and conservative treatment of myofacial pain dysfunction syndrome, Oral Surg. **44:**844, 1977.

Butler, J. H., Folke, L. E. A., and Brandt, C. L.: A descriptive survey of signs and symptoms associated with the myofacial pain-dysfunction syndrome, J. Am. Dent. Assoc. **90**:635, 1975.

Cherrick, H. M.: Trigeminal neuralgia, Oral Surg. **34**:714, 1972.

Clark, G. T., Beemsterboer, P. L., Solberg, W. K., and Rugh, J. D.: Nocturnal electromyographic evaluation of myofacial pain dysfunction in patients undergoing occlusal splint therapy, J. Am. Dent. Assoc. **99**:607, 1979.

Cohen, S. R.: Follow-up evaluation of 105 patients with myofacial pain-dysfunction syndrome, J. Am. Dent. Assoc. **97**:825, 1978.

Domnitz, J. M., Swintak, E. F., Schriver, W. R., and Shereff, R. H.: Myofacial pain syndrome masquerading as temporomandibular joint pain, Oral Surg. **43**:11, 1977.

Duncan, D. J.: Bell's palsy: a review of current treatment, J. Am. Osteopath. Assoc. **73**:144, 1973.

Eagle, W. W.: Elongated styloid process: symptoms and treatment, Arch Otolaryngol. **67**:127, 1958.

Finelli, P. F.: Herpes simplex virus and the human nervous system: current concepts and review, Milit. Med. **140**:765, 1975.

Gessel, A. H.: Electromyographic biofeedback and tricyclic antidepressants in myofacial pain-dysfunction syndrome: psychological predictors of outcome, J. Am. Dent. Assoc. **91**:1048, 1975.

Greene, C. S., and Laskin, D. M.: Long-term evaluation of conservative treatment for myofacial pain-dysfunction syndrome, J. Am. Dent. Assoc. **89**:1365, 1974.

Laskin, D., and Dohrmann, R. J.: An evaluation of electromyographic biofeedback, in the treatment of myofacial pain-dysfunction syndrome, J. Am. Dent. Assoc. **96**:656, 1978.

Laskin, D. M. and Greene, C. S.: Influence of the doctor-patient relationship on placebo therapy for patients with myofacial pain-dysfunction (MPD) syndrome, J. Am. Dent. Assoc. **85**:892, 1972.

Lerman, M. D.: A unifying concept of the TMJ pain-dysfunction syndrome, J. Am. Dent. Assoc. **86**:833, 1973.

Olson, R. E., and Laskin, D. M.: Relationship between allergy and bruxism in patients with myofacial pain-dysfunction syndrome, J. Am. Dent. Assoc. **100**:209, 1980.

Russell, T. E.: Eagle syndrome: diagnostic considerations and report of a case, J. Am. Dent. Assoc. **94**:548, 1977.

Sanders, B., and Weiner, J.: Eagle's syndrome, J. Oral Med. **32**:44, 1977.

Sapiro, S. M.: Bell's palsy associated with acute herpetic gingivostomatitis, Oral Surg. **39**:403, 1975.

Winter, A. A., and Yavelow, I.: Oral considerations of the myofacial pain-dysfunction syndrome, Oral Surg. **40**:720, 1975.

Index